穴位

Xué Wèi

Point Location

& Channel Pathways

Handbook

Jim Cleaver LAc.

Muddy Bottom Press

Table of Contents

© 1990–2016   Jim Cleaver LAc.

Organization of the Eastern Energetic Anatomy System

I. 經 Jīng = Channels:

A. 12 Primary Channels · are likened to Rivers [that circulate qi & blood]
B. 8 Extraordinary Vessels · are likened to Lakes (resevoirs) [that store qi & blood]
C. 4 Seas (not channels) · are likened to Oceans [that represent the true source of qi & blood]

- **12 Primary Channels:** · named & associated with the 11 **Organs** & Triple Burner (San Jiao)
  正 經 zhèng **jīng** · bilateral distribution
  (lit. regular/ordinary channels) · have points (total = 309 pts x 2 = 618)

- **8 Extraordinary Vessels:** · **Ren, Du / Chong, Dai // Yin & Yang Wei / Yin & Yang Qiao**
  奇經 八脈 Qí Jīng Bā Mài (Conception, Governing, Thoroughfare, Belt, // Linking Heel or Motility)
  (irregular channels, 8 vessels) · associated with ba gua (8 trigrams)
  (lit. odd, strange, curious, extraordinary channels) · two are unilateral (Ren/CV & Du/GV) and have their own pts (52 pts)
  · the other six vessels are bilateral
  these vessels share their points with the primary channels (~60 pts)
  · There are ~112 pts altogether on the 8 vessels (see p. 124)
  · In addition, there are 8 points, called **master pts** (1 for each vessel)
  These open, or control access to the vessel,
  but are not necessarily on the channel, or part of its trajectory.

- **4 Seas   :** · **Sea of Qi, Blood, Marrow, & Nourishment** (lit. water & grains)
  四 海 Sì Hǎi · 10 points, shared with primary channels (see p. 31)
  (lit. 4 seas or oceans) · Qi (3 pts), Blood (3 pts) // Marrow (2 pts), Nourishment (2 pts)

II. 穴 Xué = Point(s): · **3 Types:** Channel, Extra, & A-shi points

A. **Channel pts:** · Total number on the 14 channels that have points = 361 (309 + 52)
   正經穴 · alpha-numeric designation [channel abbreviation + #] [my system of abbrev.]
   zhèng jīng xué · numbering also reflects the direction qi flows in that channel
   · all 361 have Chinese names, most are two characters [35 have 3]

B. **Extra pts:** · not part of the channel system of points, (though some are on those channels)
   經外穴 · discovered after the channel system was set (smt. called new or misc. pts)
   jīng wài xué · they are named, but there is no set number, (& no universal numbering)
   · we will learn ~ 85 of the most important ones, (mostly during Spring term)

C. **A-shi pts:** · literally *that's it* points ('that's the spot', or 'ouch/sensitive' point)
   阿是穴 · potentially infinite number
   ā shì xué · represent the body's ability to create points as it needs to
   · correlate with 'trigger' points (western rediscovery of acupuncture)

The Main Subdivisions of the Channel System

經 絡 jīng-luò = channels & collaterals (the main channels (jing) and their network (luo) of tributaries.

經 脈 jīng-mài = channels & vessels (the main channels (jing) and the extraordinary vessels (mai))

絡 脈 luò mài = nework vessels (another name for the network of connecting vessels)

• **Primary/Regular Channels**   正 經 (zhèng jīng)   [Qi flow is described in LS 16]

    a. external pathways: (like rivers)   this is where the points are
         • follow relatively superficial course between muscles and bones
         • hands/fingers are perfect tools to locate them (not electron microscopes)
    b. internal pathway: (like ocean currents)
         proceed to various organs and tissues

屬 shǔ   • 'homes to'   its pertaining organ – circulates qi to & from the organ

絡 luò   • 'wraps/nets' its yin/yang phase paired organ, connecting them internally

• **Connecting/Network Vessels**   絡 脈 (luò mài)   [locus classicus LS 10]

     • A short connecting bridge from one channel to its element paired channel.
     • connect from the luo pt of one channel to the yuan pt on the paired channel.
     these points are on the limbs (wrists & ankles)
     • Connects the yin/yang (phase paired) channels externally.

• **Channel Divergences**   經 別 (jīng bié)   [locus classicus LS 11]

     • again one diverging channel is associated with each primary channel
     • they diverge from their primary channel on the upper aspect of the limbs
     (proximal to the knee or elbow) and then continue internally.

• **Channel Sinews** or **Muscle/Tendon channels**   經 筋 (jīng jīn)   [locus classicus LS 13]

     • channels representing individual & groups of muscles – connect from joint to joint
     • account for both structure and function (anatomy & kinesiology)

• **Cutaneous Regions / Skin Zones**   皮 部 (pí bù)   [locus classicus SW 56]

     • essentially the 6 divisions (analogous to valleys in which the main channel/river flows)
     • anatomically includes the skin and superficial fascia, subcutaneous regions, and pores.
     • wei qi circulates here

For further investigation, I recommend the following books:

The Channels of Acupuncture	Maciocia	(2006)	esp. Parts 3–6 pp.217–369
Manual of Acupuncture	Deadman	(1998)	p. 11–27 and beginning of each channel section
Meridian Style Acupuncture	Pirog	(1996)	chapter 4 and section 3
Navigating the Channels	Ni	(1996)	p.1–12 and individual channel chapters

Abbreviations:

     LS = Ling Shu # = chapter   Ling Shu = Spiritual Axis or Pivot
     SW = Su Wen # = chapter   Su Wen = Plain or Simple Questions

Historical Development of the Number of Regular Acu-Points

The system of channels and points has been an evolving one. It did not attain its current number until 1871, even though it was essentially complete by about 300. That being said, it is not known how many points were part of the system during the Nei Jing era, but only 160 are mentioned by name in the surviving text.

Date	Text	Author	Number of Points			
			Midline	Bilateral	Total	adds
–200	Nei Jing	unknown (attributed to Huang Di)	25	135	160	
						+ 189
282	Jia Yi Jing	Huang Fu-mi	49	300	349	
						+ 5
1026	Tong Ren	Wang Wei-yi	51	303	354	
						+ 5
1601	Da Cheng	Yang Ji-zhou	51	308	359	
						+ 2
1871	Feng Yuan	Li Xue-chuan	52	309	**361**	
				618 +52 = 670		Total

Key to Abbreviations

Nei Jing = the Yellow Emperor's **Classic of Internal Medicine** or **Inner Classic**
(Huang Di Nei Jing)
2 parts: Su Wen = SW = Plain or Simple Questions (81 chapters)   Ling Shu = LS (Spiritual Pivot/Axis) (81 chapters)

Jia Yi Jing = Acu-Moxa AB Classic (the **Systematic Classic**)
(Zhen Jiu Jia Yi Jing)

Tong Ren = the **Bronze Man** Acu-Moxa Illustrated Classic
(Tong Ren Zhen Jiu Shu Xue Tu Jing)

Da Cheng = the **Great Compendium** of Acu-Moxa Therapy
(Zhen Jiu Da Cheng)

Feng Yuan = **Meet(ing) the Source** of Acu-Moxa Therapy
(Zhen Jiu Feng Yuan)

Sources: Needham   *Celestial Lancets*   p. 100
              Li Ding   *Acupuncture Meridian Theory & Points*   p. 35
              Omura   *Acupuncture Medicine*   p. 41-44

Development of Extraordinary Vessel Theory

Date	Text	Author	Contribution
− 200	**Nei Jing** (Su Wen & Ling Shu) Inner Classic (Simple Questions & Spiritual Axis)	(attrib. Huang Di)	pathways first described esp. LS 10
+300	**Nan Jing** Classic of Difficulties	(attrib. Bian Que) (Wang Shu-he's commentary on)	pathways clarified symptoms and pulses described
~1295	Zhen Jing Zhi Nan Needle Classic, Pointing South (south=light=clear) = South Pointing Needle Classic	???	4 pairs of points 1st described
1341	Shi-si Jing Fa Hui Elaboration of the 14 Channels	Hua Shou	
1439	**Da Quan** Complete Book of Acupuncture	Xu Feng	first complete description with master pts delineated & correlated w/ trigrams biorhythmic treatment approach
1529	Ju Ying Gleanings from Eminent Acupuncturists (aka Glorious Anthology)	Gao Wu	
~ 1570	**Qi Jing Ba Mai Kao** Examination of the 8 Extraordinary Vessels	Li Shi-zhen	
1601	**Da Cheng** Great Compendium	Yang Ji-zhou	thorough delineation of points alone & in pairs
1624	Lei Jing Classic of Categories	Zhang Jie-bing	
Source:	*Extraordinary Vessels*	Matsumoto & Birch	p. 4-7 & 25-63 1986

Introduction
to
Eastern
Anatomy

☯ *Body Surfaces & Directions* ☯

Yīn	Yáng
陰	陽
shady side	*sunny side*
anterior (ventral)	**posterior** (dorsal)
inferior (caudal)	**superior** (cephalad)
proximal	**distal**
medial	**lateral**
interior	**exterior**
right (on the exterior)	**left** (on the exterior)
left (on the interior)	right (on the interior)

Channel Distribution & Anatomical Compartments

	Flow from/to	Triad *flow in/out*	6 YIN *flow up*	Compartment	6 YANG *flow down*	Triad *flow in/out*	Flow from/to	
6 A R M	chest to fingers	**3 Arm Yin** *flow out (CF)*	**Lu**	radial	**LI**	**3 Arm Yang** *flow in (CP)*	fingers to face	**6 A R M**
			Pc	median	**TB**			
			Ht	ulnar	**SI**			
6 L E G	toes to torso	**3 Leg Yin** *flow in (CP)*	**Sp**	anterior	**ST**	**3 Leg Yang** *flow out (CF)*	face to toes	**6 L E G**
			Lr	median	**GB**			
			Kd	posterior	**BL**			

- outward flow   = centrifugal (CF) = 3 arm yin & 3 leg yang
- inward flow   = centripetal (CP) = 3 leg yin   & 3 arm yang

CV – GV Flow: front and back midlines
- CV (yin)   flows up   from perineum to lower lip (1-24)
- GV (yang)   flows up   from tailbone to upper lip   (1-28)

Channels, Five Element Correspondences, and their Colors

		六陰 Liù Yīn **6 YIN**	五行 Wǔ Xíng **Five Elements**	六陽 Liù Yáng **6 YANG**	
6 ARM		**Lu**	金 **Jīn** **Metal** (white)	**LI**	**6 ARM**
		Pc	相火 **Xiàng Huǒ** Ministerial Fire **M. Fire** (red/orange)	**TB**	
		Ht	君火 **Jūn Huǒ** Imperial Fire **I. Fire** (red)	**SI**	
6 LEG		**Sp**	土 **Tǔ** **Earth/Soil** (yellow)	**ST**	**6 LEG**
		Lr	木 **Mù** **Wood** (green, azure)	**GB**	
		Kd	水 **Shuǐ** **Water** (black)	**BL**	

My channel abbreviations are all two letters and are yin-yang coded as follows:
Yang channels are all two words except stomach, therefore I capitalize both letters.
Technically bladder is the *urinary* bladder to distinguish it from the *gall* bladder and therefore should be UB, but I bow to convention here and just use BL.

Yin channels are all one word, the second letter is therefore lower case.
For Liver: I don't use Li to avoid confusion with LI, likewise I don't use Lv because handwritten it looks too much like Lu.

© 1990–2016   Jim Cleaver LAc.

Division Pairs – Sub-Divisions of Yin & Yang

	6 ARM/Hand 手 **Shǒu**	**Six** **Divisions** (liu jing = lit. 6 channels)	6 LEG/Foot 足 **Zú**
三 **Sān** 陽 **Yáng** **Divisions**	SI	**Tai-Yang**	BL
	TB	**Shao-Yang**	GB
	LI	**Yang-Ming**	ST
三 **Sān** 陰 **Yīn** **Divisions**	Lu	**Tai-Yin**	Sp
	Ht	**Shao-Yin**	Kd
	Pc	**Jue-Yin**	Lr

太 • **Tài** = very or **Greater** (yin or yang)

少 • **Shǎo** = diminished or **Lesser** (yin or yang) shào = young(er)

明 • **Míng** = **Bright** yang (yang flaring up)

厥 • **Jué** = diminshed to the point of disappearing (shrinking or **Faint** yin)
(smt. translated as Absolute, Terminal, or End of yin)

➢ Channel Names:
(4 parts)

Limb	**Division**	**Organ**	**Channel**
(arm or leg) (lit. hand or foot)	(yin or yang) (1 of 6)	(1 of 12)	(the word for)

example: **Shou** **Tai-Yin** **Fei** **Jing**

translation: arm/hand greater yin lung channel

Six (Sub) Divisions of the Body

color the 6 divisions

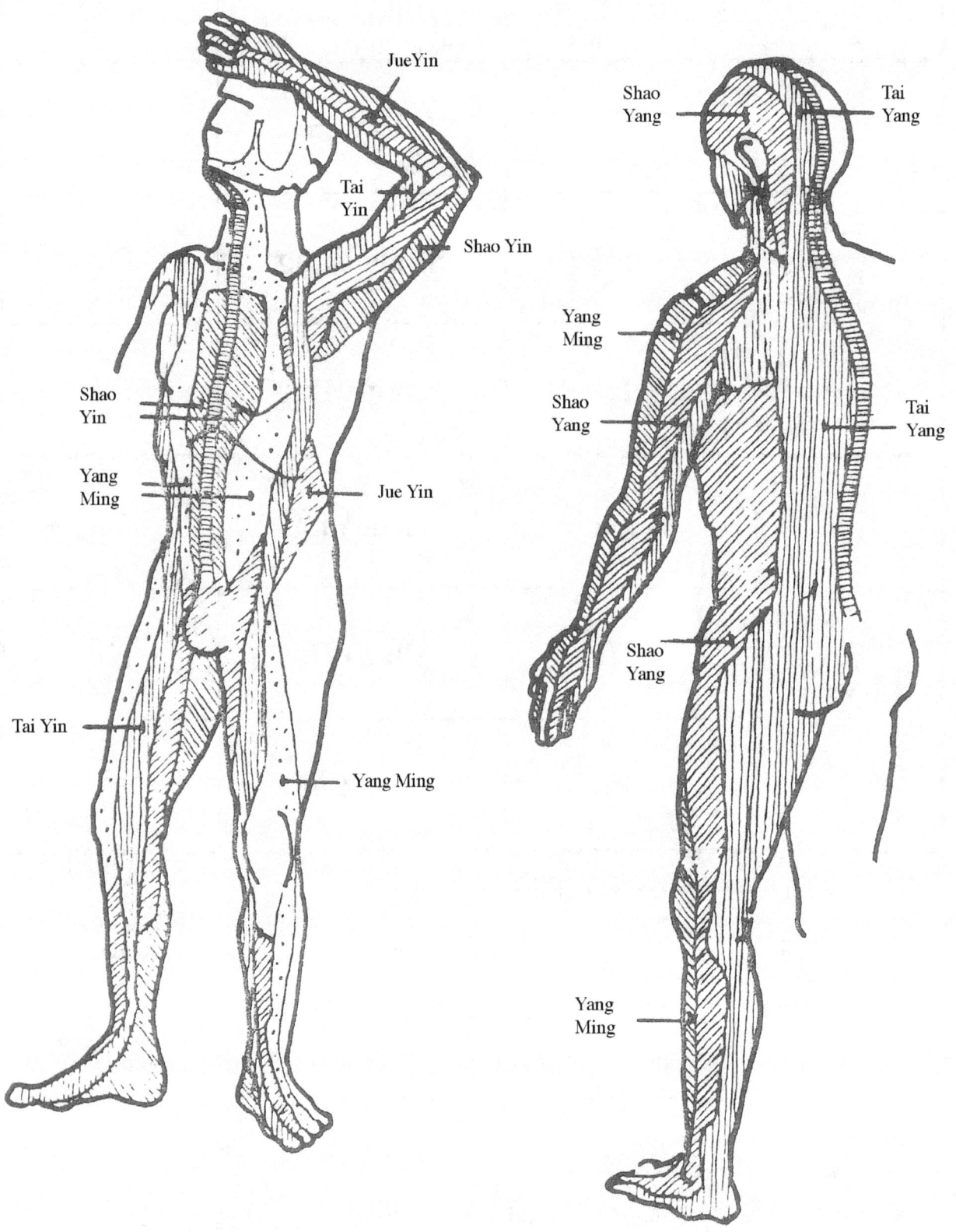

© 1990–2016   *Jim Cleaver LAc.*

Division Pairs & Anatomical Sectors

		ARM/hand 手 (Shǒu)	Six Divisions	LEG/Foot 足 (Zú)		
手三陽	Arm 3 Yang	**LI** radial dorsal	**Yáng Míng**	**ST** anterior lateral	Leg 3 Yang	足三陽
		TB median dorsal	**Shǎo Yáng**	**GB** median lateral		
		SI ulnar dorsal	**Tài Yáng**	**BL** posterior		
手三陰	Arm 3 Yin	**Lu** radial ventral	**Tài Yīn**	**Sp** anterior	Leg 3 Yin	足三陰
		Pc median ventral	**Jué Yīn**	**Lr** median		
		Ht ulnar ventral	**Shǎo Yīn**	**Kd** posterior		

Division Pairs & Digits

		ARM/Hand 手 (Shǒu)	Six Divisions	LEG/Foot 足 (Zú)		
手三陽	Shou San Yang	**SI** 5th finger ulnar	**Tài Yáng**	**BL** 5th toe lateral	Zu San Yang	足三陽
		TB 4th finger ulnar	**Shǎo Yáng**	**GB** 4th toe lateral		
		LI 2nd finger <u>radial</u>	**Yáng Míng**	**ST** 2nd toe lateral		
手三陰	Shou San Yin	**Lu** thumb radial	**Tài Yīn**	**Sp** big toe medial	Zu San Yin	足三陰
		Pc 3rd finger radial	**Jué Yīn**	**Lr** big toe <u>lateral</u>		
		Ht 5th finger radial	**Shǎo Yīn**	**Kd** 5th toe medial		

* the two exceptions to yin-yang rule are bold & underlined

The Circadian Clock

Cycle of Energy through the Channels
The sequence of flow, and the time/hours of Maximum Qi in each channel

	6 YIN	Circulation of Qi	6 YANG	
	Lu 3-5 am (0400)	→	**LI** 5-7 am (0600)	
	Sp 9-11 am (1000)	←	**ST** 7-9 am (0800)	
	Ht 11-1 pm (1200)	→	**SI** 1-3 pm (1400)	
	Kd 5-7 pm (1800)	←	**BL** 3-5 pm (1600)	
	Pc 7-9 pm (2000)	→	**TB** 9-11 pm (2200)	
	Lr 1-3 am (0200)	←	**GB** 11-1 am (2400)	

* I refer to the time of maximum flow as ***high tide*** in the channel.

Notice the ancient Chinese double-hour, when mapped onto the western clock, always goes from odd number to odd number
The number in parentheses is military time, and emphasizes the midpoint of the two hour time frame, (and therefore is even).

The 24 Hour Clock – Elements & Channels

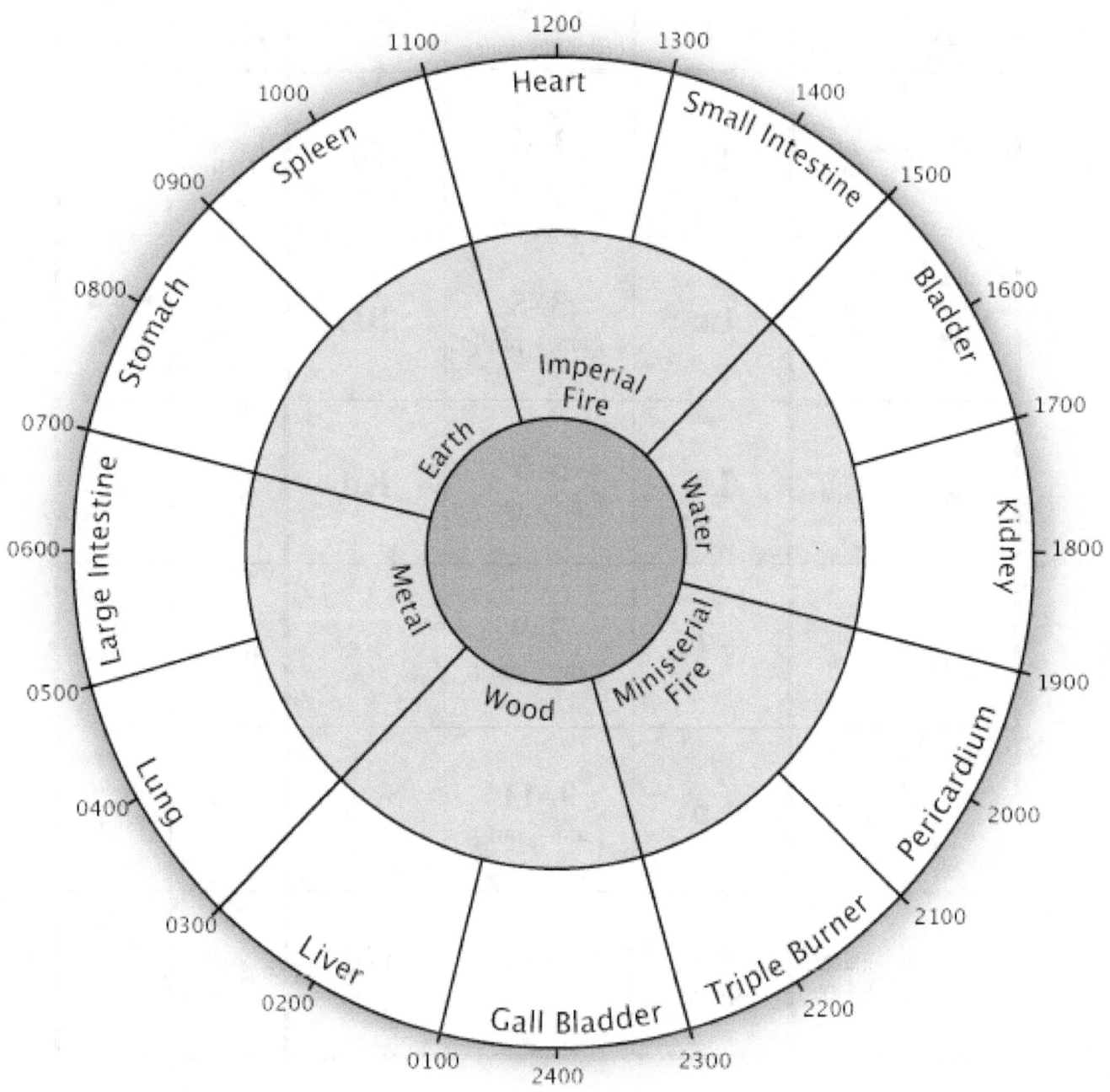

- There are twelve hours in the Chinese day. Thus a Chinese 'hour' is two Western hours.
- Each two hour period represents maximum qi flow or 'high tide' for a particular channel.
- Each channel experiences both a maximum and minimum, or high and low tide each day.
- The Chinese hour is always from odd hour to odd hour, with the even hour at the midpoint.
- By using military time each channel has a unique time of day. (compare with next page)

Clock Pairs/Partners

Using Western hours we see 'six times of day' and two channels paired, differentiated by am & pm (= yin/yang)

Order Original Current	Polarity Element	AM	High Tide (double-hour)	PM	Polarity Element	Order Original Current
2nd 12th	yin Wood	Lr	1–3 { am / pm }	SI	yang I. Fire	8th 6th
3rd 1st	yin Metal	Lu	3–5 { am / pm }	BL	yang Water	9th 7th
4th 2nd	yang Metal	LI	5–7 { am / pm }	Kd	yin Water	10th 8th
5th 3rd	yang Earth	ST	7–9 { am / pm }	Pc	yin M. Fire	11th 9th
6th 4th	yin Earth	Sp	9–11 { am / pm }	TB	yang M. Fire	12th 10th
7th 5th	yin I. Fire	Ht mid-day	11–1 { am / pm }	GB mid-night	yang Wood	1st 11th

The original order based on the 12 terrestrial branches sequence begins at mid-night with the GB.
In Chinese medicine we typically start the cycle with the Lungs (first breath).

Worsley trained practitioners start with the Heart and use Roman numerals to designate the channels.
Thus:

Ht = I	**SI = II**	**BL = III**	**Kd = IV**	**Pc = V**	**TB = VI**
GB = VII	**Lr = VIII**	**Lu = IX**	**LI = X**	**ST = XI**	**Sp = XII**

CV = XIII   GV = XIV   Most Chinese sources put GV before CV.
This is because the circulation of qi through these two channels runs up the back and down the front, despite both being numbered upward.

Circulation of Qi / Cycle of Energy

Placing them in a circle we see the two paired channels *180° apart*.
When one is at high tide its partner is at low tide, and vice versa.
In terms of circulation, we see a centrifugal (outward flow), followed by a centripetal (inward flow) of qi.

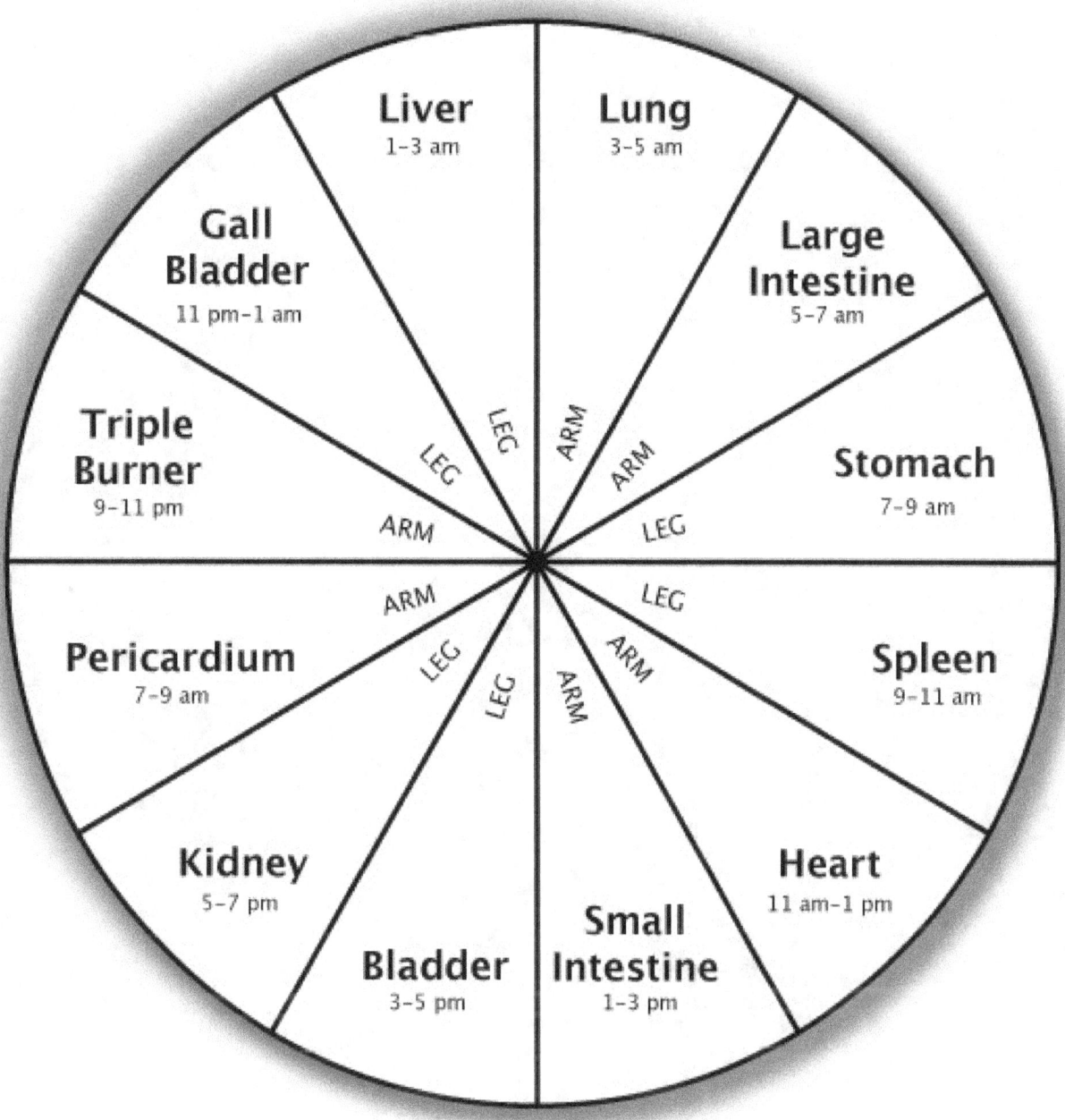

Color this page

特 定 穴

Tè Dìng Xué

(literal translation = Special Designation Points)

Point

Category

Tables

Point categories are essential elements of knowing about points and how to use them.
They are important in a couple of related ways. They provide reminders of a point's energetic nature, which in turn helps us to know how to use it clinically.

It is best to learn these attributes when first introduced to a point, much like getting someone's phone number. In fact, the three components we are going to study in
Points I & II can be likened to learning someone's name, address, and phone number.
The third step will be to learn a point's therapeutic actions, i.e. their occupation (what they do).

Not every point will have a category associated with it, some points will have several.

• **12 Primary Categories associated with each of the 12 Organ channels**
      a.   Every organ has a (front) **mu** pt & a (back) **shu** pt.
          • six (i.e. half) of the mu pts are on the Conception vessel / Ren mai, and thus unilateral
              Only 3 mu pts are on their respective channel (Lu, Lr, & GB)
          • all of the organ shu pts are on the Bladder channel (on the posterior torso).

The following are all on their respective channel pathways:
      b.   1 of each: **yuan**/source, **luo**/connecting, & **xi**/cleft pt   =   [3 per channel]

      c.   **5 transport**/5 element points   =   [5 per channel]
          These 8 are sometimes referred to as command points.   *[8 x 12 = 96 pts]*
          (however the yuan pt and one of the transport pts are redundant on yin channels, making only 90 different pts)
          The points of command are all distal to the elbows and knees. [except ST-34]

      d.   an **entry** & an **exit** point (usually the first & last pts, but there are at least 6 exceptions)

• **9 Misc. Categories not found on every channel**

      a.   8 "Influential" pts   influence particular tissues of the body

      b.   8 "Master" pts   'open' the 8 extraordinary vessels

      c.   6 Lower-uniting pts   powerful pts for each of the 6 fu organs

      d.   4-8 "Rulers"   strongly effect 6 general regions of the body

      e.   4 Group-luo pts   influence all 3 yin or yang channels on a limb

      f.   9 pts/needles that Rescue Yang   (abbreviated as 9N)

      g.   10 pts for controlling the 4 Seas of the body (Qi, Blood, Marrow & Nourishment)

      h.   10 or 12 Celestial Windows (aka windows of the sky)
          (all in the upper body, most of which have 天 Tiān = sky/heaven/celestial in their name)

      i.   13 Ghost pts   for psychotic behavior, epileptic disorders, etc. *aka 'possession'*
          (all have alternate names with 鬼 Guǐ = ghost/demon/spirit in them)

• These total ~75 points, but some of the points are in more than one category.

募 腧 穴
Mù Shū Xué = Mu & Shu Points

What does the order of channels in this list derive from?   Fill in the missing information.

Channel	*front* **Mu pts**	*back* **Shu pts**
Lu	name } **Lu-1** *location:*	name } **BL-13** *location:*
LI	name } **ST-25** *location:*	name } **BL-25** *location:*
ST	name } **CV-12** *location:*	name } **BL-21** *location:*
Sp	name } **Lr-13** *location:*	name } **BL-20** *location:*
Ht	name } **CV-14** *location:*	name } **BL-15** *location:*
SI	name } **CV-4** *location:*	name } **BL-27** *location:*
BL	name } **CV-3** *location:*	name } **BL-28** *location:*
Kd	name } **GB-25** *location:*	name } **BL-23** *location:*
Pc	name } **CV-17** *location:*	name } **BL-14** *location:*
TB	name } **CV-5** *location:*	name } **BL-22** *location:*
GB	name } **GB-24** *location:*	name } **BL-19** *location:*
Lr	name } **Lr-14** *location:*	name } **BL-18** *location:*

原 絡 隙穴
Yuán, Luò, & Xì Xué (Points)

郗 is the character *Grasping the Wind* uses for xi-cleft pts. It is the name of a city, but is used as a substitute for 隙

郗 is pronounced què in the Apple dictionary, and is only found in the simplified dictionary) In Mathews it is hsi #2474.

Xi is sometimes translated as 'accumulating or accumulation' pts. I usually translate luo as net-like or network, but here use 'connecting'.

Channel	(12) Yuan-source pts	(15/16) Luo-connecting pts	(16) Xi-cleft pts
Lu	Lu-9	Lu-7	Lu-6
LI	LI-4	LI-6	LI-7
Pc	Pc-7	Pc-6	Pc-4
TB	TB-4	TB-5	TB-7
Ht	Ht-7	Ht-5	Ht-6
SI	SI-4	SI-7	SI-6
Sp	Sp-3	Sp-4	Sp-8
ST	ST-42	ST-40	ST-34
Lr	Lr-3	Lr -5	Lr -6
GB	GB-40	GB-37	GB-36
Kd	Kd-3	Kd-4	Kd-5
BL	BL-64	BL-58	BL-63
CV		CV-15	
GV		GV-1	
Yin Qiao			Kd-8
Yang Qiao			BL-59
Yin Wei			Kd-9
Yang Wei			GB-35
Great Luo of Sp		Sp-21	
Great Luo of ST		(ST-18)	

The 5 Transport Points
五 輸 穴 Wǔ Shū Xué

Character	Pīn-Yīn	literal meaning	Image	Abbreviation	Phase-element association	
					Yin chan.	*Yang chan.*
井	**Jǐng**	a **well,** water welling up, emerging	**well**	J/W	**Wood**	*Metal*
熒 榮 湧	**Yíng** **Xíng** **Yǒng**	ying/sparkle = xing = brook, rivulet, rapids/riffles and interpreted as yǒng = to bubble up, **gush,** rush forth	(spring) **brook** (babbling brook)	Y/B	**Fire**	*Water*
俞	**Shū**	big and smooth enough to float a boat and **transport** things	**stream**	S/S	**Earth Soil**	*Wood*
經	**Jīng**	**a river** big enough to carry large vessels over long distances (traverse)	**river**	J/R	**Metal**	*Fire*
合	**Hé**	to **unite**; merge the river's **confluence** with the sea (the channel goes internal)	**sea**	H/S	**Water**	*Earth Soil*

	Body Region	**Sequence of Points moving proximally**
J/W pts:	nail pts	the most distal & terminal pt (first or last pt on the channel)
Y/B pts:	distal to MP joints	the penultimate pt
S/S pts:	hand or foot	the third point from the terminus
J/R pts:	arm or leg	# varies, but always between wrist & elbow or ankle & knee
H/S pts:	elbow or knee	# varies, but always the point closest to the elbow or knee joint

Intro to Point Categories

Color code this page:

Wu Shu Xue = _____

on **Yin Channels**					
Channel	J/W–wood	Y/S–fire	S/S–earth	J/R–metal	H/S–water
Ht	**Ht-9**	**Ht-8**	**Ht-7**	**Ht-4**	**Ht-3**
Pc	**Pc-9**	**Pc-8**	**Pc-7**	**Pc-5**	**Pc-3**
Lu	**Lu-11**	**Lu-10**	**Lu-9**	**Lu-8**	**Lu-5**
Sp	**Sp-1**	**Sp-2**	**Sp-3**	**Sp-5**	**Sp-9**
Lr	**Lr-1**	**Lr-2**	**Lr-3**	**Lr-4**	**Lr-8**
Kd	**Kd-1**	**Kd-2**	**Kd-3**	**Kd-7**	**Kd-10**

Wu Shu Xue = _____

on **Yang Channels**					
Channel	J/W–metal	Y/S–water	S/S–wood	J/R–fire	H/S–earth
LI	**LI-1**	**LI-2**	**LI-3**	**LI-5**	**LI-11**
TB	**TB-1**	**TB-2**	**TB-3**	**TB-6**	**TB-10**
SI	**SI-1**	**SI-2**	**SI-3**	**SI-5**	**SI-8**
ST	**ST-45**	**ST-44**	**ST-43**	**ST-41**	**ST-36**
GB	**GB-44**	**GB-43**	**GB-41***	**GB-38**	**GB-34**
BL	**BL-67**	**BL-66**	**BL-65**	**BL-60**	**BL-54**

* Ling Shu 2 identifies the points in each category for each channel.

Tonification & Dispersion Points
Bǔ Xiè Xué

• Each organ/channel is associated with a particular phase-element.

  • Each channel has a point that is the same phase as its organ (ex: fire pt on fire channel).
  I refer to these as the **Phase pt** on the channel (aka the horary point)

  • Each organ/channel is tonified by a point that corresponds to the preceeding phase in the Sheng cycle
  i.e. its mother (ex: wood is the mother of fire, therefore the wood pt on a fire channel is its **Tonification pt**)

  • Each organ/channel is dispersed or drained by a point that corresponds to the subsequent phase in the
  Sheng cycle, i.e. its child (ex: earth is the child of fire, therefore the earth pt on a fire channel is its **Dispersion pt**)

  • Each organ/channel has a **Control** point, one that corresponds to the phase of the element that
  inhibits it via the Ke cycle, i.e. its grandparent (ex: metal controls wood, therefore the metal pt on a wood chan will curtail it)

補 穴 bǔ xué = to **supplement**, or tonification pts   (most Chinese sources translate as ***reinforce***, Rf)

瀉 穴 xiè xué = to **drain**, or dispersion pts   (most Chinese sources translate as ***reduce***, Rd)

(Worsley practitioners refer to the latter as sedation)

Color code this table   *I will often use the abbreviations T, D, P, & C for these four points*

Phase / element	**Channel**	母 *mǔ =mother pt* **Tonification pt**	子 *zǐ = child pt* **Dispersion pt**	*same element pt* **Phase pt**	*grandparent pt* **Control pt**
wood	**Lr**	Lr-8 (water)	Lr-2 (fire)	Lr-1 (wood)	Lr-4 (metal)
wood	**GB**	GB-43 (water)	GB-38 (fire)	GB-41 (wood)	GB-44 (metal)
fire	**Ht**	Ht-9 (wood)	Ht-7 (earth)	Ht-8 (fire)	Ht-3 (water)
fire	**SI**	SI-3 (wood)	SI-8 (earth)	SI-5 (fire)	SI-2 (water)
fire	**Pc**	Pc-9 (wood)	Pc-7 (earth)	Pc-8 (fire)	Pc-3 (water)
fire	**TB**	TB-3 (wood)	TB-10 (earth)	TB-6 (fire)	TB-2 (water)
earth	**Sp**	Sp-2 (fire)	Sp-5 (metal)	Sp-3 (earth)	Sp-1 (wood)
earth	**ST**	ST-41 (fire)	ST-45 (metal)	ST-36 (earth)	ST-43 (wood)
metal	**Lu**	Lu-9 (earth)	Lu-5 (water)	Lu-8 (metal)	Lu-10 (fire)
metal	**LI**	LI-11 (earth)	LI-2 (water)	LI-1 (metal)	LI-5 (fire)
water	**Kd**	Kd-7 (metal)	Kd-1 (wood)	Kd-10 (water)	Kd-3 (earth)
water	**BL**	BL-67 (metal)	BL-65 (wood)	BL-66 (water)	BL-54 (earth)

24 入 出 Rù Chū = Entry & Exit Points
12 Entry & 12 Exit

• Entry & Exit points map the specific flow of qi from one channel to the next following the cycle of energy.

• Usually, the Entry pt is the first point & the Exit pt is the last point of the channel.

• Generally, 6 exceptions are usually counted, I note 7 (see footnotes). • The **Exceptions** are shaded in the chart below.

• LI-4 is the only exception to the first point being the entry point, all the other exceptions are exit points.

Region }	chest	hand	hand	face	face	foot	foot	chest
Entry/Exit	entry	exit	entry	exit	entry	exit	entry	exit
Circuit I	Lu-1	Lu-7 (not Lu-11)	LI-4 (not LI-1)	LI-20	ST-1	ST-42 (not ST-45)	Sp-1	Sp-21
II	Ht-1	Ht-9	SI-1	SI-18 (vs. SI-19)	BL-1	BL-67	Kd-1 (actually Kd-0)	Kd-22 (not Kd-27)
III	Pc-1	Pc-8 (not Pc-9)	TB-1	TB-23	GB-1	GB-41 (not GB-44)	Lr-1	Lr-14

Some considerations are as follows:
The end of one channel (its exit pt) and the beginning of the next (its entry pt), are always in close proximity to one another.

Lung: Some sources consider Lu-2 to be the entry pt. *(the channel flows from the lung to the throat, then downward under the clavicle arriving at Lu-2 first)*

Lg. Intestine: Many sources describe the route from LI-20 to ST-1 as going through BL-1 at the inner canthus.

Sm. Intestine: I consider SI-18, on the cheek, to be the exit pt, instead of SI-19, by the ear. *(next entry point is BL-1, SI-18 is closer by half a face)*

Spleen: Sp-20 connects to Lu-1 (one intercostal space up) to link the Tai-Yin channels before descending to Sp-21, and then flowing on to Ht-1 in the axilla.

Kidney: The actual entry point is the nail point (Kd-0) on the medial aspect of the little toe, from there it proceeds across the ball of the foot to Kd-1.

Entry / Exit Sequence of Channels & Points

previous channel	Primary Channel	next channel	previous channel exit pt	Primary Channel entry ⇒ exit	next channel entry pt
Lr	Lung	LI	Lr-14 →	Lu-1 ⇒ Lu-7	→ LI-4
Lu	Lg. Intestine	ST	Lu-7 →	LI-4 ⇒ LI-20	→ ST-1
LI	Stomach	Sp	LI-20 →	ST-1 ⇒ ST-42	→ Sp-1
ST	Spleen	Ht	ST-42 →	Sp-1 ⇒ Sp-21	→ Ht-1
Sp	Heart	SI	Sp-21 →	Ht-1 ⇒ Ht-9	→ SI-1
Ht	Sm. Intestine	BL	Ht-9 →	SI-1 ⇒ SI-18	→ BL-1
SI	Bladder	Kd	SI-18 →	BL-1 ⇒ BL-67	→ Kd-0
BL	Kidney	Pc	BL-67 →	Kd-0 ⇒ Kd-22	→ Pc-1
Kd	Pericardium	TB	Kd-22 →	Pc-1 ⇒ Pc-8	→ TB-1
Pc	Triple Burner	GB	Pc-8 →	TB-1 ⇒ TB-23	→ GB-1
TB	Gall Bladder	Lr	TB-23 →	GB-1 ⇒ GB-41	→ Lr-1
GB	Liver	Lu	GB-41 →	Lr-1 ⇒ Lr-14	→ Lu-1

* Underline means it's not the first or last point on the channel

© 1990–2016   Jim Cleaver LAc.

Channel Pairings and Number of Points

Phase	Yin	Yang	Total Points
Wood	Lr = **14**	GB = **44**	= 58
I. Fire	Ht = **9**	SI = **19**	= 28
M. Fire	Pc = 9	TB = 23	= 32
Earth	Sp = 21	ST = 45	= 66
Metal	Lu = 11	LI = 20	= 31
Water	Kd = **27**	BL = **67**	= 94
Total # of Pts }	91	218	309

Bold # = a kind of symmetry between phase pairs in which the **same last digit** occurs in both. (Wood, I. Fire, & Water)
Total # of Fire Pts = 60 (Imperial + Ministerial Fire)
(making wood, fire and earth all about 60, with metal at 30 & water at 90)

Division	Arm	Leg	Total Points
Tai Yin	Lu = 11	Sp = 21	= 32
Jue Yin	Pc = 9	Lr = 14	= 23
Shao Yin	Ht = 9	Kd = 27	= 36
Tai Yang	SI = 19	BL = 67	= 86
Yang Ming	LI = 20	ST = 45	= 65
Shao Yang	TB = 23	GB = 44	= 67
Total # of Pts }	91	218	309

Clock	Yin	Yang	Total Points
11 – 1	Ht = 9	GB = 44	= 53
1 – 3	Lr = 14	SI = 19	= 33
3 – 5	Lu = 11	BL = 67	= 78
5 – 7	Kd = 27	LI = 20	= 47
7 – 9	Pc = 9	ST = 45	= 54
9 – 11	Sp = 21	TB = 23	= 44

Interestingly the total number of yin channel points is the same as the total for all the arm channel points (91 pts).
Likewise for the six yang & six leg channels (218 pts).
This means there are an equal number of points on the 3 arm yang as on the 3 leg yin (62 pts).

The leg yang total is 156 pts, and the arm yin total is 29 pts.
Adding the Ren & Du changes this slightly because GV has four more points (CV=24, GV=28) making yang 246 pts & yin 115 pts.

下 合 穴 Xià Hé Xué
(6) Lower-Uniting Points

All six are located on the lower body
Of key importance is that the arm channel organs have a point on the legs

Point	Organ (bold = arm channels)
ST-36	stomach
ST-37	**lg. intestine**
ST-39	**sm. intestine**
GB-34	gall bladder
BL-53/39	**triple burner**
BL-54/40	bladder

* The 3 leg channel Xia-He points are the same as their channels' He/sea pt (Hé is the same character)

總 穴 Zǒng Xué
(4-8) Rulers (aka Dominant or Command Points)
zǒng can mean 1) to assemble, put together, sum up; 2) general, overall, total; 3) main, chief, head, general

Point	Region of Rulership
Lu-7 &/or SI-3	back of the neck and head
LI-4	face and mouth
ST-36	abdomen
BL-54/40	back
Pc-6	chest & diaphragm
GB-34	sides, esp. of the torso
Sp-6	pelvic cavity (lower jiao)

* These points have such a strong influence over the entire region, that they are designated as 'Rulers' of them.

(4) Group Luo Points

Point	*Name*	*Translation*	Group
Pc-5	Jian Shi	Go Between Messenger / Ambassador	3 arm yin
TB-8	**San Yang Luo**	3 Yang Connect	3 arm yang
Sp-6	**San Yin Jiao**	3 Yin Junction/Intersect	3 leg yin
GB-39	Xuan Zhong	Hanging Bell	3 leg yang

Note that two of the four tell you this is their category with their name, and that this category was considered significant enough to name the point according to it.   Also notice that the group luo pt will always be on the middle of the three channels on that aspect of the limb.

© 1990–2016   Jim Cleaver LAc.

八會穴 Bā Huì Xué (lit. 8 meeting/confluent points)
Eight Influential Points

Influential Point	Characters	Pinyin	Tissue Influenced
Lr-13	臟	Zàng	Yin organs (viscera)
CV-12	腑	Fǔ	Yang organs (bowels)
CV-17	氣	Qì	宗 zōng qi = ancestral qi 胸 xiōng qi = chest qi
BL-17	血	Xuè	**blood**
Lu-9	脈	Mài	blood **vessels** & the **pulse**
BL-11	骨	Gǔ	**bones**
GB-39	髓	Suǐ	**marrow**
GB-34	筋	Jīn	**sinews** / (tendons, ligaments, muscles, big nerves)

* These eight points possess a powerful influence over the named tissue type, throughout the body.

八交會穴 Bā Jiāo-huì Xué = 8 intersection-meeting pts (aka **Confluent pts**)
Eight Master Points (of the 8 Extraordinary Vessels)

Master Point	Characters	Vessel	Translation
Lu-7	任	**Ren mai**	Conception (Controlling) vessel
SI-3	督	**Du mai**	Governing vessel
Pc-6	陰維	**Yin Wei mai**	Yin Linking vessel
TB-5	陽維	**Yang Wei mai**	Yang Linking vessel
Sp-4	衝	**Chong mai**	Thoroughfare (Pulsing) vessel *most sources call this the* Penetrating vessel
GB-41	帶	**Dai mai**	Belt (Girdling) vessel
Kd-6	陰蹺	**Yin Qiao mai**	Yin Heel/Motility vessel
BL-62	陽蹺	**Yáng Qiao mai**	Yang Heel/Motility vessel

* These eight points control access to the energetic layer of the body under the auspices of the 8 vessels
and may be thought of as 'opening' them like a key, or combination (they are used in pairs) that unlocks that layer.

回 陽 九 針 Huí Yáng Jiǔ Zhēn
9 Points/Needles to Return/Restore/Rescue Yang

Arm		Leg		Torso	
yin	*yang*	*yin*	*yang*	*front*	*back*
Pc-8 *(palm)*	**LI-4** *(hand)*	**Kd-1** *(sole)* **Kd-3** *(ankle)* **Sp-6** *(lower leg)*	**GB-30** *(hip)* **ST-36** *(knee)*	**CV-12** *(abd)*	**GV-15** *(occiput)*

* These points alone or in combination are used to rescue yang in conditions diagnosed as yang collapse or yang desertion. (亡陽 wáng yáng, or 陽脫 yáng tuó) These conditions are characterized by sweating, cold skin, and cold limbs.

四 海 穴 Sì Hǎi Xué
4 Seas Points (10 pts)

Sea of ...	Points
水穀 **Shuǐ Gǔ** (lit. water & grain) ~ **Nourishment**	**ST-30 & 36**
血 **Xuè = Blood**	**ST-37 & 39, BL-11**
氣 **Qì = Energy**	**CV-17, ST-9, BL-10** Some sources substitute **GV-15** for BL-10 the classics are unclear, saying the neck betw GV-14 & 15 Bl-10 is in the trapezius, level with GV-15 I think BL-10 is a better pairing with ST-9
髓 **Suǐ = Marrow**	**GV-16 & 20**

* These points are given in the Ling Shu / Spirit Pivot part of the Nei Jing as ones to regulate the four seas.
Again we may think of them as providing access to these energetic layers of the body.
In a general way:
the Sea of Marrow may be thought of as the brain, and mental function,
the Sea of Qi as being associated with the chest, which controls respiration and more importantly, heart rate & rhythm,
the Sea of Blood pertains to all the blood in the body,
while the Sea of Nourishment is exactly that, and closely associated with the stomach.

To confuse things just a little, the Chong mai / Penetrating Vessel is sometimes referred to as the Sea of the Twelve Channels.

天牖穴 Tiān Yǒu Xué				
Celestial Windows (aka Windows of/to the Sky/Heaven) (10 or 12 pts)				

Point	Characters	Name	Translation	Location
Lu-3*	天府	Tiān Fu	Celestial Official	*upper arm:*
Pc-1 (men)	天池	Tiān Chi	Celestial Pool	*chest:*
Pc-2 (women)	天泉	Tiān Quan	Celestial Spring	*upper arm:*
CV-22	天突	Tiān Tu	Celestial Projection	*throat:*
ST-9*	人迎 aka 天五會	*Ren Ying* aka Tiān Wu Hui	*Person's Prognosis* Celestial 5 Meet	*throat:*
LI-18*	扶突	*Fu Tu*	*Aid the Prominence*	*neck:*
SI-16	天窗	Tiān Chuang	Celestial Vent	*neck:*
SI-17	天容	Tiān Rong	Celestial Look	*neck:*
or **GB-9**	天衝	Tiān Chong	Celestial Thoroughfare	*head:*
TB-16*	天牖	**Tiān You**	Celestial Window	*neck:*
BL-10*	天柱	Tiān Zhu	Celestial Pillar	*neck:*
GV-16	風府	*Feng Fu*	*Wind Official/Mansion*	*occiput:*

* in the Nei Jing these 5 are listed with specific symptomology (LS 21:7)

• BL-7, LI-17, SI-11, TB-15 & 10; Sp-18 & ST-25 also have Tiān in their names. = 16 altogether (all are in the upper body)

十三鬼穴 Shí Sān Guǐ Xué
13 Ghost Points / 13 Points for Ghosts/Possession (from **Sun Si-miao** circa 625 CE)

* Each of these points has an alternate name with the character gui/ghost in it

Order	Point	Characters	Ghost Name	**Translation**: **Ghost**; Demon; Phantom; Spirit
1.	**GV-26**	鬼宮	Guǐ Gōng	Ghost Palace (Temple; Womb; Earth-Note)
2.	**Lu-11**	鬼信	Guǐ Xìn	Ghost Message (strange, nonsensical speech) Ghost Evidence/Certified (Proof of Possession)
3.	**Sp-1**	鬼壘	Guǐ Lěi	Ghost Ramparts/Fortress/Base
4.	**Pc-7**	鬼心	Guǐ Xīn	Ghost Heart
5.	**BL-62**	鬼路	Guǐ Lù	Ghost Road/Highway
6.	**GV-16**	鬼枕	Guǐ Zhěn	Ghost Pillow (the occiput is the pillow bone)
7.	**ST-6**	鬼床	Guǐ Chuáng	Ghost Bed
8.	**CV-24**	鬼市	Guǐ Shì	Ghost Marketplace
9.	**Pc-8**	鬼窟	Guǐ Kū	Ghost Den (Hole/Cave/Grotto)
10.	**GV-23**	鬼堂	Guǐ Táng	Ghost Hall/Court
11.	**CV-1**	鬼藏	Guǐ Cáng	Concealed/Hidden Ghost
12.	**LI-11**	鬼臣	Guǐ Chén	Ghost's Vassal/Minister/Ambassador
13.	**Hǎi Quán**	鬼封	Guǐ Fēng	Enclosed/Sealed/Trapped Ghost

General Distribution of Ghost Points

Head & Torso (7 pts) (6 head, 1 torso) *6 midline (3 GV, 3 CV)* *6 are unilateral*		**Limbs** (6 pts) (4 arm, 2 leg) *4 yin, 2 yang* *all 6 are bilateral*
Head 6. **GV-16** *occiput* 10. **GV-23** *vertex* 1. **GV-26** *philtrum* 8. **CV-24** *chin* 13. **Hǎi Quán** *tongue* 7. **ST-6** *jaw/masseter* ------------------------- *Torso* 11. **CV-1** *perineum*		*Arm* 4. **Pc-7** *wrist* 9. **Pc-8** *palm* 2. **Lu-11** *thumb* 12. **LI-11** *elbow* ------------------------- *Leg* 3. **Sp-1** *big toe* 5. **BL-62** *ankle*

* The seven bilateral points are distributed on the following channels:
  2 are Taiyin (1 Lu; 1 Sp);   2 are Yangming (1 LI, 1 ST);   2 are Jueyin (both Pc);   1 is Taiyang (BL)
* The one extra pt is on the midline under the tongue (I counted it as a CV pt)   (there are no Lr or SI; Shaoyin, or Shaoyang pts)

* These points are for bizarre, unexplainable behavior and mental disease, including schizophrenia and psychosis, as well as disorders of the brain & nervous system such as epilepsy, autism, and mental retardation. They could be summarized as insanity.
All are poorly understood disorders, even today, and could easily be culturally explained as being caused by ghosts.
If ghosts are understood to be invisible, mystery agents, the effects of some neurotoxins, might fit into this treatment approach as well.

Anatomical Measurement

Anatomical Measurement is a Proportional Measurement System

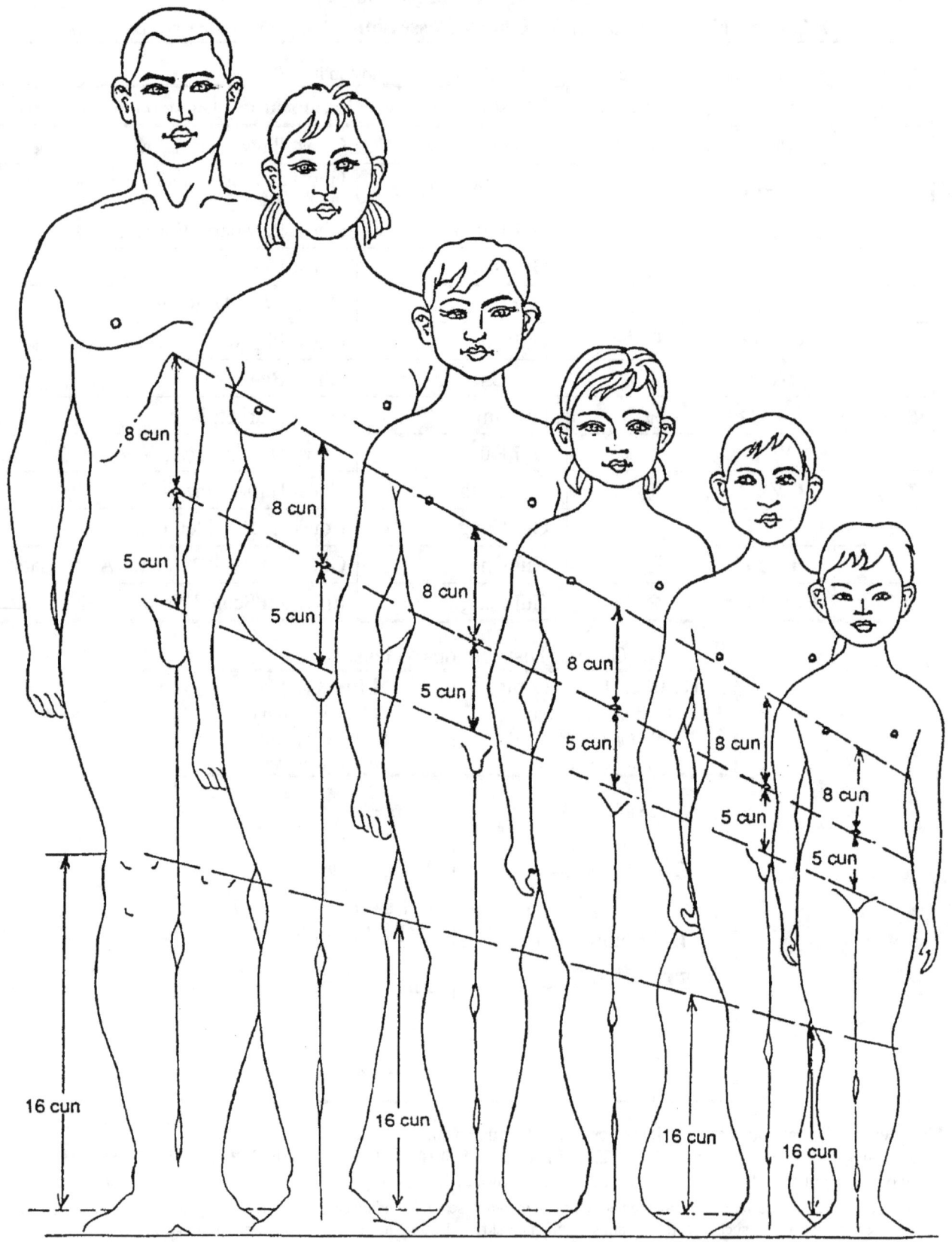

骨度法 Gǔ Dù Fǎ = Bone-Measuring Method

Cun Measurements

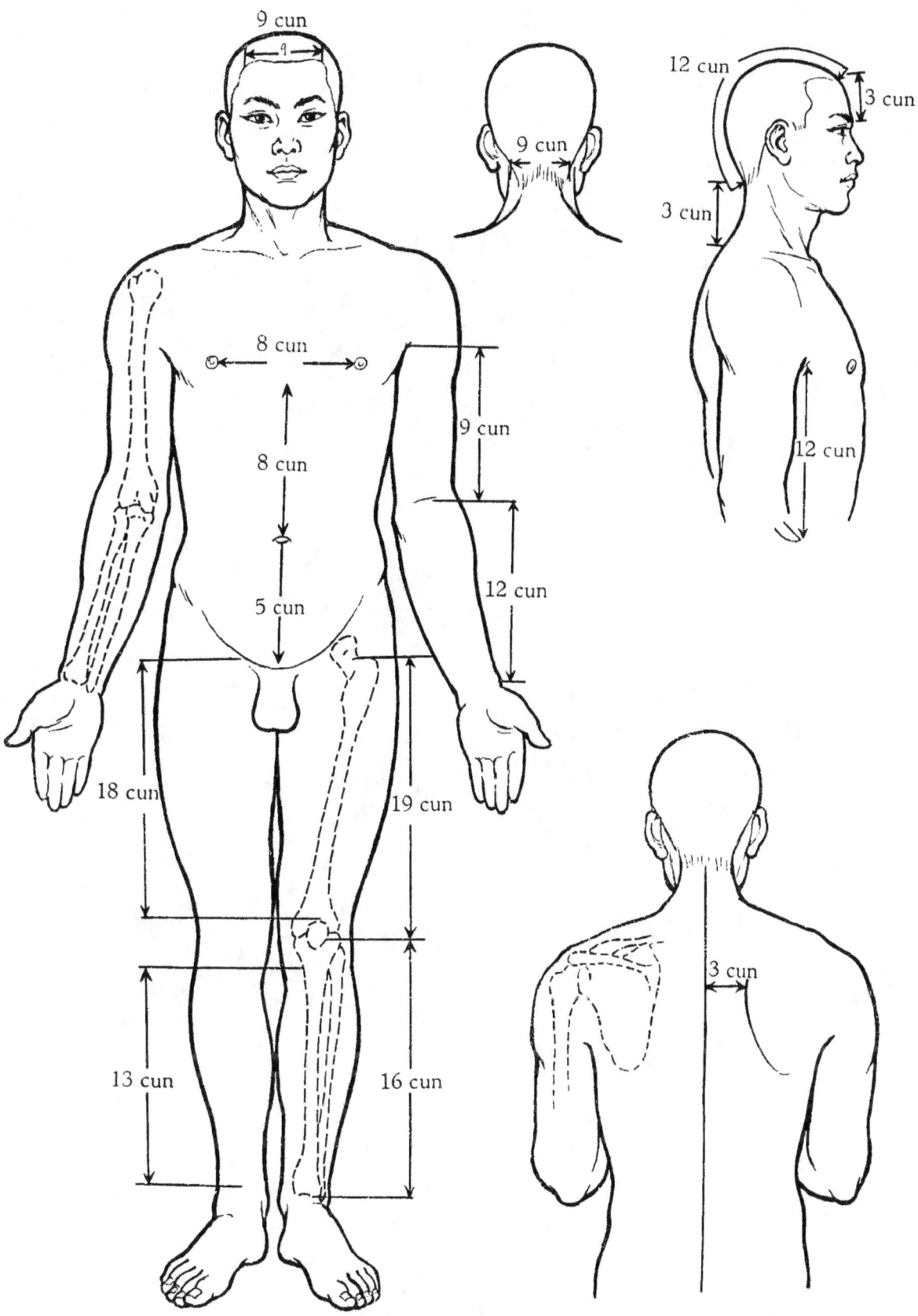

寸 Cùn = the anatomical inch (a thumb width)

© 1990–2016   *Jim Cleaver LAc.*

Points 1

- Six Arm Channels (91 pts)

- Two Midline Vessels (52 pts)

- Total = 143 pts

Channel Pathways, Point Locations, Categories, & Names

General Channel Flow Pattern

The 3 Yin Channels of the Arm

• begin on the chest   • end at the hands/fingertips

(centrifugal / outward flow of yin)

The 3 Yang Channels of the Arm

• begin on the fingertips   • end on the face

(centripetal / inward flow of yang)

The 3 Yang Channels of the Leg

• begin on the face   • end at the feet/toes

(centrifugal / outward flow of yang)

The 3 Yin Channels of the Leg

• begin on the toes   • end on the torso

(centripetal / inward flow of yin)

The 3 Yin Channels of the Arm
Ht – Pc – Lu (29 pts)

• begin on the chest   • end at the hands/fingertips

(centrifugal / outward, flow of yin)

Fill in the 3 pairings of each channel: Heart is done for you.

Channel	*compartment*	Phase	Division	Time
Heart	*ulnar*	yin I. Fire	shou Shao Yin	11 am–1 pm
	3 pairings }	**SI**	**Kd**	**GB**
Pericardium	*middle*	yin M. Fire	shou Jue Yin	7–9 pm
	3 pairings }			
Lung	*radial*	yin Metal	shou Tai Yin	3–5 am
	3 pairings }			

心 經 Xīn Jīng = Heart Channel

- **Division:** (Arm) **Shao Yin**
- **Phase/Element:** (Yin) Imperial **Fire**
- **High Tide: 11am–1pm**

---

begins: **in the armpit**

ends: **on the radial side of the little finger**

❖ *The Heart Channel external pathway:*

· begins in center of the axilla   **(Ht-1)**

· proceeds along the ulnar side of the bicep to the elbow   (Ht-3)

· follows the ulnar aspect of the forearm (flexor carpi ulnaris) to the wrist   (Ht-4–7)

· across the palm between the 4th & 5th metacarpals   (Ht-8)

· along the radial side of the little finger

· to end at the radial nail point on the little finger   **(Ht-9)**

心 經 **Heart Channel** (9 pts)

Axilla
Ht-1
• in the center (deepest part) of the axilla (adjacent to the axillary artery)
    Tip: place clients palm behind, or on top of their head

Upper Arm   ➤ *9 cun are measured between the anterior axillary fold and the cubital fold*

Ht-2
• in the brachial groove, (medial/ulnar side of the biceps)
  3 cun proximal to the cubital crease/medial epicondyle/Ht-3

Elbow
Ht-3
• between the ulnar end of the cubital crease and the medial epicondyle
    Tip: flex the arm at least 90°, full flexion (hand touching shoulder) is also good

Forearm   ➤ *12 cun are measured between the cubital fold and the wrist fold*

Ht-4
• **1.5 cun proximal** to the wrist, in the groove on the radial side of the flexor carpi ulnaris tendon

Ht-5
• **1 cun proximal** to the wrist, in the groove on the radial side of the flexor carpi ulnaris tendon

Ht-6
• **0.5 cun proximal** to the wrist, in the groove on the radial side of the flexor carpi ulnaris tendon

Wrist
Ht-7
• at the ulnar end of the wrist fold, proximal to the pisiform,
  on radial side of the flexor carpi ulnaris

Hand
Ht-8
• on the palm, between the shafts of the 4th & 5th metacarpals, proximal to their heads

Ht-9
• the nail point on the radial side of the little finger

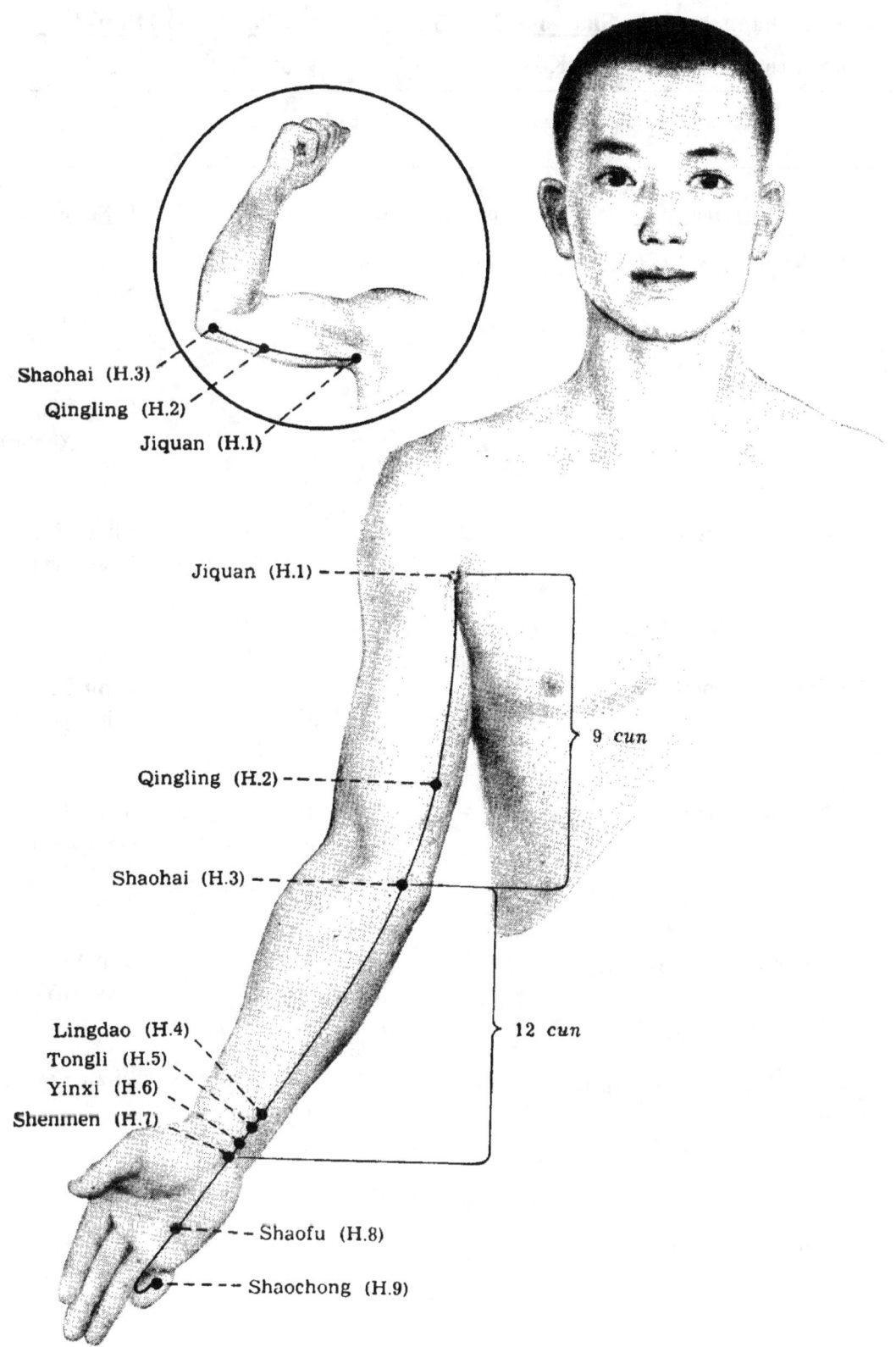

Shaohai (H.3)
Qingling (H.2)
Jiquan (H.1)

Jiquan (H.1)

Qingling (H.2)

Shaohai (H.3)

9 cun

12 cun

Lingdao (H.4)
Tongli (H.5)
Yinxi (H.6)
Shenmen (H.7)

Shaofu (H.8)

Shaochong (H.9)

手少陰心經
Shou Shao-Yin Xin Jing
Arm Lesser-Yin Heart Channel

Heart Channel = Shǒu **Shǎo-Yīn** Xīn Jīng		**I. Fire**	**11am–1pm**
paired channels }	Kd	SI	GB

Mu pt = CV-14	**Shu pt** = BL-15

	• Main Categories	• Misc. Categories	Pt Name & Translation
	on every channel		
Ht-1	• entry pt: *from Sp-21*		Jí Quán 極泉 Summit Spring Spring at the Summit
Ht-2			Qīng Líng 青靈 Azure (Yin/Rain) Spirits
Ht-3	• he/sea–water–Control pt.		**Shǎo Hǎi** 少海 Lesser (Yin) Sea
Ht-4	• jing/river–metal		**Líng Dào** 靈道 (Yin) Spirits Path(way)
Ht-5	• **luo/connecting**		**Tōng Lǐ** 通里 Open the Interior Through the Village
Ht-6	• **xi/cleft**		**Yīn Xī** 陰隙 (Lesser) Yin Cleft
Ht-7	• shu/stream–earth–Disp. pt. • **yuan/source**		**Shén Mén** 神門 Spirit/Mind/Consciouness Gate
Ht-8	• ying/brook–fire–Phase pt.		Shǎo Fǔ 少府 Lesser (Yin) Official
Ht-9	• jing/well–wood–Tonif. pt. • exit pt: *to SI-1*		Shǎo Chōng 少衝 Lesser (Yin) Thoroughfare

• *Memorize All Categories, On All Channels*   • *Quizzes Test Bold Names Only*

心包經 Xīn Bāo Jīng = Pericardium Channel

- **Division:** (Arm) **Jue Yin**
- **Phase/Element:** (Yin) Ministerial **Fire**
- **High Tide:** 7–9 pm

---

begins: on the chest, near the nipple

ends: on the middle finger

❖   *The Pericardium Channel external pathway:*

· begins supra-lateral to the nipple, in the 4th ICS   **(Pc-1)**

· arcs over the axillary fold (inferior to the Lu channel)

· flows between the two bellies of the biceps to the elbow   (Pc-2)
   (ulnar to the biceps tendon at the cubital fold)   (Pc-3)

· from elbow to the wrist it follows the middle of the forearm between the radius and the ulna
   more precisely; between the two prominent tendons (flexor carpi radialis & palmaris longus)   (Pc-4–7)

· across the palm between the 2nd & 3rd metacarpals   (Pc-8)

· along the radial side of the middle finger

· to end at the radial nail point on the middle finger (or the tip of the middle finger)   **(Pc-9)**

心包經 **Pericardium Channel**   (9 pts)

Chest

Pc-1
- • **~1 cun supralateral** to the areola (~5 cun lateral to the midline)
 over the 4th IC space (in, or just inferior to the pectoralis major)

Upper Arm   ➤ *9 cun are measured between the anterior axillary fold and the cubital fold*

Pc-2
- • **2 cun inferior** to the axillary fold, between the two bellies of the biceps

Elbow

Pc-3
- • at the cubital fold, on the ulnar side of the biceps tendon

* The two tendons in the middle of the anterior forearm are:
* flexor carpi radialis } the more radial of the two (make a fist and flex the wrist to isolate)
* palmaris longus } the more ulnar (some people don't have this one)

Forearm   ➤ *12 cun are measured between the cubital fold and the wrist fold*

Pc-4
- • **5 cun proximal** to the wrist, on the ulnar side of the flexor carpi radialis tendon

Pc-5
- • **3 cun proximal** to the wrist, on the ulnar side of the flexor carpi radialis tendon

Pc-6
- • **2 cun proximal** to the wrist, on the ulnar side of the flexor carpi radialis tendon

Wrist

Pc-7
- • at the center of the wrist fold, on the ulnar side of the flexor carpi radialis tendon
 distal to the arm bones, between them and the carpal bones

Hand

Pc-8
- • on the palm, between the 2nd & 3rd metacarpals, proximal to their heads

Pc-9
- • the nail point on the radial side of the middle finger
Alt Loc }   • *at the center of the tip of the middle finger*   • *Know both locations*

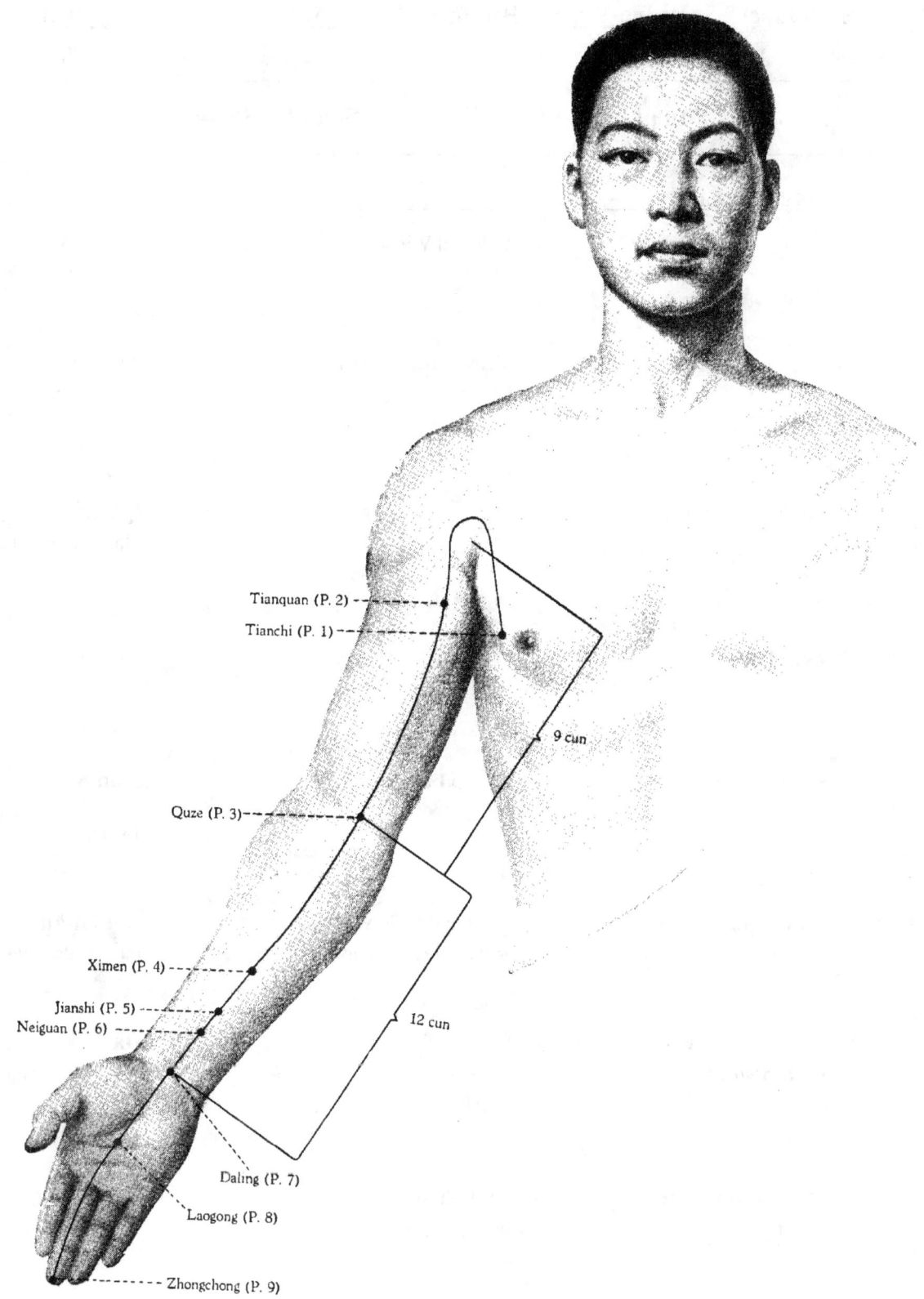

Tianquan (P. 2)

Tianchi (P. 1)

9 cun

Quze (P. 3)

Ximen (P. 4)

Jianshi (P. 5)

Neiguan (P. 6)

12 cun

Daling (P. 7)

Laogong (P. 8)

Zhongchong (P. 9)

手厥陰心包經
Shou Jue-Yin Xin-Bao Jing
Arm Faint-Yin Pericardium Channel

Pc Channel = Shǒu **Jué-Yīn** Xīn-Bāo Jīng	**M. Fire**	**7–9 pm**
paired channels } Lr	TB	ST

Mu pt = CV-17	**Shu pt** = BL-14

	• Main Categories <small>on every channel</small>	• Misc. Categories	Pt Name & Translation
Pc-1	• entry pt: *from Kd-22*	• Celestial Window	Tiān Chí 天池 Celestial Pond/Pool/Moat
Pc-2		• alt. celestial window	Tiān Quán 天泉 Celestial Spring
Pc-3	• he/sea–water–Control pt.		**Qū Zé** 曲澤 Marsh at the Crook
Pc-4	• **xi/cleft**		**Xī Mén** 隙門 Cleft Gate
Pc-5	• jing/river–metal	• **Group Luo**: (3 arm yin)	**Jiān Shǐ** 間使 Between, Messenger The Envoy/Ambassador/Minister
Pc-6	• **luo/connecting**	• **Master Pt**: Yin Wei mai • **Ruler**: chest & diaphragm	**Nèi Guān** 內關 Inner Gateway
Pc-7	• shu/stream–earth–Disp. pt. • **yuan/source**	• (4th) Ghost pt	**Dà Líng** 大陵 Big Mound/Tomb
Pc-8	• ying/brook–fire–Phase pt. • **exit pt**: *to TB-1*	• (9th) Ghost pt • 9N (to Rescue Yang)	**Láo Gōng** 勞宮 Labor's Palace / Palace of Labor Palace of Toil/Fatigue
Pc-9	• jing/well–wood–Tonif. pt.		Zhōng Chōng 中衝 Middle Thoroughfare

肺 經 Fèi Jīng = Lung Channel

- **Division:** (Arm) **Tai Yin**
- **Phase/Element:** (Yin) **Metal**
- **High Tide: 3–5 am**

begins: **on the upper, lateral chest**

ends: **on the thumb**

❖ *The Lung Channel external pathway:*

· begins below the clavicle, in the delto-pectoral triangle (medial to the coracoid)   **(Lu-1–2)**

· arcs over the axillary fold following the anterior deltoid

· proceeds along the radial side of the bicep to the elbow (cubital fossa)   (Lu-3–5)

· follows the radial aspect of the forearm (brachioradialis) to the wrist   (Lu-6–9)

· across the thenar eminence   (Lu-10)

· along the radial side of the thumb

· to end at the radial nail point on the thumb   **(Lu-11)**

肺經 **Lung Channel** (11 pts)

Chest

Lu-1
> *there are ~ 8 cun from the anterior midline to the axillary fold / acromial head of clavicle*
- on the upper chest, just inferior to the delto-pectoral triangle
  1.6 cun inferior to the clavicle, (i.e. Lu-2), in the upper fibers of the pectoralis major muscle
  (~ level with the 1st ICS as palpated next to the sternum), **6 cun lateral** to the midline

Lu-2
- in the delto-pectoral triangle, immediately inferior to the clavicle,
  just medial to the coracoid process, = 6 cun lateral to the midline

Upper Arm

Lu-3
> *9 cun are measured between the anterior axillary fold and the cubital fold*
- on the upper arm, **3 cun inferior** to the axillary fold
  in the groove on the radial side of the biceps / anterior edge of the humerus
  at the jct of the biceps and the anterior deltoid
  (sl. proximal to the level of the deltoid insertion)

Lu-4
- on the upper arm, **4 cun inferior** to the axillary fold (1 cun distal to Lu-3)
  almost halfway between the axillary & cubital folds
  (both Lu-3 & 4 lie alongside the cephalic vein)

Elbow

Lu-5
- at the cubital fold, in the depression on the radial side of the biceps tendon

Forearm

Lu-6
> *there are 12 cun between the cubital fold and the wrist fold*
- **5 cun distal** to the cubital crease (near the distal end of the brachioradialis muscle body)

Lu-7
- on the radial edge of the radius, just proximal to the styloid process,
  1.5 cun proximal to the wrist fold / Lu-9

Lu-8
- on the anterior surface of the radial styloid process, 1 cun proximal to the wrist fold

Wrist

Lu-9
- at the radial end of the wrist fold,
  in the space between the flexor carpi radialis & the abductor pollicis longus tendons
  locate on the ulnar side of the abductor pollicis tendon, & radial side of the artery

Hand

Lu-10
- at the midpoint of the 1st metacarpal,
  in the space between the muscles of the thenar eminence and the bone
  (at the skin change, i.e. jct of the red & white skin)

Lu-11
- the nail point on the radial side of the thumb

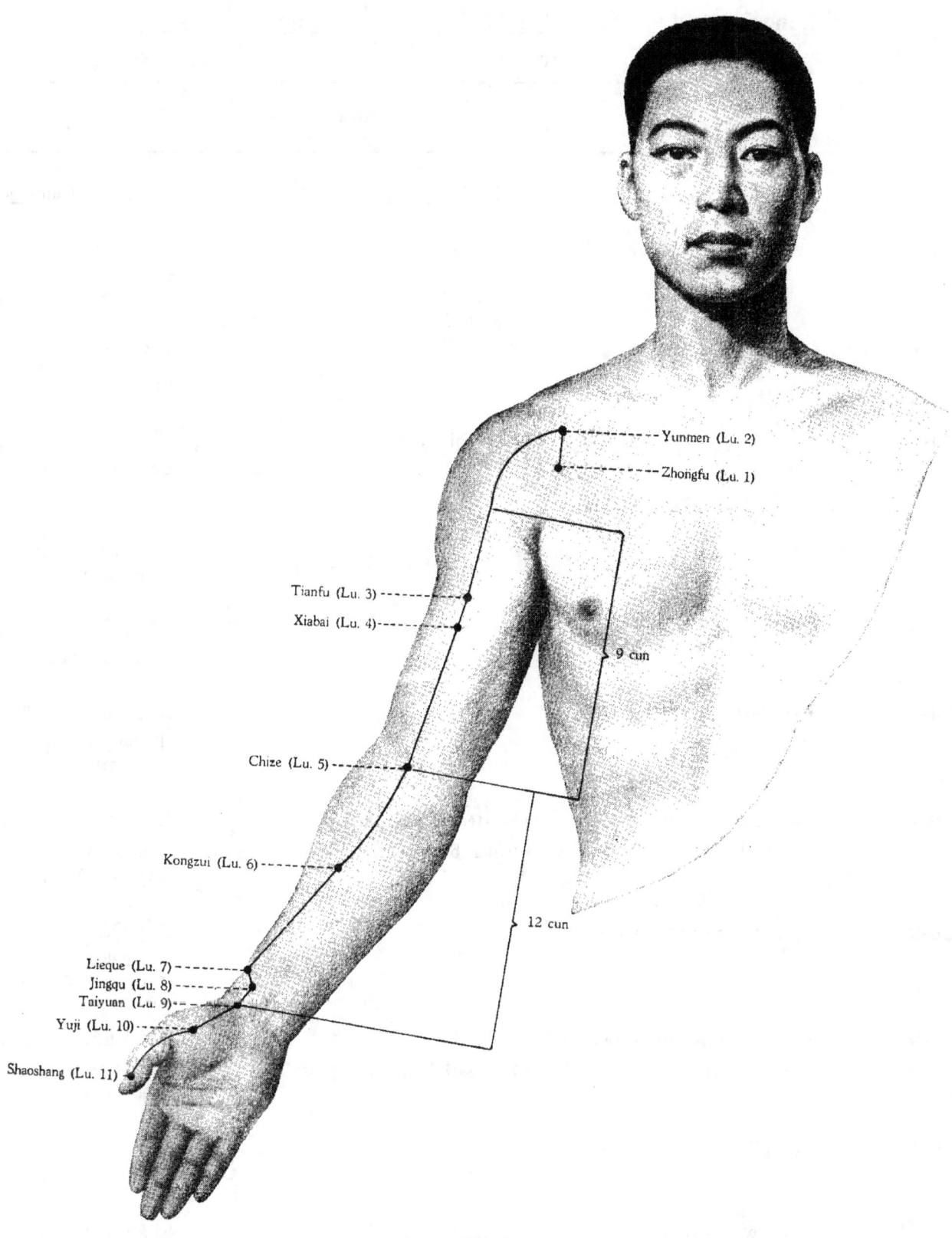

Yunmen (Lu. 2)
Zhongfu (Lu. 1)

Tianfu (Lu. 3)
Xiabai (Lu. 4)

9 cun

Chize (Lu. 5)

Kongzui (Lu. 6)

12 cun

Lieque (Lu. 7)
Jingqu (Lu. 8)
Taiyuan (Lu. 9)
Yuji (Lu. 10)

Shaoshang (Lu. 11)

手太陰肺經
Shou Tai-Yin Fei Jing
Arm Greater-Yin Lung Channel

Lung Channel = Shǒu **Tài-Yīn** Fèi Jīng		**Metal**	**3–5 am**
paired channels }	Sp	LI	BL

Mu pt = Lu-1	**Shu pt** = BL-13

	• Main Categories on every channel	• Misc. Categories	Pt Name & Translation
Lu-1	• entry pt: *from Lr-14*	• lung mu	**Zhōng Fǔ**　中府 Central Official Central Archive/Repository
Lu-2	• alternate entry pt		**Yún Mén**　雲門 Cloud Gate
Lu-3		• Celestial Window	Tiān Fǔ　天府 Celestial Official
Lu-4			Xiá Bái　俠白 Bold/Gallant/Heroic White (White Knight / Guard Metal)
Lu-5	• he/sea–water–Disp. pt.		**Chǐ Zé**　尺澤 Marsh at the Cubit
Lu-6	• **xi/cleft**		Kǒng Zuì　孔最 Humongous Hole Most Open
Lu-7	• **luo/connecting** • **exit pt**: *to LI-4*	• **Master pt**: Ren mai • **Ruler**: back of head & neck	**Liè Quē**　列缺 Sequence Gap/Jog (Lightning Bolt)
Lu-8	• jing/river–metal–Phase pt.		Jīng Qú　經渠 Channels/Rivers & Canals (River pt on Channel)
Lu-9	• shu/stream–earth–Tonif. pt. • **yuan/source**	• **Influential pt**: vessels/pulse	**Tài Yuān**　太淵 Very Deep-Pool Great Abyss (source of water)
Lu-10	• ying/brook–fire–Control pt.		Yú Jì　魚際 Edge of the Fish
Lu-11	• jing/well–wood	• (2nd) Ghost pt	Shǎo Shāng　少商 Lesser Metal-Note Minor Metal-Note

The 3 Yang Channels of the Arm
LI – TB – SI (62 pts)

• begin on the fingertips   • end on the face

(centripetal / inward, flow of yang)

Fill in the 3 pairings of each channel:

Channel	compartment	Phase	Division	Time
Lg Intestine	*radial*	yang Metal	shou Yang Ming	5–7 am
	3 pairs }			
Triple Burner	*middle*	yang M. Fire	shou Shao Yang	9–11 pm
	3 pairs }			
Sm. Intestine	*ulnar*	yang I. Fire	shou Tai Yang	1–3 pm
	3 pairs }			

大腸經 Dà Cháng Jīng = Large Intestine Channel

- **Division:** (Arm) **Yang Ming**
- **Phase/Element:** (Yang) **Metal**
- **High Tide: 5–7 am**

---

begins: **on the radial side of the index finger**

ends: **beside the nose** (same or opposite side)

❖ *The Large Intestine Channel external pathway:*

- begins at the radial nail point on the index finger   **(LI-1)**

- follows the radial side of the index finger & 2nd metacarpal to the anatomical snuffbox   (LI-5)

- follows the radius to the elbow (just anterior to the lateral epicondyle)   (LI-11)

- ascends the upper arm to the deltoid insertion   (LI-14)

- flows through the deltoid to the anterior end of the acromion   (LI-15)

- over the shoulder into the space between the clavicle and the scapula   (LI-16)

- it then flows along the anterior margin of the trapezius to the neck

- ascends the side of the neck, crossing the SCM, to the jaw   (LI-17–18)

- crosses the mandible (~ midway between the chin and the angle of the jaw) and

- proceeds to the upper jaw/lip, inferior to the nostril   (LI-19)

- ending beside the nose (same or opposite side) in the naso labial groove
  (level with the midpoint of the ala nasi)   **(LI-20)**

大腸經 **Large Intestine Channel** (20 pts)

Hand
LI-1   • the radial nail pt, on the index finger
LI-2   • on the radial side of the index finger, just **distal to the base** of the proximal phalanx
LI-3   • on the hand, just **proximal to the head** of the 2nd metacarpal
LI-4   • between the thumb & forefinger, at the midpoint of the 2nd metacarpal

Wrist
LI-5   • in the anatomical **snuffbox** (the 2 tendons are the extensor pollicis longus & brevis)

Forearm   ➤ *12 cun are measured between the snuffbox and the lateral epicondyle / LI-11*
        LI points on the forearm lie along a line connecting LI-5 and LI-11

LI-6   • **3 cun proximal** to the wrist/snuffbox (on the radius)
LI-7   • **5 cun proximal** to the wrist/snuffbox (on the radius)

LI-8   • **4 cun distal** to LI-11 (on the extensor carpi radialis longus)   *8 cun proximal*
LI-9   • **3 cun distal** to LI-11 (on the extensor carpi radialis longus)   *9 cun proximal*
LI-10   • **2 cun distal** to LI-11 (on the extensor carpi radialis brevis)   *10 cun proximal*

Elbow
LI-11   • (with arm bent 90°), midway between the lateral epicondyle & the cubital crease
LI-12   • ~ **1 cun proximal** to the lateral epicondyle
        on the anterior edge of the supracondylar ridge (supralateral to LI-11)

Upper Arm   ➤ *points lie along a line connecting LI-11 and LI-15*

LI-13   • **3 cun proximal** to LI-11 – in the depression between the brachioradialis & triceps

LI-14   • ~ 1 inch proximal to the deltoid insertion (slightly inferior to the top of the anterior axillary crease)

Shoulder
LI-15   • lateral aspect of the shoulder, inferior to the acromion,
        at the anterior end of the bone (in the anterior depression when the arm is abducted)
LI-16   • on top of the shoulder, in the 'V' formed by the jct of the scapular spine and the clavicle
        (posterior to the acromial head of the clavicle)

Neck
LI-17   • on the side of the neck, ~**1 cun inferior** to LI-18, but posterior to the SCM
LI-18   • level with the laryngeal prominence, between the two heads of the SCM

Face
LI-19   • on the upper lip, inferior to the lateral side of the nostril
LI-20   • in the naso-labial groove, level with the midpoint of the ala nasi

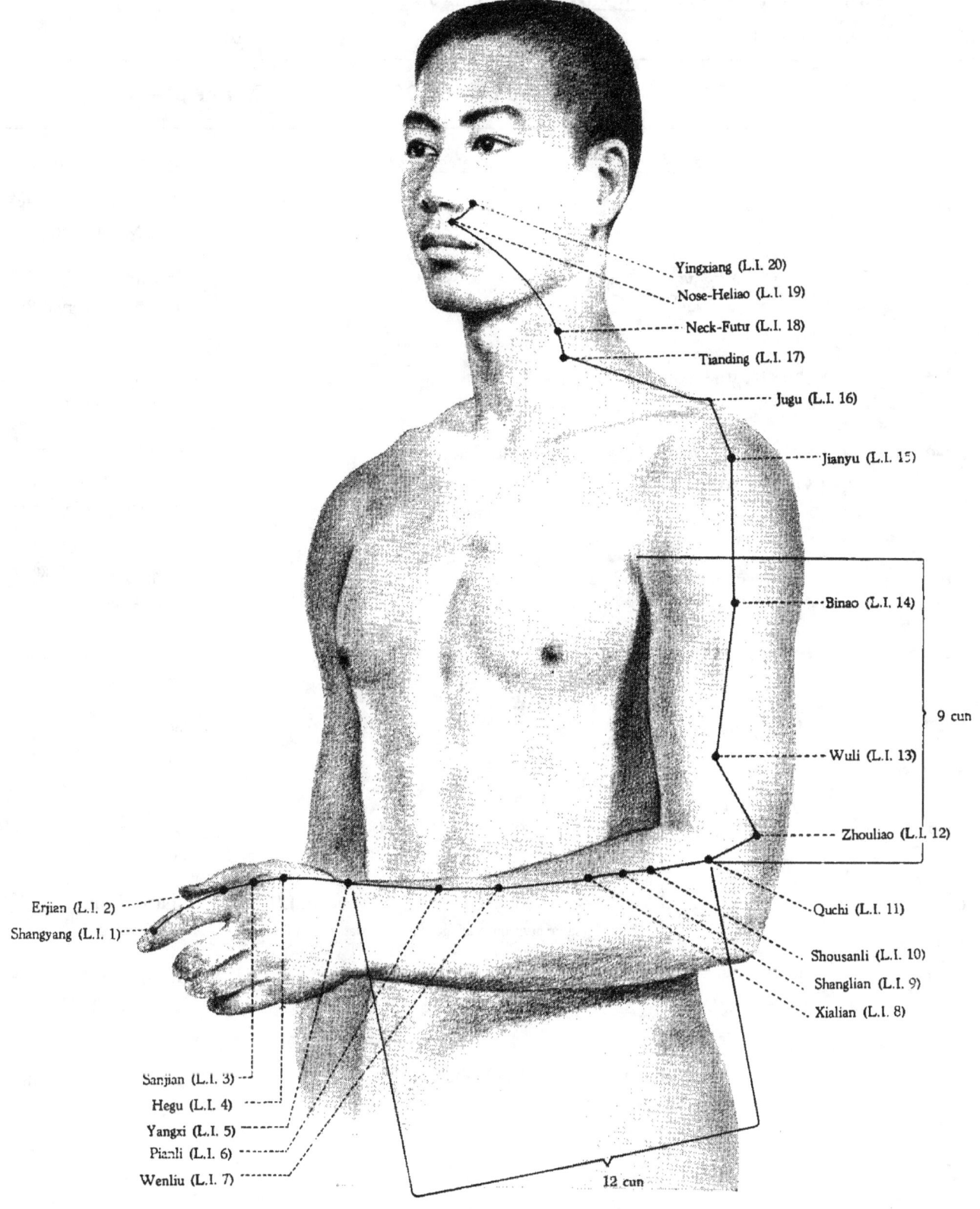

Yingxiang (L.I. 20)

Nose-Heliao (L.I. 19)

Neck-Futu (L.I. 18)

Tianding (L.I. 17)

Jugu (L.I. 16)

Jianyu (L.I. 15)

Binao (L.I. 14)

9 cun

Wuli (L.I. 13)

Zhouliao (L.I. 12)

Quchi (L.I. 11)

Erjian (L.I. 2)

Shangyang (L.I. 1)

Shousanli (L.I. 10)

Shanglian (L.I. 9)

Xialian (L.I. 8)

Sanjian (L.I. 3)

Hegu (L.I. 4)

Yangxi (L.I. 5)

Pianli (L.I. 6)

Wenliu (L.I. 7)

12 cun

手陽明大腸經

Shou Yang-Ming Da-Chang Jing

Arm Bright-Yang Large Intestine Channel

Lg.Int. Channel = Shǒu **Yáng-Míng** Dà Cháng Jīng		**Metal**	**5–7 am**
paired channels } ST		Lu	Kd

Mu pt = ST-25	**Shu pt** = BL-25	**Xia-he pt** = ST-37

	• Main Categories _{on every channel}	• Misc. Categories	Pt Name & Translation
LI-1	• jing/well–metal–Phase pt.		**Shāng Yáng** 商陽 Yang Metal (Note)
LI-2	• ying/brook–water–Disp. pt.		Èr Jiān 二間 2nd Space/Interval/Pt
LI-3	• shu/stream–wood		Sān Jiān 三間 3rd Space/Interval/Pt
LI-4	• **entry pt**: *from Lu-7* • **yuan/source**	• **Ruler**: face & mouth • 9N (to Rescue Yang) • *Cx: pregnancy*	**Hé Gǔ** 合谷 EnClosed Valley [where the] Valley Unites
LI-5	• jing/river–fire–Control pt.		Yáng Xī 陽谿 Yang Stream(bed)
LI-6	• **luo/connecting**		Piān Lì 偏歷 Offset Passage
LI-7	• **xi/cleft**		Wēn Liū 溫溜 Warm Flow/Current
LI-8		• corollary to ST-39 (xia-he for SI) _(same division; analogous name, location, & function)	Xià Lián 下廉 Lower Ridge
LI-9		• corollary to ST-37 (xia-he for LI) _(same division; analogous name, location, & function)	Shàng Lián 上廉 Upper Ridge
LI-10		• corollary to ST-36 (xia-he for ST) _(same division; analogous name, location, & function)	**Shǒu Sān Lǐ** 手三里 Arm/Hand 3 Li
LI-11	• he/sea–earth–Tonif. pt.	• (12th) Ghost pt	**Qū Chí** 曲池 Pond at the Crook
LI-18		• Celestial Window	Fú Tū 扶突 Aid the Prominence
LI-20	• exit pt: *to ST-1*		**Yíng Xiāng** 迎香 Welcome Fragrance

---

小 腸 經 Xiǎo Cháng Jīng = Small Intestine Channel

• **Division:** (Arm) **Tai Yang**

• **Phase/Element:** (Yang) Imperial **Fire**

• **High Tide: 1–3 pm**

---

begins: **on the ulnar side of the little finger**

ends: **in front of the ear** (tragus)

❖ *The Small Intestine Channel external pathway:*

· begins at the ulnar nail point on the little finger   **(SI-1)**

· follows the ulnar side of the little finger & 5th metacarpal to the wrist (ulno-carpal joint)   (SI-2–5)

· then follows the edge of the ulna (between the bone and the flexor compartment)   (SI-7)
  to the elbow (between the medial epicondyle & the olecranon)   (SI-8)

· ascends the upper arm following the long head of the triceps to the posterior axillary fold
  continues upward to the angle of the scapula   (SI-9-10)

· drops into the infra-spinous fossa   (SI-11)

· rises into the middle of the supra-spinous fossa   (SI-12)

· then proceeds medially to the supraspinatus origin   (SI-13)

· then onto the upper back   (SI-14-15)

· arcing upward across the back to the neck (trapezius to posterior SCM)   (SI-16)

· crosses the SCM to the angle of the mandible   (SI-17)

· continues upward across the cheek to the zygoma/maxilla
  at the anterior edge of the masseter, below the outer canthus of the eye   (SI-18)

· reverses direction to end in front of the ear anterior to the midpoint of the tragus   **(SI-19)**

小 腸 經 **Small Intestine Channel**   (19 pts)

Hand
SI-1   • the ulnar nail pt on the little finger

SI-2   • on the ulnar side of the little finger, distal to the base of the phalanx

SI-3   • on the ulnar side of the hand, proximal to the head of the 5th metacarpal

SI-4   • ulnar side of the hand, between the base of the 5th metacarpal and the triquetral bone

Wrist
SI-5   • on the side of the wrist, between the triquetral bone and the ulna

SI-6   • in the depression on the radial side of the ulna, just proximal to the styloid process

Forearm   ➤ *there are 12 cun from the ulno-carpal joint to the medial epicondyle of the humerus*

SI-7   • in the groove between the flexor compartment and the ulna, 5 cun proximal to the wrist

Elbow   • draw a line connecting the tip of the olecranon and the **medial** epicondyle,
SI-8   SI-8 is in a shallow depression slightly distal to the midpoint of that line.

Shoulder
SI-9   • **1 cun superior** to the end of the posterior axillary fold (inferior edge of the teres m.)

SI-10   • inferior to the lateral end of the scapular spine (medial to the acromial angle)
       on the line projected upward from the axillary fold   (~ a hand width above SI-9)

Scapula
SI-11   • in the infraspinous fossa   (level is ~ midway between SI-9 & 10)   (~ T4)
       (~ midway between the axillary fold vertical and the vertebral border of the scapula)

SI-12   • in the center of the supraspinous fossa, directly superior to SI-11

SI-13   • on the scapula, in the depression at the medial end of the supraspinous fossa

Back
SI-14   • level with T1, **3 cun lateral** to the midline, at the medial border of the scapula

SI-15   • level with C7, **2 cun lateral** to the midline

Neck
SI-16   • posterior to the SCM, level with the laryngeal prominence

SI-17   • anterior to the SCM,   level with the angle of the mandible

Face
SI-18   • below the outer orbit, inferior to the maxilla, at the anterior edge of the masseter

SI-19   • anterior to the midpoint of the tragus

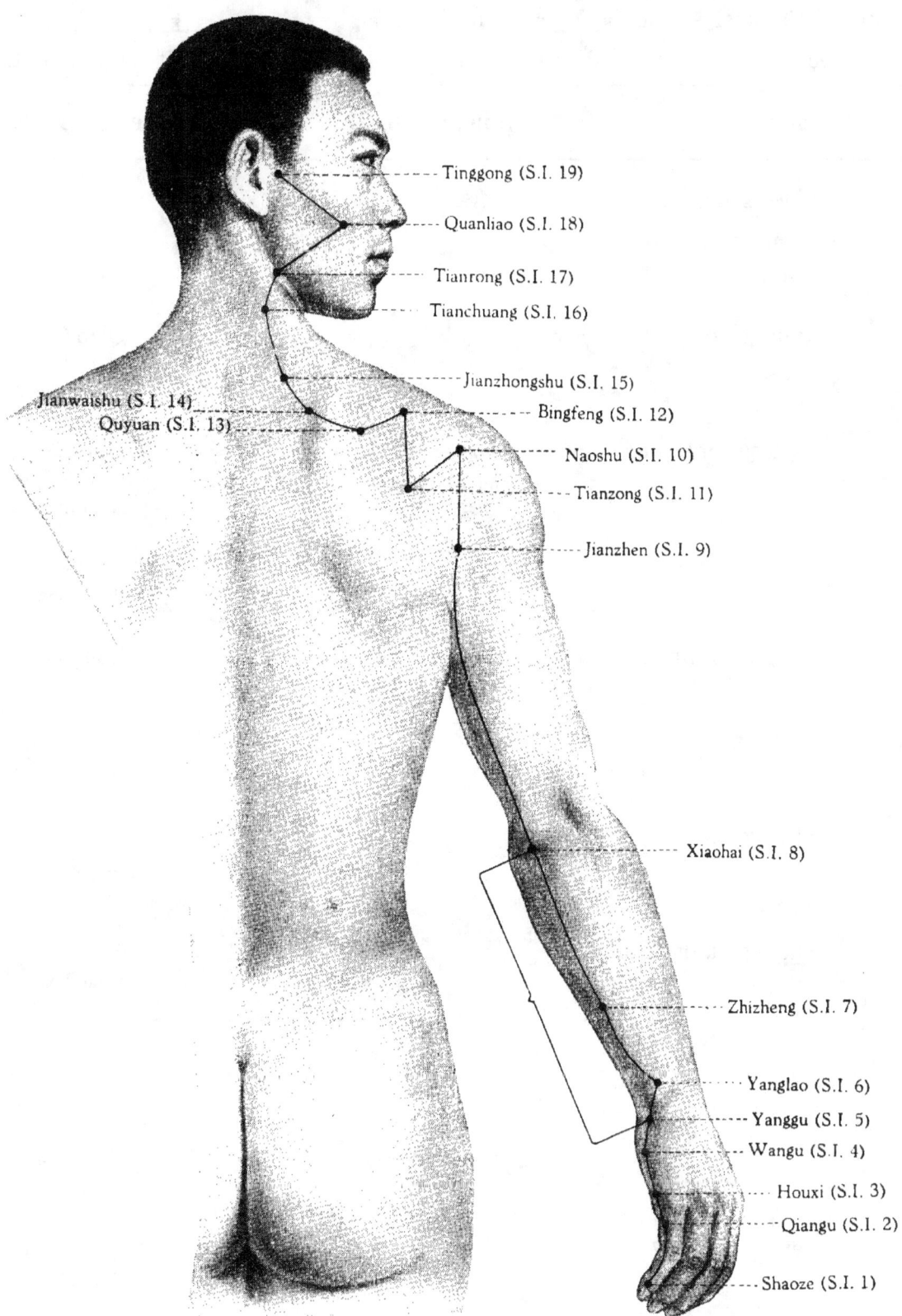

Tinggong (S.I. 19)

Quanliao (S.I. 18)

Tianrong (S.I. 17)

Tianchuang (S.I. 16)

Jianzhongshu (S.I. 15)

Jianwaishu (S.I. 14)

Bingfeng (S.I. 12)

Quyuan (S.I. 13)

Naoshu (S.I. 10)

Tianzong (S.I. 11)

Jianzhen (S.I. 9)

Xiaohai (S.I. 8)

Zhizheng (S.I. 7)

Yanglao (S.I. 6)

Yanggu (S.I. 5)

Wangu (S.I. 4)

Houxi (S.I. 3)

Qiangu (S.I. 2)

Shaoze (S.I. 1)

手太陽小腸經
Shou Tai-Yang Xiao-Chang Jing
Arm Greater-Yang Small Intestine Channel

Sm.Int. Channel = Shǒu **Tài-Yáng** Xiǎo Cháng Jīng		**I. Fire**	**1–3 pm**
paired channels } BL		Ht	Lr

Mu pt = CV-4	**Shu pt** = BL-27	**Xia-he pt** = ST-39

	• <u>Main Categories</u> on every channel	• Misc. Categories	<u>Pt Name & Translation</u>
SI-1	• entry pt: *from Ht-9* • jing/well–metal		**Shǎo Zé** 少澤 Lesser/Little (finger) Marsh
SI-2	• ying/brook–water–Control pt.		Qián Gǔ 前谷 Distal Valley Before the Valley
SI-3	• shu/stream–wood–Tonif. pt.	• **Master pt**: Du mai • alt. Ruler for back of head & neck	**Hòu Xī** 後谿 Proximal Streambed After the Streambed
SI-4	• **yuan/source**		Wàn Gǔ 腕骨 Wrist Bone
SI-5	• jing/river–fire–Phase pt.		Yáng Gǔ 陽谷 (Tai) Yang Valley
SI-6	• **xi/cleft**		**Yǎng Lǎo** 養老 Nourish the Elderly
SI-7	• **luo/connecting**		Zhī Zhèng 支正 Branch to the Primary Correct the Limb(s)
SI-8	• he/sea–earth–Disp. pt.		Xiǎo Hǎi 小海 Small Sea
SI-16		• Celestial Window	**Tiān Chuāng** 天窗 Celestial (roof) Window/Vent
SI-17		• Celestial Window	Tiān Róng 天容 Sky Look / Look Skyward
SI-18	***exit pt**: *to BL-1*		Quán Liáo 顴髎 Cheek Bone-hole
SI-19	• last pt *(exit: to BL-1)*		**Tīng Gōng** 聽宮 Hearing Palace

---

三焦經 Sān Jiāo Jīng = Triple Burner Channel
aka Triple Warmer, Heater, Energizer

• **Division:** (Arm) **Shao Yang**

• **Phase/Element:** (Yang) Ministerial **Fire**

• **High Tide: 9–11 pm**

---

begins: **on the ulnar side of the ring finger**

ends: **at lateral end of the eyebrow**

❖ *The Triple Burner Channel external pathway:*

• begins at the ulnar nail point on the ring finger   **(TB-1)**

• follows the ulnar side of the ring finger

• flows between the 4th & 5th metacarpals on the dorsum of the hand   (TB-2 & 3)

• to the wrist (ulno-carpal joint), just ulnar to the extensor digitorum tendons   (TB-4)

• flows between the radius & ulna to the elbow   (TB-5–9)
     (between the lateral epicondyle & olecranon) into the olecranon fossa   (TB-10–11)

• ascends between the heads of the triceps to the shoulder
     (posterior end of the acromion)   (TB-12–14)

• traverses the posterior shoulder, just above the superior angle of the scapula   (TB-15)
     to the neck

• follows the posterior edge of the SCM to the space between the mandible and the
     mastoid process (under the earlobe)   (TB-17)

• upward behind and around the ear, then across the temple   (TB-18–22)

• ending at lateral end of the eyebrow (posterior edge of the fronto-zygomatic bones)   **(TB-23)**

三 焦 經 **Triple Burner Channel**   (23 pts)

Hand
TB-1   • the ulnar nail pt on the ring finger
TB-2   • between the 4th & 5th fingers, 0.5 cun proximal to the web margin (distal to the MP joint)
TB-3   • between the 4th & 5th metacarpals, proximal to their heads (proximal to the MP joint)
Wrist
TB-4   • at the wrist, slightly distal & radial to the dorsal prominence of the ulnar styloid
                  between the extensor digitorum and extensor digiti minimi tendons (radial edge of triquetral bone)

Forearm   ➤ *there are 12 cun between the wrist joint and the lateral epicondyle/tip of olecranon*

TB-5   • between the radius & ulna, **2 cun proximal** to the wrist, on the radial side of the ext. digitorum
TB-6   • between the radius & ulna, **3 cun proximal** to the wrist, on the radial side of the ext. digitorum
TB-7   • between the radius & ulna, **3 cun proximal** to the wrist, on the radial side of the ulna, (prox to SI-6)
TB-8   • between the radius & ulna, **4 cun proximal** to the wrist
TB-9   • between the radius & ulna, **5 cun distal** to the tip of the olecranon (TB-10)
                  (more like 3-4 cun from the lateral epicondyle)
          (in the groove between the extensor digitorum and the extensor carpi ulnaris muscles)

Elbow   *the channel flows between the lateral epicondyle & the olecranon process into the olecranon fossa*
TB-10   • in the olecranon fossa, **1 cun proximal** to the tip of the olecranon
TB-11   • in the olecranon fossa, **2 cun proximal** to the tip of the olecranon

Upper Arm   ➤ *9 cun divide the space between the olecranon and the posterior axillary fold*

TB-12   • on the posterior arm, level with the bulge of the lateral head of the triceps, midway between TB-11 & TB-13
TB-13   • on the posterior arm, between the lateral and long heads of the triceps, at the edge of the posterior deltoid
                  (should be slightly above the level of the posterior axillary fold)

Lateral Shoulder
TB-14   • inferior to the [postero-lateral end of the] acromion (the posterior depression when the arm is abducted)

Posterior Shoulder
TB-15   • at the superior angle of the scapula (midway between SI-13 & GB-21)

Neck
TB-16   • on the posterior edge of the SCM, level with the angle of the mandible
TB-17   • lift the earlobe, between the ramus of the mandible and the mastoid process (ant. to SCM)

Around the Ear   *TB pts are anterior to the post-auricular hairline, at the perimeter of the helix when the*
                      ear is pressed flat against the head or ~ midway betw the auricular attachment and the hairline.
TB-18   • behind the ear, **1/3** of the arc distance between lobe and apex (TB-17 & TB-20)
TB-19   • behind the ear, **2/3** of the arc distance between lobe and apex (TB-17 & TB-20)
TB-20   • above the ear, on the side of the head, immediately superior to the apex of the ear

Front of the Ear
TB-21   • anterior to the ear, (on the vertical line just anterior to the tragus), level with the supra-tragic notch
TB-22   • at the pre-auricular hairline, level with the superior root of the ear

Face
TB-23   • the depression at the lateral end of the eyebrow (on the post. edge of the fronto-zygomatic bone at level of suture)

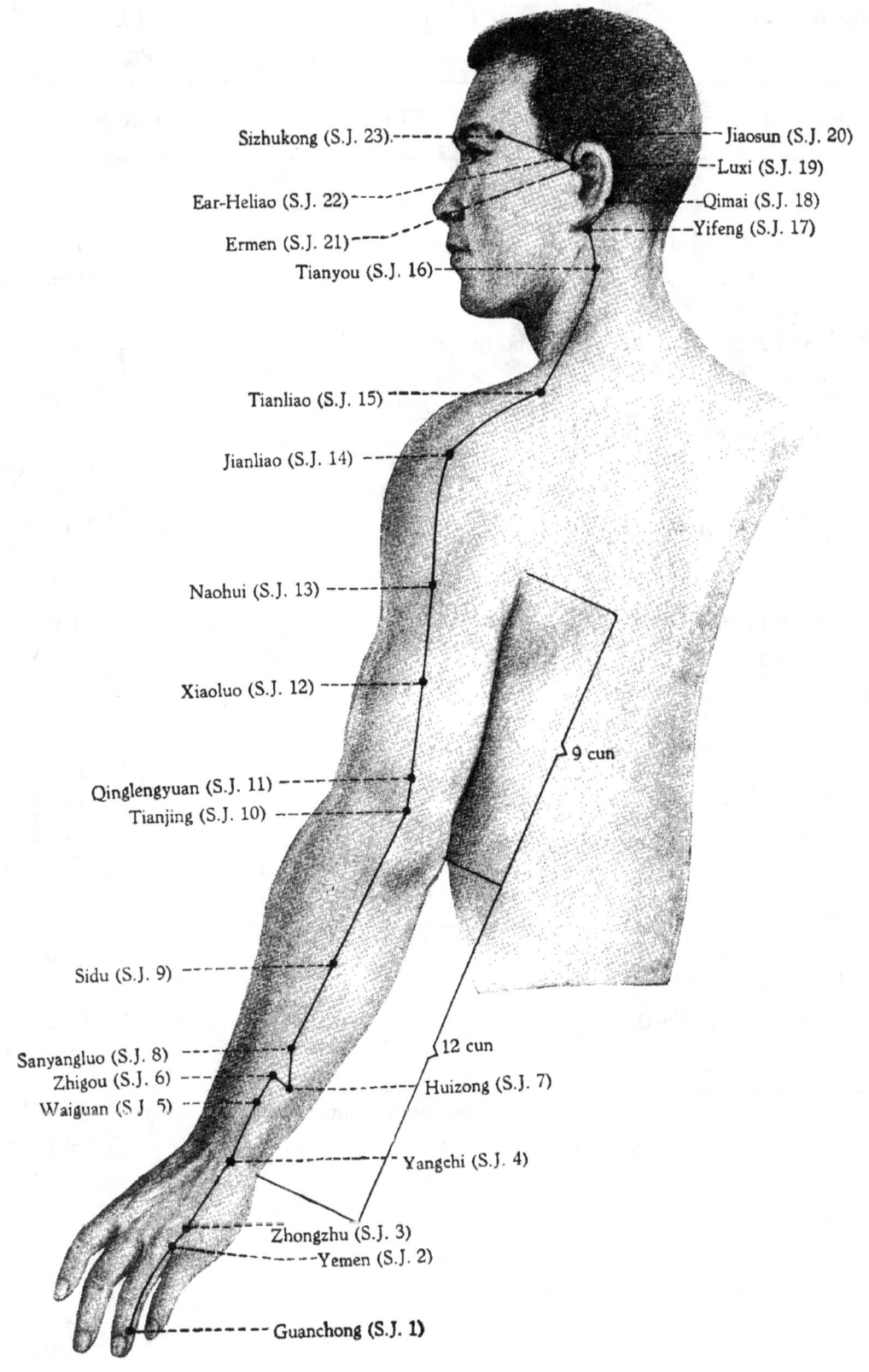

Sizhukong (S.J. 23)
Jiaosun (S.J. 20)
Luxi (S.J. 19)
Ear-Heliao (S.J. 22)
Qimai (S.J. 18)
Ermen (S.J. 21)
Yifeng (S.J. 17)
Tianyou (S.J. 16)

Tianliao (S.J. 15)

Jianliao (S.J. 14)

Naohui (S.J. 13)

Xiaoluo (S.J. 12)

9 cun

Qinglengyuan (S.J. 11)
Tianjing (S.J. 10)

Sidu (S.J. 9)

Sanyangluo (S.J. 8)
Zhigou (S.J. 6)
Huizong (S.J. 7)
Waiguan (S J 5)

12 cun

Yangchi (S.J. 4)

Zhongzhu (S.J. 3)
Yemen (S.J. 2)

Guanchong (S.J. 1)

手少陽三焦經
Shou Shao-Yang San-Jiao Jing
Arm Lesser-Yang Triple Burner Channel

3 Burners Channel = Shǒu **Shǎo-Yáng** Sān Jiāo Jīng		**M. Fire**	**9–11 pm**
paired channels } GB		Pc	Sp

Mu pt = CV-5	**Shu pt** = BL-22	**Xia-he pt** = BL-53/39

	• <u>Main Categories</u> on every channel	• <u>Misc. Categories</u>	<u>Pt Name & Translation</u>
TB-1	• entry pt: *from Pc-8* • jing/well–metal		Guān Chōng 關衝 Gateway Thoroughfare
TB-2	• ying/brook–water–Control pt.		Yè Mén 液門 (yin) Fluids Gate
TB-3	• shu/stream–wood–Tonif. pt.		**Zhōng Zhǔ** 中渚 Central (small) Island
TB-4	• **yuan/source**		Yáng Chí 陽池 Yang Pond
TB-5	• **luo/connecting**	• **Master pt**: Yang Wei mai	**Wài Guān** 外關 Outer Gateway
TB-6	• jing/river–fire–Phase pt.		Zhī Gōu 支溝 Limb Trough/Groove
TB-7	• **xi/cleft**		Huì Zōng 會宗 Meet & Gather Meeting of Ancestors
TB-8		• **Group Luo**: (3 arm yang)	**Sān Yáng Luò** 三陽絡 3 Yang Connect
TB-10	• he/sea–earth–Disp. pt.		Tiān Jǐng 天井 Celestial Well
TB-16		• Celestial Window	Tiān Yǒu 天牖 Celestial (wall) Window (compare SI-16)
TB-17			**Yì Fēng** 翳風 Screen the Wind
TB-21			**Ěr Mén** 耳門 Ear Gate
TB-23	• exit pt: *to GB-1*		Sī Zhú Kōng 系竹空 Silk Bamboo Hollow

The 2 Midline Channels
Ren & Du Mai   (52 pts)

- begin at the floor of the pelvis
  (bottom of the torso)
- end on the face
  (above & below the mouth)

(externally both flow upward, internally both flow down)

Vessel	relative position	in charge of:	# of Points	Master pt
Ren (CV)	anterior midline	controls yin	24 pts	**Lu-7**
function pair: *Yin Qiao*	*medial leg*	*mobilizes yin*	*6 pts*	***Kd-6***
Du (GV)	posterior midline	governs yang	28 pts	**SI-3**
function pair: *Yang Qiao*	*lateral leg*	*mobilizes yang*	*13 pts*	***BL-62***

Structural Pairs: *Ren & Du constitute a yin/yang pair, controlling or governing yin & yang respectively.*

Functional Pairs: *Ren & Yin Qiao are both yin*   *(analogous to division pairs)*
Du & Yang Qiao are both yang.

任 脈 Rèn Mài = Conception Vessel
(*old spelling* – Jen Mo)
aka Controlling or Directing Vessel

anterior midline

begins: **the perineum**

ends: **below the lower lip**

❖ *The Conception Vessel external pathway:*

· beginning at the center of the perineum (midway between anus and genitalia)   **(CV-1)**

· it flows upward to the pubis symphysis   (CV-2)

· then follows the anterior midline up the abdomen   (CV-2–15)

· ascending onto the chest to the sternal notch   (CV-16–22)

 · upward on the throat to the chin   (CV-23)

· ending in the mento-labial groove below the lower lip   **(CV-24)**
       (energetically it correlates with the tip of the tongue)

· *Internally* it flows down: from the tip of the tongue to the throat and then downward through
           the center of the body to the anus & connects to the Governing Vessel at GV-1.

任 脈 Rèn Mài = Conception Vessel   (24 pts)

Perineum
CV-1   • the center of the perineum (midway between the genitals and the anus)

Lower Abdomen   ➤ *5 cun are measured between the umbilicus and the pubis*

CV-2   • **5 cun inferior**   to the umbilicus, immediately superior to the pubic symphysis

CV-3   • **4 cun inferior**   to the umbilicus

CV-4   • **3 cun inferior**   to the umbilicus   ~ level with the anterior projection of the ASIS

CV-5   • **2 cun inferior**   to the umbilicus

CV-6   • **1.5 cun inferior** to the umbilicus

CV-7   • **1 cun inferior**   to the umbilicus

CV-8   • **the center of the umbilicus**   (this pt is not needled, use moxa)

Upper Abdomen   ➤ *8 cun are measured between the umbilicus and the xipho-sternal jct*

CV-9   • **1 cun superior** to the umbilicus

CV-10   • **2 cun superior** to the umbilicus

CV-11   • **3 cun superior** to the umbilicus

CV-12   • **4 cun superior** to the umbilicus   (midway between the umbilicus and the xipho-sternal jct)

CV-13   • **5 cun superior** to the umbilicus

CV-14   • **6 cun superior** to the umbilicus

CV-15   • **7 cun superior** to the umbilicus   (on or below the xiphoid process)

Chest   ➤ *8 cun can be measured between the xiphosternal jct and the sternal notch (1.6 cun between ribs)*

CV-16   • **at the xipho-sternal junction**   level with the **5th** intercostal space

CV-17   • on the sternum   level with the **4th** intercostal space   (~ level with the nipples)

CV-18   • on the sternum   level with the **3rd** intercostal space   (midway between the 3rd IC spaces)

CV-19   • on the sternum   level with the **2nd** intercostal space

CV-20   • on the manubrium   level with the **1st** intercostal space

CV-21   • on the manubrium, midway between CV-20 & 22   (between Kd-27's)

Throat
CV-22   • immediately superior to the sternal notch   (point is actually behind the manubrium)

CV-23   • immediately superior to the hyoid bone   (hyoid is immediately superior to the laryngeal prominence)

Chin
CV-24   • inferior to the lower lip, anterior midline, in the mento-labial groove/sulcus

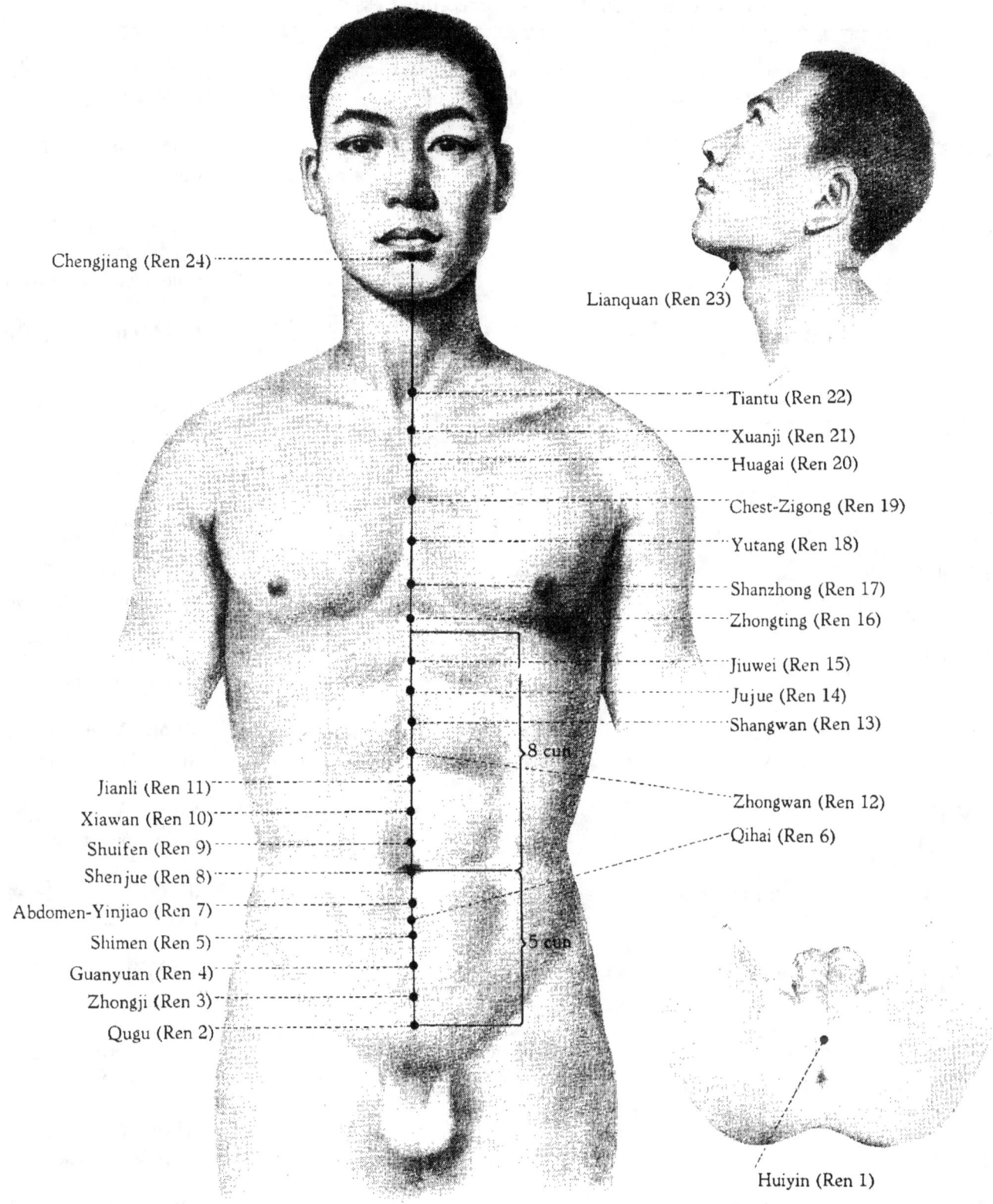

Chengjiang (Ren 24)

Lianquan (Ren 23)

Tiantu (Ren 22)

Xuanji (Ren 21)

Huagai (Ren 20)

Chest-Zigong (Ren 19)

Yutang (Ren 18)

Shanzhong (Ren 17)

Zhongting (Ren 16)

Jiuwei (Ren 15)

Jujue (Ren 14)

Shangwan (Ren 13)

8 cun

Jianli (Ren 11)

Xiawan (Ren 10)

Shuifen (Ren 9)

Shenjue (Ren 8)

Abdomen-Yinjiao (Ren 7)

Shimen (Ren 5)

Guanyuan (Ren 4)

Zhongji (Ren 3)

Qugu (Ren 2)

Zhongwan (Ren 12)

Qihai (Ren 6)

5 cun

Huiyin (Ren 1)

任 脈
Ren Mai
Conception/Controlling Vessel

Conception/Controlling/Directing Vessel = Rèn Mài

CV-1	• alt. luo pt • *exit pt: to GV-1*	• Jct pt: (Ren, Du & Chong) • (11th) Ghost pt	**Huì Yīn**	會陰 Converging Yin/Yin Meeting
CV-3	• **BL mu pt**		**Zhōng Jí**	中極 Central Pole
CV-4	• **SI mu pt**		**Guān Yuán**	關元 Original Gateway Gateway to the Source 關原
CV-5	• **TB mu pt**		**Shí Mén**	石門 Stone Gate
CV-6	• key pt for LJiao	• pt most associated with lower dan tian	**Qì Hǎi**	氣海 Sea of Qi
CV-7	• alt mu pt for TB & LJiao	• Jct pt: (Ren & Chong)	**Yīn Jiāo**	陰交 Yin Junction
CV-8		• portal of pre-natal qi	**Shén Què**	神闕 Spirit Portal/Watchtower
CV-10			**Xià Wǎn**	下脘 Lower Epigastrium
CV-12	• **ST mu pt** • key pt for MJiao	• **Influential pt**: Fu organs • 9N (to Rescue Yang)	**Zhōng Wǎn**	中脘 Middle Epigastrium
CV-13			**Shàng Wǎn**	上脘 Upper Epigastrium
CV-14	• **Ht mu pt**		**Jù Què**	巨闕 Huge Portal/Archway
CV-15	• **luo point**		**Jiū Wěi**	鳩尾 Dove's Tail
CV-17	• **Pc mu pt** • key pt for UJiao	• **Influential pt**: Qi • Sea of Qi pt	**Dàn Zhōng**	膻中 Chest Center
CV-22		• Celestial Window	**Tiān Tū**	天突 Celestial Prominence
CV-24	• last point • *entry pt: from GV-28*	• (8th) Ghost pt	**Chéng Jiāng**	承漿 Catch Drool (For Drooling)
Extra Pt:		• (13th) Ghost pt	Hǎi Quān	海泉 Ocean & Spring

督脈 Dū Mài = Governing Vessel
(*old spelling* – Tu Mo)

---

posterior midline
(mid-sagittal plane)

---

begins: **at the tip of the tailbone**

ends: **on the gum, under the upper lip**

❖ *The Governing Vessel external pathway:*

· begins at the tip of the coccyx (midway between the anus & the coccyx)   **(GV-1)**

· it ascends the posterior midline following the spine up to the occiput   (GV-2-16)

· up and over the top of the head   (GV-17-24)

· down the face to the phliltrum   (GV-26-27)

· ending on the gum under the upper lip   **(GV-28)**
        (energetically this correlates with a spot just behind the two front teeth on the hard palate)

· *Internally* it flows down: flowing along the roof of the mouth and back of the throat,
                    it descends through the center of the body to the perineum,
                    where it connects to the Conception Vessel at CV-1.

督 脈 **Dū Mài = Governing Vessel**   (28 pts)

Tailbone
GV-1   • midway between the tip of the coccyx and the anus

Sacrum
GV-2   • at the sacral hiatus   ~S$_4$ *Note: GV-1, 2, & 3 are too low on the illustration

Ex Pt: • *inferior to the spinous process of S$_2$*   *Yao Qi = Lumbar Strange*

Low Back
Ex Pt: • *lumbo-sacral jct*   *L$_5$*   *Shi-Qi Zhui Xia = 17 vertabra, Below*

GV-3   • inferior to the spinous process of **L$_4$**

GV-4   • inferior to the spinous process of **L$_2$**

GV-5   • inferior to the spinous process of **L$_1$**

Lower Mid Back
GV-6   • inferior to the spinous process of **T$_{11}$**

GV-7   • inferior to the spinous process of **T$_{10}$**

GV-8   • inferior to the spinous process of **T$_9$**

Mid Back
GV-9   • inferior to the spinous process of **T$_7$**

GV-10   • inferior to the spinous process of **T$_6$**

GV-11   • inferior to the spinous process of **T$_5$**

Upper Back
GV-12   • inferior to the spinous process of **T$_3$**

GV-13   • inferior to the spinous process of **T$_1$**

GV-14   • inferior to the spinous process of **C$_7$**

* Note the pattern of omitted spinous processes: **T-2, 4, 8, 12**

L-3, 5

(S-1, 2, 3)

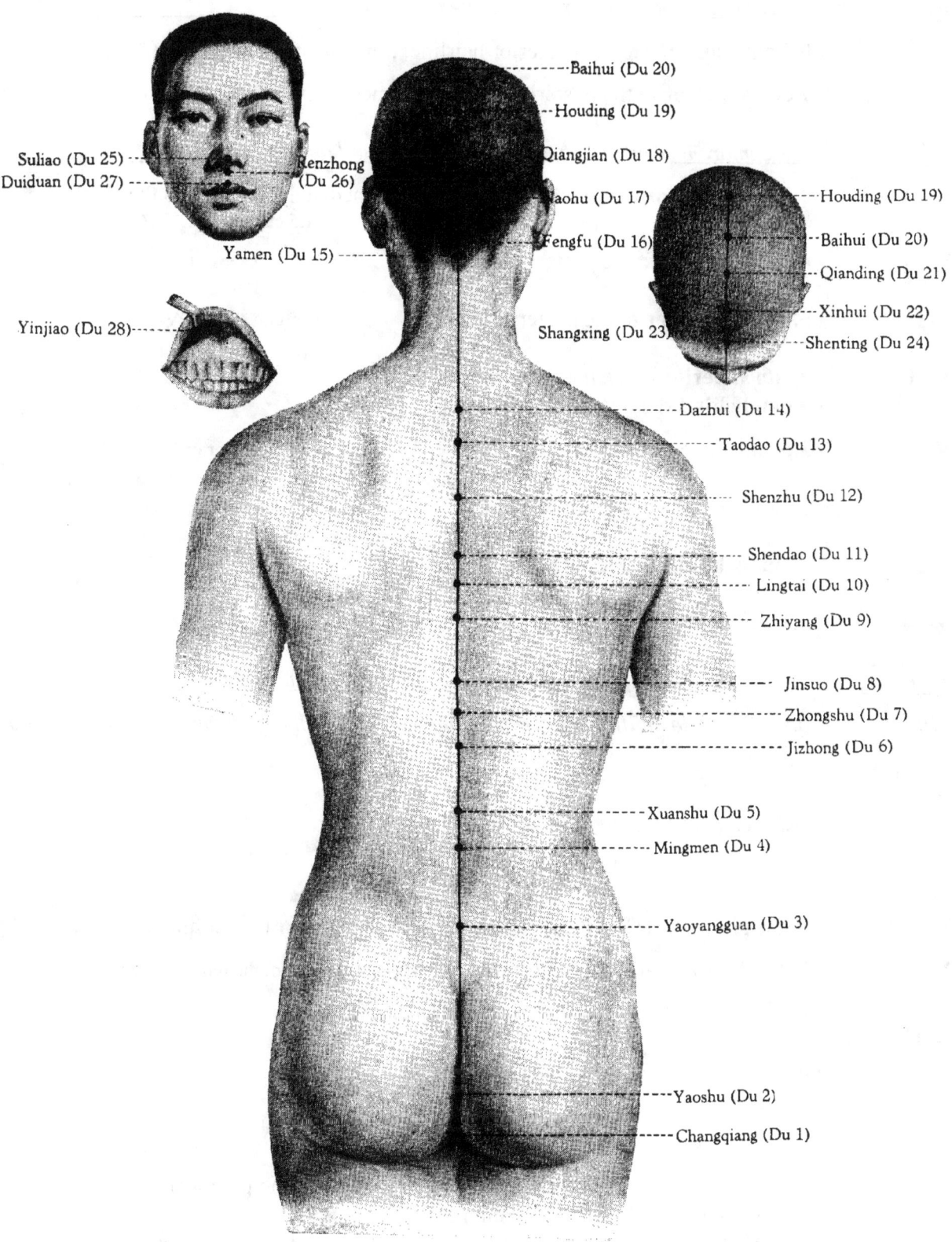

- Baihui (Du 20)
- Houding (Du 19)
- Qiangjian (Du 18)
- Naohu (Du 17)
- Fengfu (Du 16)
- Houding (Du 19)
- Baihui (Du 20)
- Qianding (Du 21)
- Xinhui (Du 22)
- Shangxing (Du 23)
- Shenting (Du 24)
- Suliao (Du 25)
- Renzhong (Du 26)
- Duiduan (Du 27)
- Yamen (Du 15)
- Yinjiao (Du 28)
- Dazhui (Du 14)
- Taodao (Du 13)
- Shenzhu (Du 12)
- Shendao (Du 11)
- Lingtai (Du 10)
- Zhiyang (Du 9)
- Jinsuo (Du 8)
- Zhongshu (Du 7)
- Jizhong (Du 6)
- Xuanshu (Du 5)
- Mingmen (Du 4)
- Yaoyangguan (Du 3)
- Yaoshu (Du 2)
- Changqiang (Du 1)

督 脈

Du Mai

Governing Vessel

Neck	➤ *There are 3 cun between C7 and the posterior hairline*
GV-15	• **0.5 cun superior** to the posterior hairline, immediately superior to C2
GV-16	• **1 cun superior** to the posterior hairline, immediately inferior to the occiput

Scalp	➤ *12 cun are measured between the posterior and anterior hairlines*
GV-17	• **2.5 cun superior** to the posterior hairline, immediately superior to the EOP
	1.5 cun above GV-16
GV-18	• **4 cun superior** to the posterior hairline 1.5 cun above GV-17
GV-19	• **5.5 cun superior** to the posterior hairline 1.5 cun above GV-18
GV-20	• **7 cun superior** to the posterior hairline 1.5 cun above GV-19
or	• **5 cun behind the anterior hairline**
GV-21	• **3.5 cun behind** the anterior hairline 1.5 cun anterior to GV-20
GV-22	• **2 cun behind** the anterior hairline 1.5 cun anterior to GV-21
GV-23	• **1 cun behind** the anterior hairline 1.0 cun anterior to GV-22
GV-24	• **0.5 cun behind** the anterior hairline 0.5 cun anterior to GV-23

Forehead	➤ *There are 3 cun between the anterior hairline and the glabella*
Ex Pt:	• *at the glabella, midway between the medial ends of the eyebrows* *Yin Tang = Seal Hall*

Nose	
GV-25	• at the center of the tip of the nose

Upper Lip	
GV-26	• in the philtrum, 1/3 of the distance between the base of the septum and the upper lip
GV-27	• in the philtrum, at the junction with the upper lip (jct of the red & white skin)

Upper Gum	
GV-28	• on the upper gum, immediately inferior to the attachment of the frenum

* Note:
- Un-dot-able points (mostly scalp pts.) will **Not** be on the practical final, but will be fair game on the written final.
- The un-dot-able pts are: GV-15 to 24   (TB-20 & 22 can be difficult, but OK)
                                              GV-1 & 28
                                              CV-1   = 13 pts (143 – 13 = 130 pts)

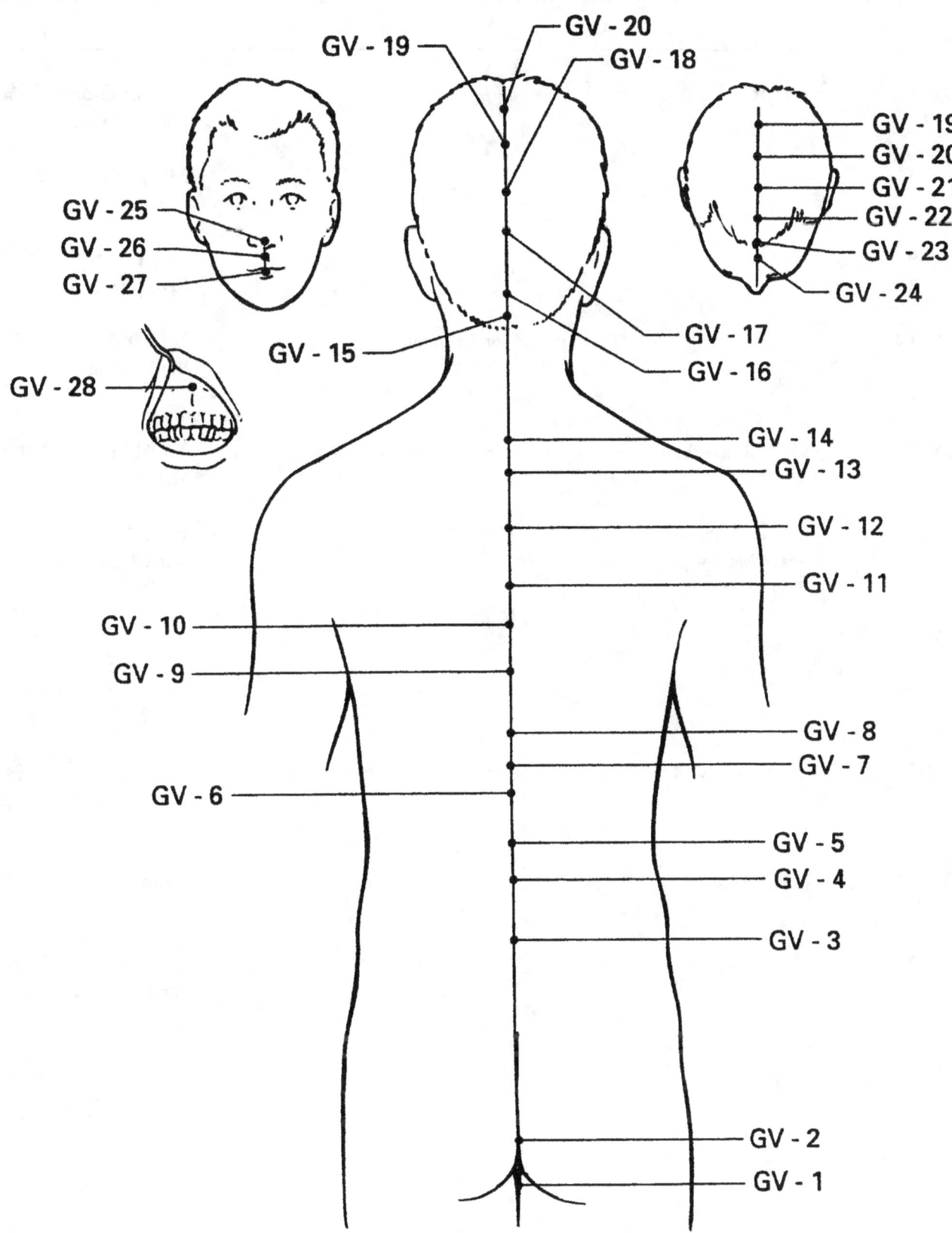

Dū Mài Schematic Diagram

Governing Vessel = Dū Mài			

GV-1	• luo pt	• *entry pt: from CV-1*	**Cháng Qiáng** 長強 Long & Strong
GV-4			**Mìng Mén** 命門 Life/Destiny/Fate Gate
GV-9			**Zhì Yáng** 至陽 Reach the Yang
GV-14		• major Jct pt: (all yang channels)	**Dà Zhuī** 大椎 Big Vertebra
GV-15	• 9N (to Rescue Yang)	(some sources say this is a Sea of Qi pt)	**Yǎ Mén** 瘂門 Mute Gate
GV-16	• Celestial Window • Sea of Marrow pt • (6th) Ghost pt		**Fēng Fǔ** 風府 Wind Repository Wind Official
GV-17			Nǎo Hù 腦戶 Brain Door Doorway to the Brain
GV-20	• Sea of Marrow pt	• major Jct pt: (BL, TB, GB, Lr)	**Bǎi Huī** 百會 100 Converge/Converging
GV-23	• (10th) Ghost pt		**Shàng Xīng** 上星 Upper Star
GV-24			**Shén Tíng** 神庭 Spirit Courtyard
GV-26	• (1st) Ghost pt		**Rén Zhōng** 人中 Human (Realm) Central *aka* **Shuǐ Gōu** 水溝 Water Trough
GV-28	• last point	• *exit pt: to CV-24*	Yín Jiāo 齦交 Gum Junction

Governing Vessel = Dū Mài

Points 2

Six Leg Channels

(218 pts)

Channel Pathways,
Point Locations,
Categories, & Names

Synopsis of Leg Channels

The 3 Yang Channels of the Leg
ST – GB – BL (156 pts)

• begin on the face   • end at the toes

(centrifugal / outward flow of yang)

Channel	compartment	Phase	Division	Time
Stomach	anterior	Earth	Yang Ming	7–9 am
Gall Baldder	lateral	Wood	Shao Yang	11 pm–1 am
Bladder	posterior	Water	Tai Yang	3–5 pm

The 3 Yin Channels of the Leg
Sp – Lr – Kd (62 pts)

• begin on the toes   • end on the torso

(centripetal / inward flow of yin)

Channel	compartment	Phase	Division	Time
Spleen	anterior	Earth	Tai Yin	9–11 am
Liver	medial	Wood	Jue Yin	1–3 am
Kidney	posterior	Water	Shao Yin	5–7 pm

The 2 Water Channels (94 pts)

Bladder = Zu Tai-Yang **Pang-Guang** Jing

- The **Bladder** flows downward
- from head to toes

(centrifugal / outward flow of yang)

(67 pts)

Kidney = Zu Shao-Yin **Shen** Jing

- The **Kidney** flows upward
- from toes to torso

(centripetal / inward flow of yin)

(27 pts)

Fill in the 3 pairings of each channel:

Channel	compartment	Phase	Division	Time
Bladder	posterior lateral	yang Water	zu Tai Yang	3–5 pm
	3 pairings }			
Kidney	posterior medial	yin Water	zu Shao Yin	5–7 pm
	3 pairings }			

<u>Problem:</u>
- There are two methods of numbering points on the Bladder channel.
- One derives from the Beijing College of TCM, the other from the Shanghai College of TCM.
- 19 points have 2 different numbers.   • Neither system is convenient.
- The numbers are arbitrary and do not reflect the flow of qi, as they do other channels.

<u>Solution:</u>
- Number the point on the outer/lateral column with the same number as the Bladder point on the inner column at the same level, then add an "a".
- **The inner column being easy to memorize, correlates to clinical application.**
- Thus Fu Fen becomes 12a instead of BL-36 or 41.
  (BL-12 and 12a are both level with the space inferior to the T_2 spinous process)

<u>Advantages:</u>
- My numbering is much easier to learn and remember.
- It accurately depicts the channel pathway and flow of qi, which divides on the neck at BL-10, goes to the uppermost point of each column and flows down the inner and outer columns simaltaneously.
- Supports the connection (obvious in Chinese) that the names of points in the outer column are intended to convey their link to the inner column point via organ association.

12 Points on the Back & 2 Gluteal points = 14 pts

Beijing / Shanghai **BJ# / SH#**	**Characters**	**PīnYīn**	**Level with:**	**Back Shu**	outer column **Re-Number as:**	**Name refers to:**
BL-41 / 36	附分	**Fù Fēn**	T_2 & BL-12		**BL-12a**	
BL-42 / 37	魄戶	**Pò Hù**	T_3 & BL-13	Lu	**BL-13a**	**Lu** spirit
BL-43 / 38	膏肓	**Gāo Huāng**	T_4 & BL-14	Pc	**BL-14a**	membranes around Ht
BL-44 / 39	神堂	**Shén Táng**	T_5 & BL-15	Ht	**BL-15a**	**Ht** spirit
BL-45 / 40	譩譆	**Yì Xī**	T_6 & BL-16	GV	**BL-16a**	
BL-46 / 41	膈關	**Gé Guān**	T_7 & BL-17	Diaphragm	**BL-17a**	Diaphragm Gateway
no BL point		Yí Shū	T_8	(Pancreas)	no BL point	
BL-47 / 42	魂門	**Hún Mén**	T_9 & BL-18	Lr	**BL-18a**	**Lr** spirit
BL-48 / 43	陽綱	**Yáng Gāng**	T_{10} & BL-19	GB	**BL-19a**	**GB** as yang guide
BL-49 / 44	意舍	**Yì Shè**	T_{11} & BL-20	Sp	**BL-20a**	**Sp** spirit
BL-50 / 45	胃倉	**Wèi Cāng**	T_{12} & BL-21	ST	**BL-21a**	**ST**
BL-51 / 46	肓門	**Huāng Mén**	L_1 & BL-22	TB	**BL-22a**	central tendon umbilicus
BL-52 / 47	志室	**Zhì Shī**	L_2 & BL-23	Kd	**BL-23a**	**Kd** spirit
BL-53 / 48	胞肓	**Bāo Huāng**	S_2 & BL-28	BL	**BL-28a**	**BL &** adnexa
BL-54 / 49	秩邊	**Zhì Biān**	S_4 & BL-30		**BL-30a**	outer column end

Numbering the Bladder Channel

More Advantages:

• By renumbering the back, I avoid the huge anatomical leap from BL-40 at the knee

    to BL-41 on the upper back as in the Beijing system, and the less grievous, but still awkward,

    transition from BL-35 on the buttocks to BL-36 on the upper back in the Shanghai system.

• My numbering focuses more attention on the names of the points, and the connection

  between them that is made clear by calibrating both columns with the same number at the same level,

  rather than a linear, follow the numbers approach.

• I reunite the two columns at the gluteal fold, i.e BL-50, rather than at the knee, thereby avoiding the
  extraneous extra line that has no points (I maintain this path should belong to the sinew channel)

Possible Disadvantages: (besides flying in the face of all conventions)

• In my system, the numbers 36 through 49 are omitted, which might be confusing at first,
    of course the total number of Bladder points remains 67. (Also some levels have no "a" point)

5 Points on the Thigh				
Beijing / Shanghai **BJ# / SH#**	**Char.**	**PīnYīn**	**Location**	**Number:** same as SH#
BL-36 / 50	承扶	**Chéng Fú**	gluteal fold	**BL-50**
BL-37 / 51	殷門	**Yīn Mén**	mid thigh	**BL-51**
BL-38 / 52	浮隙	**Fú Xī**	1 cun above BL-53	**BL-52**
BL-39 / 53	委陽	**Wěi Yáng**	lateral end of popliteal crease	**BL-53**
BL-40 / 54	委中	**Wěi Zhōng**	middle of popliteal crease	**BL-54**
BL-55 / 55	合陽	**Hé Yáng**	2 cun below BL-54	**BL-55**

• I have not changed the numbering of the points on the lower extremity,
    (if one uses the Shanghai system), only the 14 points on the torso.

• I prefer the admittedly less favored enumeration typified by the Shanghai/ACT text
    and use that as my classroom convention.

• In that text, lower extremity points begin with BL-50 and continue straight through
    to BL-67 without a numerical break or an anatomical jump.

• The Shanghai method avoids counting BL-36 to 40 on the thigh, then BL-55 to 67 on the leg.

• In particular, it avoids the confusing transition from BL-40 at the knee (popliteal crease),
    to the very next point, numbered BL-55, only two cun/inches below it, on the calf.

* Most current textbooks use the Beijing system, I currently use MoA as representative of them.
BJ = MoA = *Manual of Acupuncture*   *by Deadman & Al-Khafaji*
SH = ACT = *Acupuncture: A Comprehensive Text*   *by O'Connor & Bensky*

膀 胱 經 Páng Guāng Jīng = Urinary Bladder Channel

- **Division:** (Leg) **Tai Yang**
- **Phase/Element:** (Yang) **Water**
- **High Tide:** 3–5 pm

---

begins: **at the inner canthus of the eye**

ends: **at the lateral nail point on the little toe**

❖ *The Bladder Channel external pathway:*

· begins just superior to the inner canthus of the eye	**(BL-1)**
· rises to the medial end of the eyebrow	(BL-2)
and continues upward to the hairline	(BL-3)
· jogs laterally & over the top of the head to the back of the neck (in traps, below occiput)	(BL-4–10)
· it divides into two branches (on each side) and proceeds down the back	(BL-10–49)
the two branches rejoin at gluteal fold below the ischial tuberosity	(BL-50)
(most sources show them continuing to the knee)	

a. the medial branch follows the crest of the erectors (midway between spine & scapula) to the ilium   (BL-11–26)

    then this branch splits:

the outer one [A.1] continues along the S-I joint & edge of the sacrum	(BL-27–30)
the inner one [A.2] flows through the sacral foramen ($1^{st} – 4^{th}$)	(BL-31–34)
together they sweep down to the gluteal fold below the ischial tuberosity	(BL-50)

b. the lateral branch on the back follows the line defined by vertebral border of the scapula,	(BL-36–49)
it continues thru the lumbar region and buttocks to the gluteal fold/ischial tuberosity	(BL-50)
· from the gluteal fold it proceeds down the back of the thigh between hamstrings	
to the popliteal crease(most charts show the two branches joining here at BL-54)	(BL-51–54)
· on the leg it flows between the two bellies of the gastrocnemius	(BL-55–57)
· then jogs laterally, following the achilles to the lateral malleolus	(BL-58–60)
· continues downward onto the lateral heel	(BL-61)
and follows the lateral edge of the foot to the little toe	(BL-64–66)
· ending at the lateral nail point on the little toe	**(BL-67)**

膀 胱 經 **Bladder Channel**   (67 pts)

Eye

BL-1   • in the depression just above the inner canthus
BL-2   • (superior to BL-1) in the bony depression at the medial end of the eyebrow

Scalp

level with

BL-3   • 0.5 cun behind the anterior hairline, 0.75-1.0 cun lateral to the midline   (GV-24)
BL-4   • 0.5 cun behind the anterior hairline, 1.5 cun lateral to the midline   (GV-24)
BL-5   • 1.0 cun behind the anterior hairline, 1.5 cun lateral to the midline   (GV-23)
BL-6   • 2.5 cun behind the anterior hairline, 1.5 cun lateral to the midline
BL-7   • 4.0 cun behind the anterior hairline, 1.5 cun lateral to the midline
BL-8   • 5.5 cun behind the anterior hairline, 1.5 cun lateral to the midline
     or   *6.5 cun above the posterior hairline*
BL-9   • 2.5 cun above the posterior hairline, 1.3 cun lateral to the midline   (GV-17)
          (level with the EOP)

Neck

BL-10   • 0.5 cun above the posterior hairline, 1.3 cun lateral to the midline   (GV-15)
          (in the trapezius m.)   BL-10 is where the channel divides

Back

• the inner BL line is 1.5 cun lateral to the midline, along the crest of the erectors
• the outer BL line is 3.0 cun lateral to the midline, along the vertebral border of the scapula
• all points are level with the space inferior to the spinous process of the indicated vertebra

Spine	Inner Line	Outer Line		
• T_1	**BL-11**	SI-14 <u>SH#/BJ#</u>	*(these two numbers are always different by 5)*	
• T_2	**BL-12**	**BL-12a** (**36**/41)	*(memorize all three numbers)*	
• T_3	**BL-13**	**BL-13a** (**37**/42)		(GV-12)
• T_4	**BL-14**	**BL-14a** (**38**/43)		
• T_5	**BL-15**	**BL-15a** (**39**/44)		(GV-11)
• T_6	**BL-16**	**BL-16a** (**40**/45)		(GV-10)
• T_7	**BL-17**	**BL-17a** (**41**/46)		(GV-9)
• T_9	**BL-18**	**BL-18a** (**42**/47)		(GV-8)
• T_{10}	**BL-19**	**BL-19a** (**43**/48)		(GV-7)
• T_{11}	**BL-20**	**BL-20a** (**44**/49)		(GV-6)
• T_{12}	**BL-21**	**BL-21a** (**45**/50)		
• L_1	**BL-22**	**BL-22a** (**46**/51)		(GV-5)
• L_2	**BL-23**	**BL-23a** (**47**/52)		(GV-4)
• L_3	**BL-24**			
• L_4	**BL-25**			(GV-3)
• L_5	**BL-26**			

Sacrum

• S_1	**BL-27**		
• S_2	**BL-28**	**BL-28a** (**48**/53)	(level with the inferior margin of the PSIS)
• S_3	**BL-29**		
• S_4	**BL-30**	**BL-30a** (**49**/54)	(level with the sacral hiatus) (GV-2)

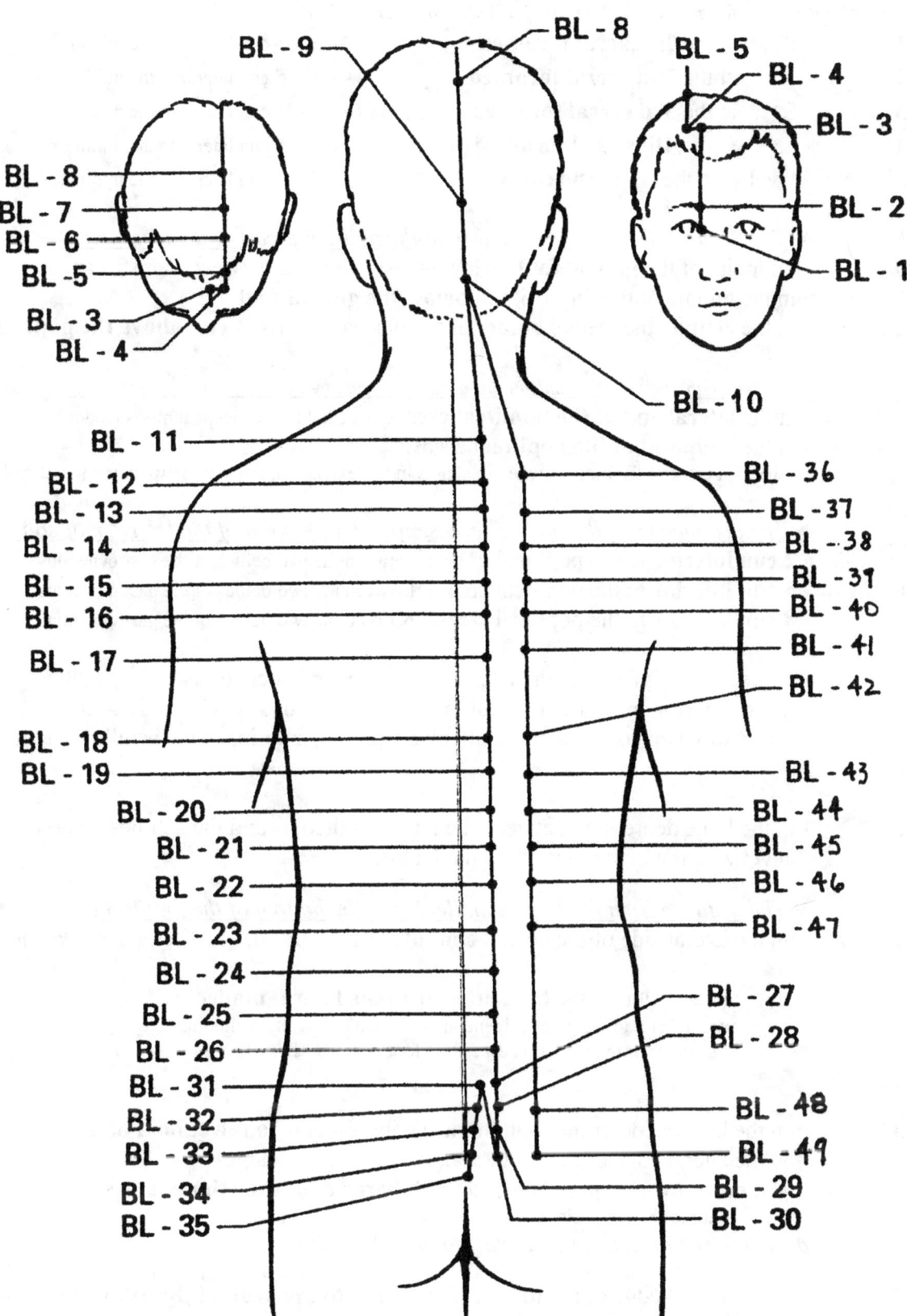

Bladder Channel
(following the Shanghai Numbering System on the Back)

Sacral Foramen		*foramen are in line with jia ji pts (jia-ji end at L5)*		*level with*
BL-31	• S$_1$	at the **1st sacral foramen**	(~ 0.5–.75 cun lateral to the midline)	
BL-32	• S$_2$	at the **2nd sacral foramen**	(~ 0.5–.75 cun lateral to the midline)	
BL-33	• S$_3$	at the **3rd sacral foramen**	(~ 0.5–.75 cun lateral to the midline)	
BL-34	• S$_4$	at the **4th sacral foramen**	(~ 0.5–.75 cun lateral to the midline)	(GV-2)
BL-35		• level with the **tip of the coccyx**	(~ 0.5–.75 cun lateral to the midline)	(GV-1)

Thigh

➤ *The distance from the gluteal fold to the politeal crease is 14 cun*

BL-50/36 • midpoint of the **gluteal fold**, below the ischium and between hamstrings

BL-51/37 • in the middle of the thigh, **6 cun below the gluteal fold**

BL-52/38 • in the cleft on the medial border of the biceps femoris, **1 cun above the popl. crease**

Knee

* *(on the thigh, the two BL numbers are always different by 14)*

BL-53/39 • at the **lateral end of the popliteal crease** (medial to the biceps femoris tendon)

BL-54/40 • at the **midpoint of the popliteal crease**
(the high point of the mound, when the leg is in full extension, midway between the two dimples)

Leg

➤ *The distance from the politeal crease to the high point of the lateral malleolus is 16 cun*

BL-55 • **2 cun inferior** to the popliteal crease, between the two bellies of the gastrocnemius

BL-56 • **5 cun inferior** to the popliteal crease, between the two bellies of the gastrocnemius

BL-57 • **8 cun inferior** to the popliteal crease, between the two bellies of the gastrocnemius

BL-58 • in the soleus, inferior to the lateral head of the gastrocnemius
1 cun inferior and ~ 1cun lateral to BL-57, or **7 cun superior** to BL-60

BL-59 • **3 cun superior** to the lateral malleolus (BL-60), anterior to the achilles tendon

Ankle

BL-60 • in the large depression between the lateral malleolus and the achilles tendon,
level with the high point of the malleolus.

Heel

➤ *The distance from the lateral malleolus to the bottom of the foot is 3 cun*

BL-61 • on the lateral side of the heel, **2 cun inferior** to BL-60, (~ 2/3 down, at the skin change)

BL-62 • on the lateral side of the foot, **inferior to the lateral malleolus**
usu. inferior to the peroneal tendon, ~ 0.5 cun below the malleolus
smt. superior to the tendon esp. if the foot is plantar flexed

Foot

BL-63 • on the lateral side of the foot, immediately **inferior to the cuboid bone**

BL-64 • on the lateral edge of the foot, (at or near the skin change)
just **posterior (i.e. proximal) to the tuberosity of the 5th metatarsal**
(not inferior to the tuberosity as many sources erroneously state)

alt loc. }   *as above, but anterior, (i.e. distal) to the tuberosity*

BL-65 • on the lateral edge of the foot, just **proximal to the head of the 5th metatarsal**

BL-66 • on the lateral side of the little toe, just **distal to the base of the 5th phalanx**

BL-67 • the lateral nail point on the little toe.

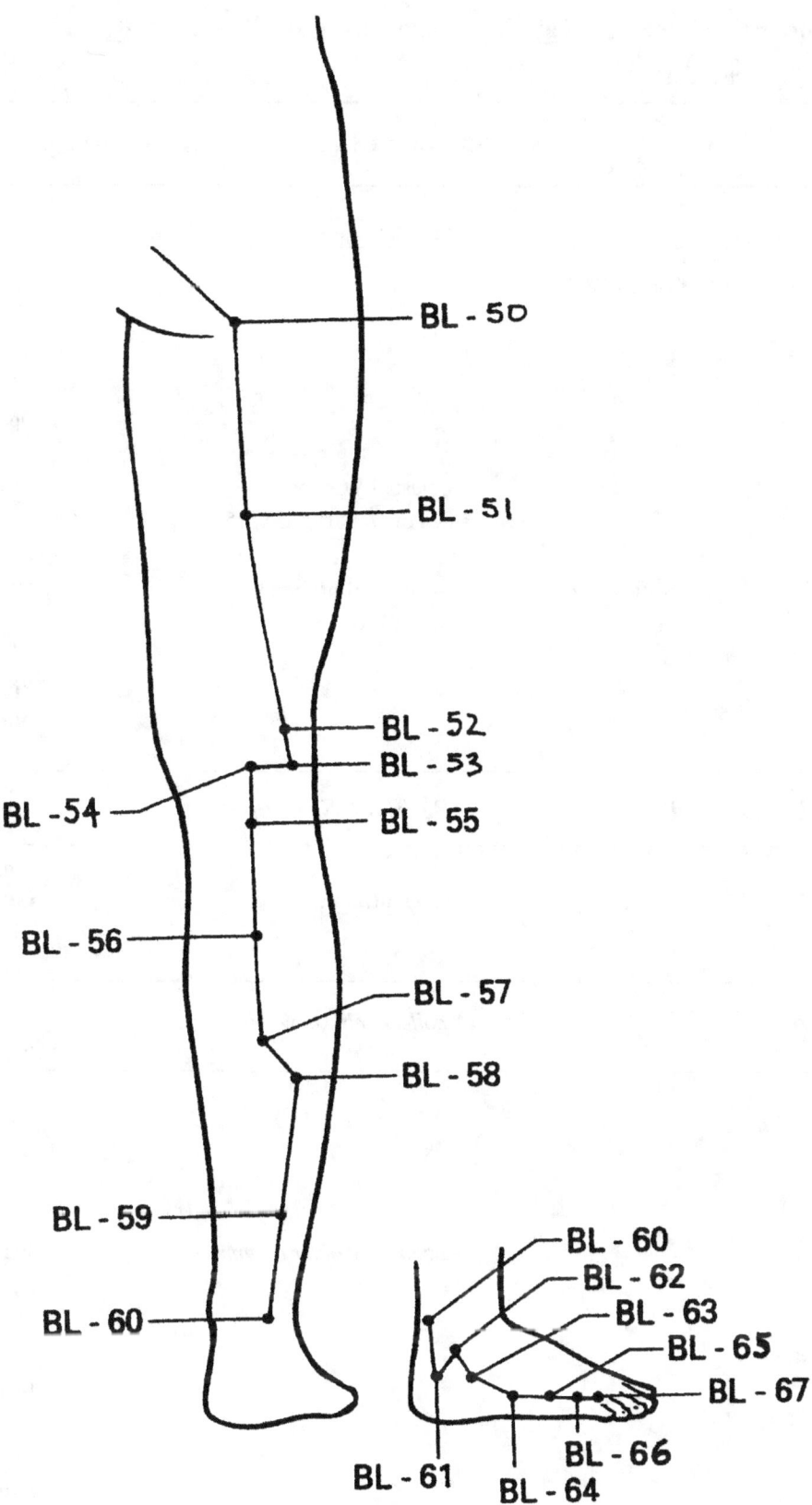

Bladder Channel
(following the Shanghai Numbering System on the Leg)

Bladder Channel = Zú **Tài-Yáng** Páng Guāng Jīng		**Water**	**3-5 pm**	
paired channels }	SI	Kd	Lu	

Mu pt = CV-3	**Shu pt** = BL-28	**Xia-he pt** = BL-54/40

	• Main Categories	• Misc. Categories	Pt Name & Translation
	on every channel		
BL-1	• entry pt: *from SI-18/19*		**Jīng Míng** 睛明 Eyes Bright/Clear
BL-7			**Tōng Tiān** 通天 Open the Celestial
BL-10		• Celestial Window • Sea of Qi pt (vs. GV-15/14)	**Tiān Zhù** 天柱 Celestial Pillar
BL-11	*aka* Bèi Shū 背腧 Back Shu	• **Influential pt**: bones • Sea of Blood pt	**Dà Zhù** 大杼 Big Shuttle
BL-12			**Fēng Mén** 風門 Wind Gate

BL-13 to 30	• *Bèi/Back Shu (pts)*	*know all 18*

BL-17		• **Influential pt**: blood	**Gé Shū** 膈腧 Diaphragm Pt

BL-31 to 34	* *collectively known as:*	***Bā Liáo*** 八髎 *8 Bone-holes*

BL-35		Huì Yáng 會陽 Yang Convergence

SH# / BJ# (JC)			
BL-36 / 41 (12a)		– *begins the outer column* –	**Fù Fēn** 附分 Appended Part
BL-37 / 42 (13a)			**Pò Hù** 魄戶 Lung Spirit Doorway
BL-38 / 43 (14a)			**Gāo Huāng Shū** 膏肓 Fatty Membrane Shu
BL-39 / 44 (15a)			**Shén Táng** 神堂 Heart Spirit Hall

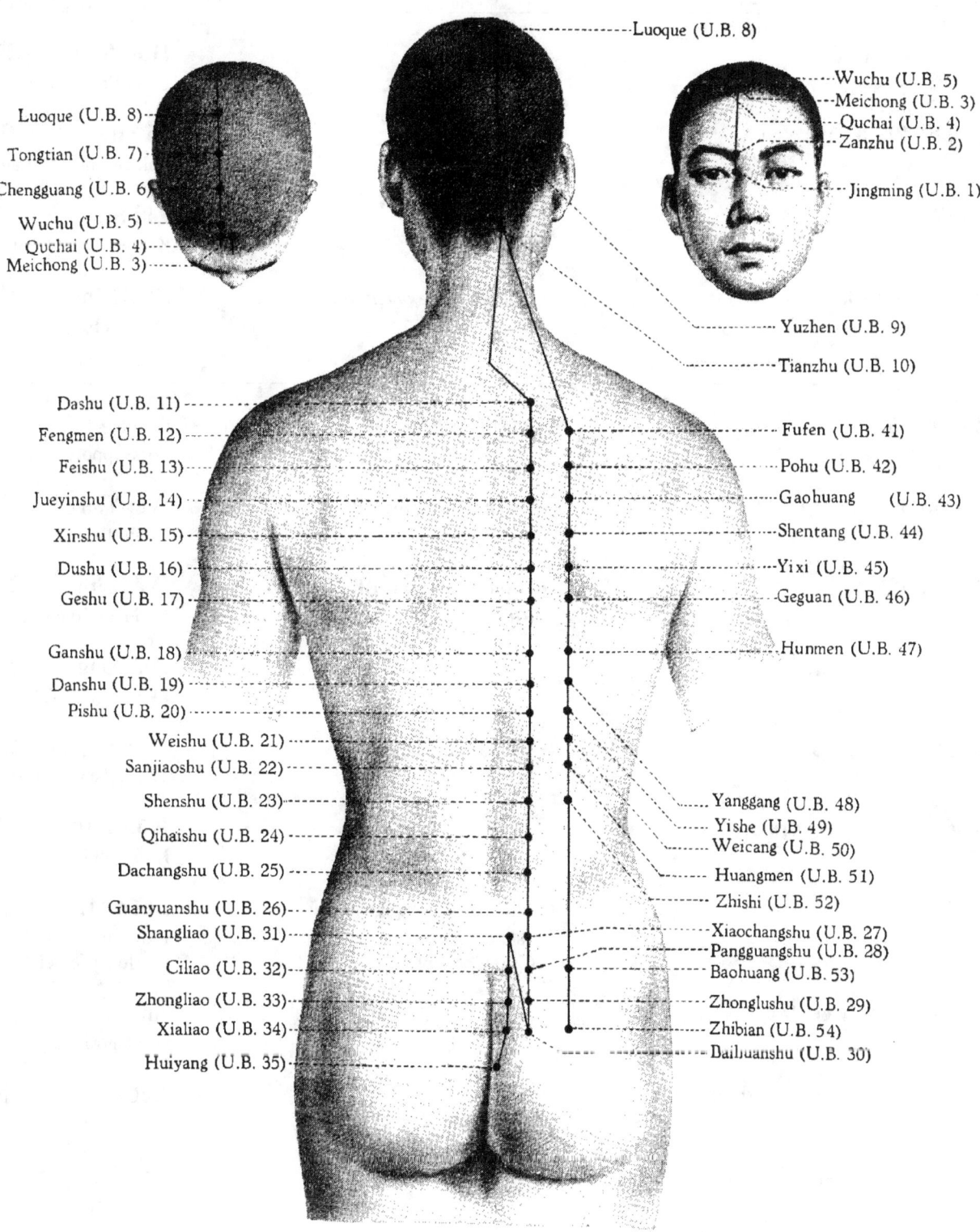

Luoque (U.B. 8)

Luoque (U.B. 8)
Tongtian (U.B. 7)
Chengguang (U.B. 6)
Wuchu (U.B. 5)
Quchai (U.B. 4)
Meichong (U.B. 3)

Wuchu (U.B. 5)
Meichong (U.B. 3)
Quchai (U.B. 4)
Zanzhu (U.B. 2)

Jingming (U.B. 1)

Yuzhen (U.B. 9)

Tianzhu (U.B. 10)

Dashu (U.B. 11)
Fengmen (U.B. 12)
Feishu (U.B. 13)
Jueyinshu (U.B. 14)
Xinshu (U.B. 15)
Dushu (U.B. 16)
Geshu (U.B. 17)

Ganshu (U.B. 18)
Danshu (U.B. 19)
Pishu (U.B. 20)
Weishu (U.B. 21)
Sanjiaoshu (U.B. 22)
Shenshu (U.B. 23)
Qihaishu (U.B. 24)
Dachangshu (U.B. 25)
Guanyuanshu (U.B. 26)
Shangliao (U.B. 31)
Ciliao (U.B. 32)
Zhongliao (U.B. 33)
Xialiao (U.B. 34)
Huiyang (U.B. 35)

Fufen (U.B. 41)
Pohu (U.B. 42)
Gaohuang   (U.B. 43)
Shentang (U.B. 44)
Yixi (U.B. 45)
Geguan (U.B. 46)

Hunmen (U.B. 47)

Yanggang (U.B. 48)
Yishe (U.B. 49)
Weicang (U.B. 50)
Huangmen (U.B. 51)
Zhishi (U.B. 52)
Xiaochangshu (U.B. 27)
Pangguangshu (U.B. 28)
Baohuang (U.B. 53)
Zhonglushu (U.B. 29)
Zhibian (U.B. 54)
Baihuanshu (U.B. 30)

足 太 陽 膀 胱 經
Zu Tai-Yang Pang-Guang Jing
Leg Greater-Yang Urinary Bladder Channel
(following the Beijing Numbering System on the Back)

	• Main Categories	• Misc. Categories	Pt Name & Translation
SH# / BJ# (JC) on every channel			
BL-42 / 47 (18a)			**Hún Mén** 魂門 Liver Spirit Gate
BL-44 / 49 (20a)			**Yì Shè** 意舍 Spleen Spirit Cottage
BL-47 / 52 (23a)			**Zhì Shì** 志室 Kidney Spirit Chamber
BL-49 / 54 (30a)		*— bottom of the outer column —*	Zhì Biān 秩邊 Order's Edge

- -

	• Main Categories	• Misc. Categories	Pt Name & Translation
BL-50 / 36		*— top of the thigh —*	**Chéng Fú** 承扶 For Support
BL-53 / 39		• **lower uniting pt: TB**	Wěi Yáng 委陽 Yang [lat. end of the] Bend
BL-54 / 40	• he/sea–earth–Control pt.	• **lower uniting pt: BL** • **Ruler**: back	**Wěi Zhōng** 委中 Middle of the Bend
BL-58	• **luo/connecting**		Fēi Yáng 飛揚 Flying Lift / Take Flight
BL-59		• Yang Qiao: xi/cleft	Fū Yáng 跗陽 Top of the Foot/Instep Yang
BL-60	• jing/river–fire		**Kūn Lún** 昆侖 Kun Lun Mt
BL-62		• **Master pt**: Yang Qiao mai • 1st pt: Yang Qiao mai • (5th) Ghost pt	**Shēn Mài** 申脈 Extension Vessel 9th Hour Vessel
BL-63	• **xi/cleft**	• 1st pt: Yang Wei mai	Jīn Mén 金門 Golden/Metal Gate
BL-64	• **yuan/source**		Jīng Gǔ 京骨 Capitol Bone
BL-65	• shu/stream–wood–Disp. pt.		Shù Gǔ 束骨 Strap Bone
BL-66	• ying/brook–water–Phase pt.		Tōng Gǔ 通谷 Unblock the Valley
BL-67	• jing/well–metal–Tonif. pt. • exit pt: *to Kd-1*		**Zhì Yīn** 至陰 Reach the Yin

---

腎 經 Shèn Jīng = Kidney Channel

- **Division:** (Leg) Shao Yin
- **Phase/Element:** (Yin) Water
- **High Tide:** 5–7 pm

---

begins: **on the little toe**

ends: **at the sternal head of the clavicle**

❖ *The Kidney Channel external pathway:*

· begins at the medial nail point on the little toe	**(Kd-0)**
· across the ball of the foot to the junction of the ball and the arch	**(Kd-1)**
· passes under the navicular toward the medial aspect of the heel	(Kd-2)
· rises posterior to the malleolus	(Kd-3)
· loops around in the space between the medial malleolus & the achilles tendon	(Kd-4–6)
· then up the leg along the anterior edge of the gastroc.	(Kd-7–9)
· to the knee, (medial end of the popliteal crease) (more precisely; between. the semi-tendinosus & semi-membranosus tendons)	(Kd-10)
· then follows the gracilis to the groin	
· whereupon it goes internally (to the kidney & bladder)	
· it reemerges at the crest of the pubis just lateral to the midline (symphysis)	(Kd-11)
· ascends the abdomen (slightly lateral to the midline) up to the costal arch	(Kd-12–21)
· jogs laterally and up onto the chest, continuing upward just lateral to the sternum	(Kd-22–26)
· ending just inferior to the sternal head of the clavicle	**(Kd-27)**

腎 經 **Kidney Channel** (27 pts)

Foot

Kd-1
• on the bottom of the foot, in the depression at the center medial to lateral;
   where the ball and the arch meet (~1/4–1/3 of the distance from the base of the toes to the heel)

Kd-2
• on the medial aspect of the foot, **inferior to the tuberosity of the navicular**

Ankle/Heel
➤ *There are 4 cun between the bottom of the heel and the high point of the medial malleolus (Kd-3)*

Kd-3
• on the inside of the ankle,
   in the space between the medial malleolus and the anterior edge of the achilles
   (level with the malleolar prominence and posterior to the artery)

Kd-4
• on the superior border of the calcaneum, at the anterior edge of the achilles
   (slightly posterior & ~**0.5 cun inferior** to Kd-3)

Kd-5
• in a depression on the medial calcaneum, ~**1 cun directly inferior** to Kd-3
   (anterior and inferior to Kd-4)

Kd-6
• ~**1 cun below** the inferior edge of the medial malleolus at its midpoint
   immediately inferior to the sustentaculum tali
   (anterior and slightly inferior to Kd-5)   (posterior and slightly superior to Kd-2)

alt loc. } as above, but slightly higher, in a depression just inferior to the medial malleolus.
   (analogous to BL-62 location)
   stay inferior/posterior to the posterior tibialis tendon to avoid confusion with Sp-5
   (some Japanese practitioners use a position analogous to BL-61)

Leg
➤ *15 cun are measured from the high point of the medial malleolus to the politeal crease*

Kd-7
• **2 cun superior** to the prominence of the medial malleolus (Kd-3),
   on the **anterior edge of the achilles**

Kd-8
• **2 cun superior** to the prominence of the medial malleolus (Kd-3),
   on the **posterior edge of the tibia**

Kd-9
• **5 cun superior** to the prominence of the medial malleolus (Kd-3),
   in the soleus, just inferior to the medial head of the gastrocnemius

Knee
locate with partner supine or sitting, and the knee bent (~90°)

Kd-10
• on the posterior-medial aspect of the knee,
   between the tendons of the semi-membranosus and semi-tendinosus.
• *when prone, or if the knee is in full extension:* the point is at the medial end of the popliteal crease,
   (in line with BL-53 & 54)

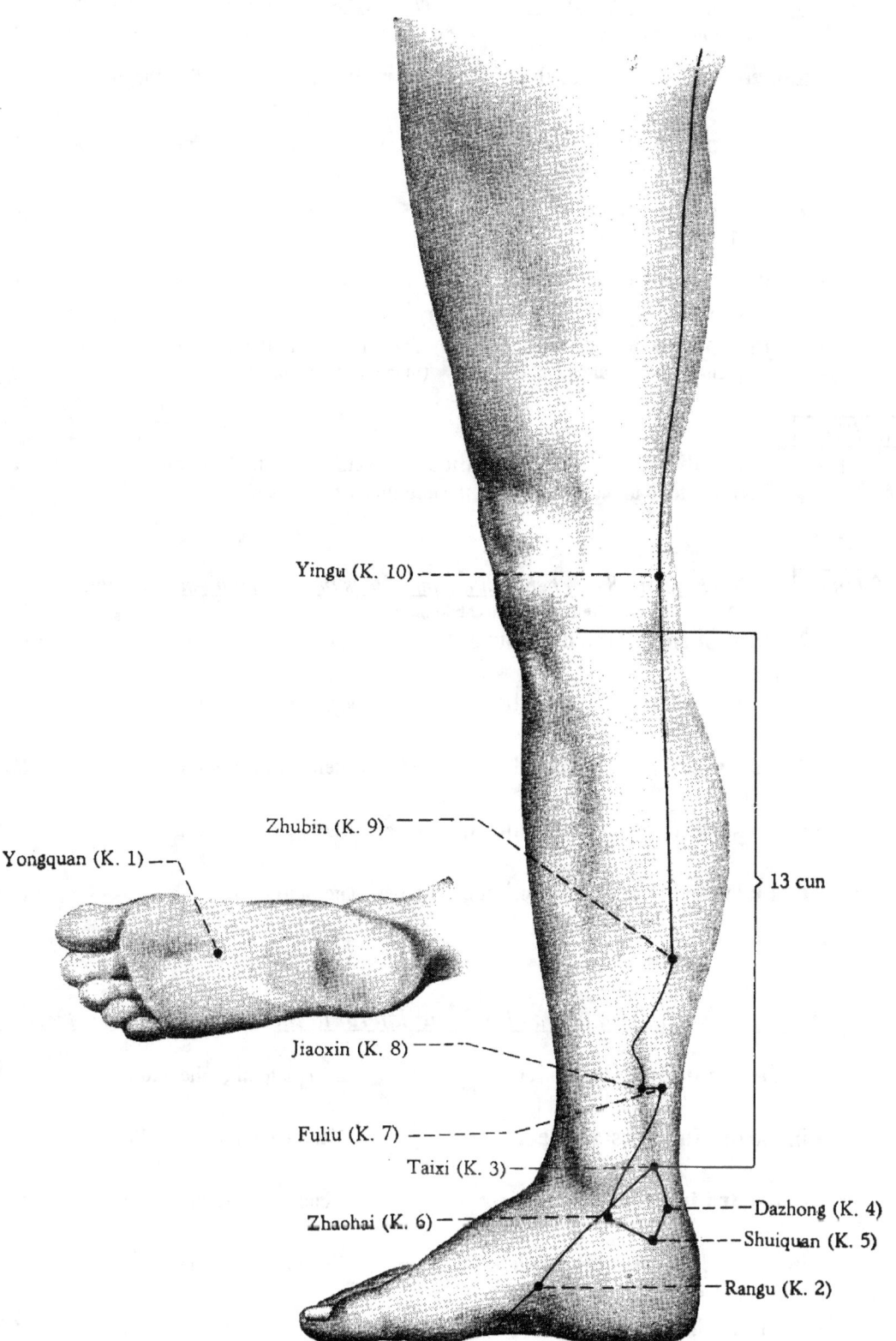

Yingu (K. 10)

Zhubin (K. 9)

Yongquan (K. 1)

13 cun

Jiaoxin (K. 8)

Fuliu (K. 7)

Taixi (K. 3)

Dazhong (K. 4)

Zhaohai (K. 6)

Shuiquan (K. 5)

Rangu (K. 2)

足少陰腎經
Zu Shao-Yin Shen Jing
Leg Lesser-Yin Kidney Channel

© 1990–2016   *Jim Cleaver LAc.*

Lower Abdomen	➤ *on the abdomen the Kd channel is defined as **0.5–1.0 cun lateral** to the midline*

*(most books say 0.5, I average it to be **0.75**)* (points are in the rectus abdominus) <u>level with</u>

Kd-11   • immediately superior to the crest of the pubis .75 cun lateral to the midline   (CV-2)
     (5 cun below the umbilicus)

Kd-12   • **1 cun superior** to the pubis,   .75 cun lateral to the midline   (CV-3)
     (4 cun below the umbilicus)

Kd-13   • **2 cun superior** to the pubis,   .75 cun lateral to the midline   (CV-4)
     (3 cun below the umbilicus)

Kd-14   • **3 cun superior** to the pubis,   .75 cun lateral to the midline   (CV-5)
     (2 cun below the umbilicus)

Kd-15   • **4 cun superior** to the pubis,   .75 cun lateral to the midline   (CV-7)
     (1 cun below the umbilicus)   (in the rectus abdominus)

Umbilical Plane

Kd-16   • level with the center of the umbilicus, .75 cun lateral to the midline   (CV-8)
     (just lateral to the perimeter of the umbilicus, this ~ 0.75)

Upper Abdomen	➤ *There are 8 cun between the umbilicus and the xipho-sternal junction*

(points are in the rectus abdominus)

Kd-17   • **2 cun superior** to the umbilicus,   .75 cun lateral to the midline   (CV-10)

Kd-18   • **3 cun superior** to the umbilicus,   .75 cun lateral to the midline   (CV-11)

Kd-19   • **4 cun superior** to the umbilicus,   .75 cun lateral to the midline   (CV-12)

Kd-20   • **5 cun superior** to the umbilicus,   .75 cun lateral to the midline   (CV-13)

Kd-21   • **6 cun superior** to the umbilicus,   .75 cun lateral to the midline   (CV-14)

Chest	➤ *on the chest the Kd channel is **2 cun lateral** to the midline* (lateral to the sternum)

Kd-22   • in the **5th intercostal space**,   2 cun lateral to the midline   (CV-16)

Kd-23   • in the **4th intercostal space**,   2 cun lateral to the midline   (CV-17)

Kd-24   • in the **3rd intercostal space**,   2 cun lateral to the midline   (CV-18)

Kd-25   • in the **2nd intercostal space**,   2 cun lateral to the midline   (CV-19)

Kd-26   • in the **1st intercostal space**,   2 cun lateral to the midline   (CV-20)

Kd-27   • immediately **inferior to the clavicle**,   2 cun lateral to the midline   (CV-21)
     slightly lateral to the sternal head

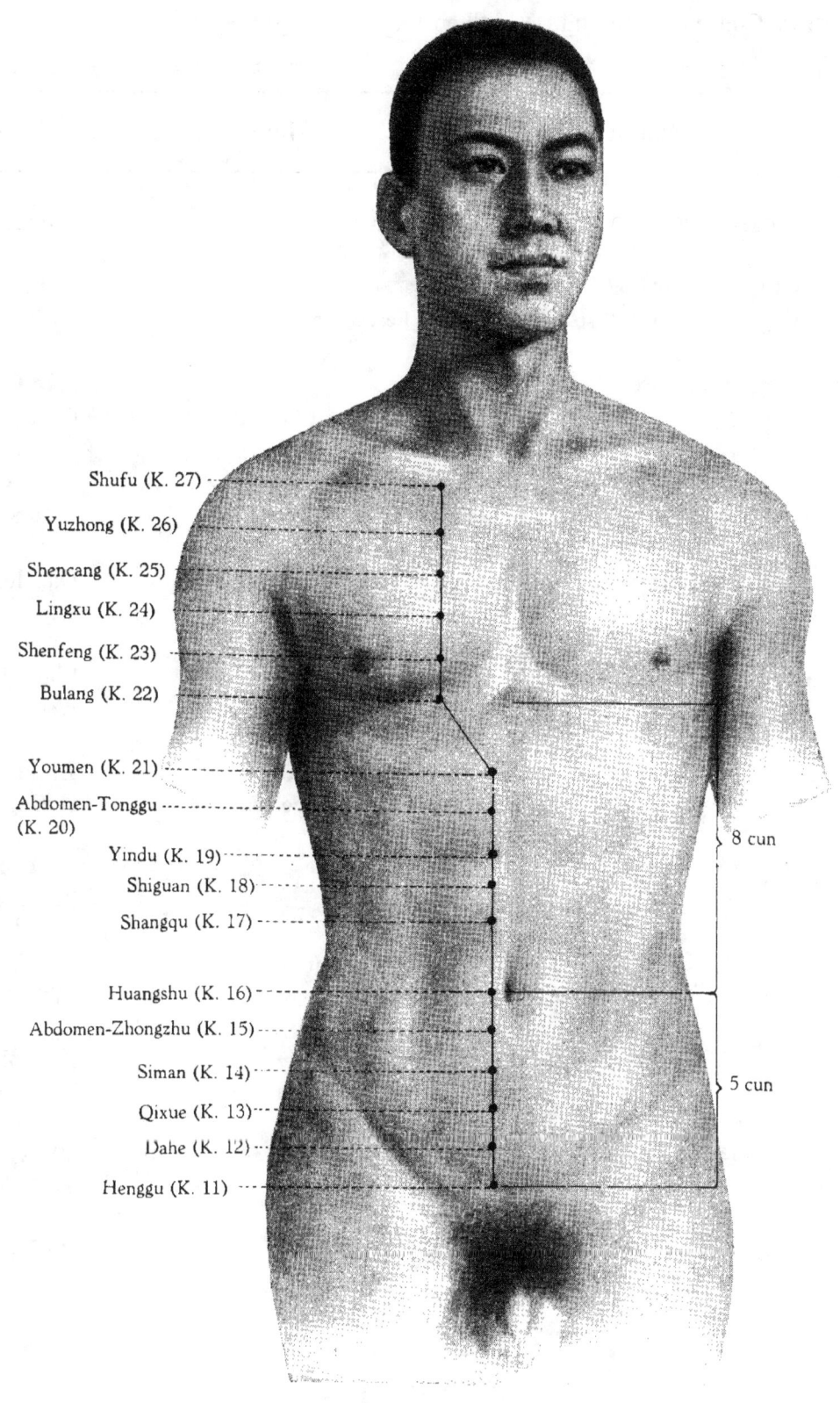

Shufu (K. 27)

Yuzhong (K. 26)

Shencang (K. 25)

Lingxu (K. 24)

Shenfeng (K. 23)

Bulang (K. 22)

Youmen (K. 21)

Abdomen-Tonggu
(K. 20)

Yindu (K. 19)

Shiguan (K. 18)

Shangqu (K. 17)

Huangshu (K. 16)

Abdomen-Zhongzhu (K. 15)

Siman (K. 14)

Qixue (K. 13)

Dahe (K. 12)

Henggu (K. 11)

8 cun

5 cun

足 少 陰 腎 經
Zu Shao-Yin Shen Jing
Leg Lesser-Yin Kidney Channel

Kidney Channel = Zú **Shǎo-Yīn** Shèn Jīng	**Water**	**5–7 pm**
paired channels } Ht	BL	LI

Mu pt = GB-25	**Shu pt** = BL-23

	• Main Categories on every channel	• Misc. Categories	Pt Name & Translation
Kd-1	• entry pt: *from BL-67* • jing/well–wood–Disp. pt.	• 9N (to Rescue Yang)	**Yǒng Quán** 湧泉 Bubbling Spring
Kd-2	• ying/brook–fire		**Rán Gǔ** 然谷 Blazing Valley
Kd-3	• shu/stream–earth–Control pt. • **yuan/source**	• 9N (to Rescue Yang)	**Tài Xī** 太谿 Great Streambed
Kd-4	• **luo/connecting**		Dà Zhōng 大鐘 Big Bell
Kd-5	• **xi/cleft**		Shuǐ Quán 水泉 Water Spring
Kd-6		• **Master pt**: Yin Qiao mai • 1st pt: Yin Qiao mai	**Zhào Hǎi** 照海 Shining Sea
Kd-7	• jing/river–metal–Tonif. pt.		**Fù Liū** 復溜 Restore Flow
Kd-8		• Yin Qiao: xi/cleft	Jiāo Xìn 交信 Faithful Junction
Kd-9		• Yin Wei: xi/cleft • 1st pt: Yin wei mai	Zhù Bīn 築賓 House Guest
Kd-10	• he/sea–water–Phase pt.		**Yīn Gǔ** 陰谷 Yin Valley
Kd-22	• **exit pt**: *to Pc-1*		Bù Láng 步廊 Step onto the/a Veranda
Kd-25		• alt. Ht mu pt	**Shén Cáng** 神藏 Spirit Stored
Kd-27		• last point	**Shū Fǔ** 俞府 Shu/Pt Official

The 2 Earth Channels (66 pts)

Stomach = Zu Yang-Ming *Wei* Jing

- The **Stomach** flows downward
- from head to toes

(centrifugal / outward flow of yang)

(45 pts)

Spleen = Zu Tai-Yin *Pi* Jing

- The **Spleen** flows upward
- from toes to torso

(centripetal / inward flow of yin)

(21 pts)

Fill in the 3 pairings of each channel:

Channel	*compartment*	**Phase**	**Division**	**Time**
Stomach	*anterior lateral*	yang Earth	zu Yang Ming	7–9 am
	3 pairings }			
Spleen	*anterior medial*	yin Earth	zu Tai Yin	9–11 am
	3 pairings }			

胃 經 Wèi Jīng = Stomach Channel

• **Division:** (Leg) **Yang Ming**

• **Phase/Element:** (Yang) **Earth**

• **High Tide: 7–9 am**

---

begins: at the midpoint of the infraorbital ridge

ends: on the 2nd toe

❖ *The Stomach Channel external pathway:*

· begins at the midpoint of the infraorbital ridge (between the eyeball & the orbit)   **(ST-1)**

· flows down the cheek to the corner of the mouth   (ST-2-4)

· a branch diverges laterally along the mandible to the masseter   (ST-5-6)
   then follows the masseter / ramus of the mandible up to the TMJ   (ST-7)
   it continues up to the corner of the forehead   (ST-8)

· the main pathway continues down along the throat (anterior edge of SCM)   (ST-9-11)
   then flows laterally to the center of the supra-clavicular fossa   (ST-12)

· descends along the mid-clavicular line, thru the nipple, to the 5th ICS   (ST-13-18)

· jogs medially and continues to descend the abdomen following the middle of the rectus
   abdominus to the pubic tubercle   (ST-19-30)

· runs laterally through the inguinal area to the thigh (below the ASIS)   (ST-31)

· then follows the anterior-lateral thigh (lateral edge of the rectus femoris) to the knee   (ST-32–34)

· passes along the lateral edge of the patella   (ST-35)

· on the leg it follows the tibialis anterior to the ankle   (ST-36–41)

· across the dorsum of the foot, between the 2nd & 3rd metatarsals & toes   (ST-42-44)

· ending at the lateral nail point on the 2nd toe   **(ST-45)**
   (a branch goes to the 3rd toe)

胃 經 Stomach Channel   (45 pts)

Face	

on the anterior face the Stomach channel follows the pupil line down to the corner of the mouth

ST-1 • between the eyeball and the midpoint of the infra-orbital ridge   (the pupil line)

ST-2 • on the maxilla, at the infra-orbital foramen   (may or may not be on the pupil line)

ST-3 • below the maxilla, on the line connecting ST-1 & ST-4, level with the lower border of the ala nasi

ST-4 • just lateral to and level with the corner of the mouth   (should, still be on the pupil line)

Lateral Face	*on the lateral face the channel follows the ramus of the mandible*

ST-5 • on the mandible, at the anterior edge of the masseter   (next to the facial artery)

ST-6 • at the high point of the masseter   (~1 finger anterior & superior to the angle of the jaw)   level with ST-4

ST-7 • in the mandibular notch, immediately inferior to the zygomatic

Head	➤ *The distance from ST-8 to ST-8 is 9 cun*

ST-8 • at the corner of the forehead; 0.5 cun within the hairline, 4.5 cun lat. to the midline (GV-24)

     Locating Tip: *extend lines up from ST-6/7, and the lateral orbit – where they intersect is ST-8*

Throat	*in the groove on the lateral edge of the thyroid cartilage (follows esophagus)*

ST-9 • level with the laryngeal prominence, on anterior edge of the SCM   (next to carotid)

ST-10 • on the anterior edge of the SCM, midway between ST-9 & ST-11

      ~ level with the cricoid cartilage   (~ 1.5 cun above the sternal head of the clavicle)

ST-11 • immediately superior to the sternal head of the clavicle, between the 2 heads of the SCM

Supraclavicular Fossa	➤ *The distance from ST-12 to ST-12 is 8 cun*

ST-12 • the center of the supraclavicular fossa, 4 cun lateral to midline   (Kd is 2, Lu is 6)

Chest	➤ *The distance between nipples (at least on males) is defined as 8 cun*
	➤ *The mid-clavicular / mid-mammillary line is 4 cun lateral to the midline* *level with*

ST-13 • **inferior to the clavicle,**   4 cun lateral to midline i.e. mid-clavicular line   (CV-21 & Kd-27)

ST-14 • **1st intercostal space,**   4 cun lateral to midline i.e. mid-clavicular line   (CV-20 & Kd-26)

ST-15 • **2nd intercostal space,**   4 cun lateral to midline i.e. mid-clavicular line   (CV-19 & Kd-25)

ST-16 • **3rd intercostal space,**   4 cun lateral to midline i.e. mid-clavicular line   (CV-18 & Kd-24)

ST-17 • **4th intercostal space,**   4 cun lateral to midline (i.e. the nipple)   (CV-17 & Kd-23)

ST-18 • **5th intercostal space,**   4 cun lateral to midline i.e. mid-clavicular line   (CV-16 & Kd-22)

       * *on males, the nipple is over the 4th IC space*

       * *on females, the 5th IC space is immediately inferior to the root of the breast*

Upper Abd	➤ *There are 8 cun between the xipho-sternal jct and the center of the umbilicus*
	On the torso the channel follows the vertical mid-line of the rectus abdominus (2 cun lateral to CV)

ST-19 • **6 cun superior** to the umbilical plane,   2 cun lateral to midline   (CV-14 & Kd-21)

ST-20 • **5 cun superior** to the umbilical plane,   2 cun lateral to midline   (CV-13 & Kd-20)

ST-21 • **4 cun superior** to the umbilical plane,   2 cun lateral to midline   (CV-12 & Kd-19)

ST-22 • **3 cun superior** to the umbilical plane,   2 cun lateral to midline   (CV-11 & Kd-18)

ST-23 • **2 cun superior** to the umbilical plane,   2 cun lateral to midline   (CV-10 & Kd-17)

ST-24 • **1 cun superior** to the umbilical plane,   2 cun lateral to midline   (CV-9 no Kd pt)

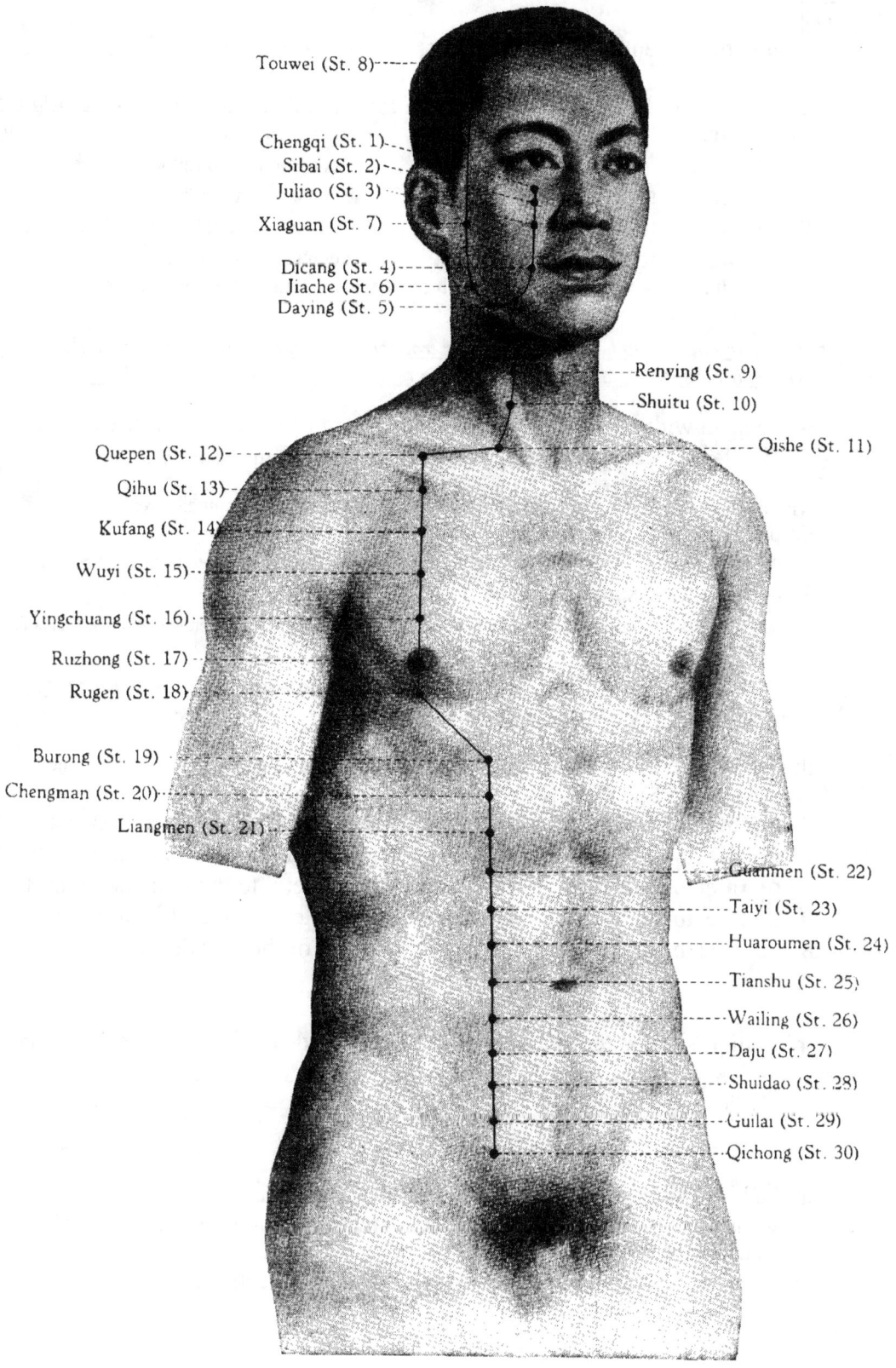

Touwei (St. 8)

Chengqi (St. 1)
Sibai (St. 2)
Juliao (St. 3)
Xiaguan (St. 7)

Dicang (St. 4)
Jiache (St. 6)
Daying (St. 5)

Renying (St. 9)
Shuitu (St. 10)

Quepen (St. 12)
Qishe (St. 11)
Qihu (St. 13)

Kufang (St. 14)

Wuyi (St. 15)

Yingchuang (St. 16)

Ruzhong (St. 17)

Rugen (St. 18)

Burong (St. 19)

Chengman (St. 20)

Liangmen (St. 21)

Guanmen (St. 22)

Taiyi (St. 23)

Huaroumen (St. 24)

Tianshu (St. 25)

Wailing (St. 26)

Daju (St. 27)

Shuidao (St. 28)

Guilai (St. 29)

Qichong (St. 30)

足 陽 明 胃 經
Zu Yang-Ming Wei Jing
Leg Bright-Yang Stomach Channel

© 1990–2016   Jim Cleaver LAc.

Umbilical Plane
ST-25   • level with the center of the umbilicus,   2 cun lateral to midline (mid rectus)   (CV-8 & Kd-16)

Lower Abd   ➤ *There are 5 cun between the umbilical plane and the superior edge of the pubis*
ST-26   • **1 cun inferior** to the umbilical plane   2 cun lateral to midline   (CV-7 & Kd-15)
ST-27   • **2 cun inferior** to the umbilical plane   2 cun lateral to midline   (CV-5 & Kd-14)
ST-28   • **3 cun inferior** to the umbilical plane   2 cun lateral to midline   (CV-4 & Kd-13)
ST-29   • **4 cun inferior** to the umbilical plane   2 cun lateral to midline   (CV-3 & Kd-12)
ST-30   • **5 cun inferior** to the umbilical plane   2 cun lateral to midline   (CV-2 & Kd-11)
          (level with the superior border of the pubic bone, just lateral to the pubic tubercle)

Thigh   ➤ *19 cun are measured between the greater trochanter and the popliteal crease / midpoint of patella*
          ST pts lie along the line connecting the ASIS and the lateral edge of the patella

ST-31   • ~ one hand width below the ASIS, on the lateral side of the sartorius
   or   • ~ at the level of the perineum   (between the sartorius & rectus femoris)

          with the leg extended, the middle of the patella is level with the popliteal crease
          the patella is considered to be 2 cun high
ST-32   • **6 cun above** the supralateral corner of the patella (on the lateral edge of the rectus femoris)
ST-33   • **3 cun above** the supralateral corner of the patella (on the lateral edge of the rectus femoris)
ST-34   • **2 cun above** the supralateral corner of the patella (on the lateral edge of the rectus femoris)

Leg   ➤ *16 cun are measured between the popliteal crease and the lateral malleolus*
          ST channel pts on the leg are in the muscle body of the tibialis anterior

ST-35   • the lateral eye of the knee (inferior to the patella and lateral to the patellar ligament)
          * when the knee is bent ST-35 is considered to be level with the popliteal crease & is used to measure from
ST-36   • **3 cun inferior** to ST-35   one finger width lateral to the tibia (in the ant tibialis m.)
ST-37   • **6 cun inferior** to ST-35   one finger width lateral to the tibia (in the ant tibialis m.)
ST-38   • **8 cun inferior** to ST-35   one finger width lateral to the tibia (in the ant tibialis m.)
ST-39   • **9 cun inferior** to ST-35   one finger width lateral to the tibia (in the ant tibialis m.)
ST-40   • **8 cun inferior** to ST-35   on the lateral edge of the tibialis anterior

Ankle
ST-41   • mid-point of the anterior ankle, on the medial side of the extensor digitorum t.
          (between the ext. digitorum & ext. hallucis longus tendons)
          (on the line connecting the high points of the malleoli)

Foot
ST-42   • at the high point of the dorsum of the foot (cuneiforms)
          between the ext. digitorum & ext. hallucis longus tendons, (alongside the dorsalis pedis artery)
          (~ midway between ST-41 & ST-43)
ST-43   • between the 2nd & 3rd metatarsals, ~ midway between their heads & bases

Toes
ST-44   • between the 2nd & 3rd toes, midway between the web margin & the knuckle prominences
ST-45   • the lateral nail pt on the 2nd toe

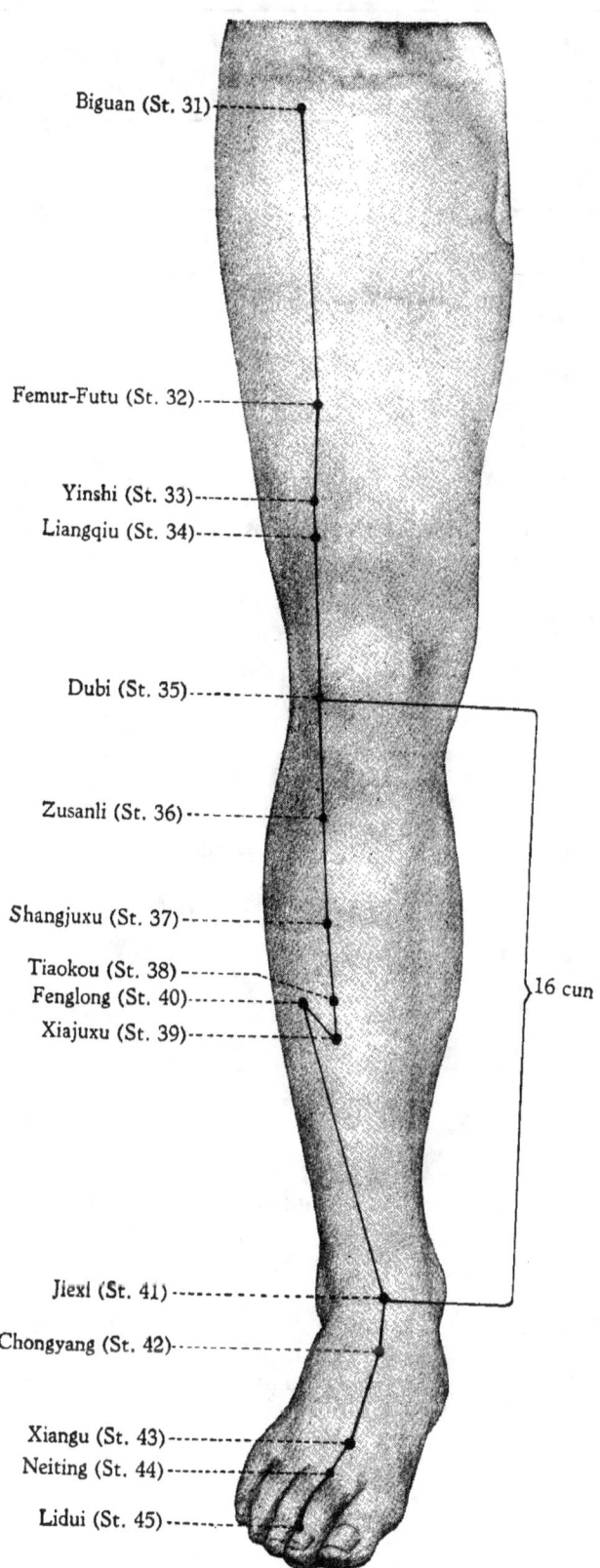

Biguan (St. 31)

Femur-Futu (St. 32)

Yinshi (St. 33)

Liangqiu (St. 34)

Dubi (St. 35)

Zusanli (St. 36)

Shangjuxu (St. 37)

Tiaokou (St. 38)

Fenglong (St. 40)

Xiajuxu (St. 39)

16 cun

Jiexi (St. 41)

Chongyang (St. 42)

Xiangu (St. 43)

Neiting (St. 44)

Lidui (St. 45)

足陽明胃經
Zu Yang-Ming Wei Jing
Leg Bright-Yang Stomach Channel

© 1990–2016   *Jim Cleaver LAc.*

Stomach Channel = Zú **Yáng-Míng** Wèi Jīng		**Earth**	**7–9 am**
paired channels } LI		Sp	Pc

Mu pt = CV-12	**Shu pt** = BL-21	**Xia-he pt** = ST-36

	• Main Categories on every channel	• Misc. Categories	Pt Name & Translation
ST-1	• entry pt: *from LI-20*		Chéng Qì 承泣 For Tearing
ST-4			**Dì Cāng** 地倉 Terrestial Granary
ST-6		• (7th) Ghost pt	Jiá Chē 頰車 Jaw Cart
ST-8			**Tóu Wéi** 頭維 Head Corner/Link
ST-9		• Sea of Qi pt • Celestial Window	**Rén Yíng** 人迎 Person's Prognosis
ST-12		• major Jct pt: (LI, SI, TB, GB)	Quē Pén 缺盆 Empty Basin
ST-17			Rǔ Zhōng 乳中 Breast Center
ST-18		• Great Luo (of ST)	**Rǔ Gēn** 乳根 Breast Root
ST-25		• **LI mu pt**	**Tiān Shū** 天樞 Celestial Axis/Pivot
ST-28			Shuǐ Dào 水道 Water Pathway
ST-30		• Sea of Nourishment pt	**Qì Chōng** 氣衝 Qi Thoroughfare Surging (Pulsing) Qi

	• Main Categories <small>on every channel</small>	• Misc. Categories	Pt Name & Translation
ST-34	• **xi/cleft**		Liáng Qiū 梁丘 Beam Hill / Bridge Hill
ST-35			Dú Bí 犢鼻 Calf's Nose
ST-36	• he/sea–earth–<small>Phase pt.</small>	• **lower uniting pt**: ST • **Ruler**: abdomen • 9N (to Rescue Yang) • Sea of Nourishment pt	**Zú Sān Lǐ** 足三里 Leg 3 Units
ST-37		• **lower uniting pt**: LI • Sea of Blood pt	**Shàng Jù Xū** 上巨虛 Upper Huge Depletion (Upper Strong Legs)
ST-39		• **lower uniting pt**: SI • Sea of Blood pt	**Xià Jù Xū** 下巨虛 Lower Large Depletion (Lower Strong Legs)
ST-40	• **luo/connecting**		**Fēng Lóng** 豐隆 Copious & Abundant
ST-41	• jing/river–fire–<small>Tonif. pt.</small>		Jiě Xī 解谿 Separating Stream(bed)s
ST-42	• **yuan/source** • **exit pt**: *to Sp-1*		Chōng Yáng 衝陽 Pulsing Yáng / Yang Surge Yang Thoroughfare
ST-43	• shu/stream–wood–<small>Control pt.</small>		Xiàn Gǔ 陷谷 Sunken Valley Soggy/boggy Valley
ST-44	• ying/brook–water		**Nèi Tíng** 內庭 Inner Courtyard
ST-45	• jing/well–metal–<small>Disp. pt.</small>	• last point	Lì Duì 厲兌 Severe/Harsh Mouth

脾 經 Pí Jīng = Spleen Channel

- **Division:** (Leg) **Tai Yin**
- **Phase/Element:** (Yin) **Earth**
- **High Tide: 9–11 am**

begins: on the medial aspect of the big toe

ends: in the 7th ICS, mid-axillary line

❖   *The Spleen Channel external pathway:*

· begins at the medial nail point on the big toe	**(Sp-1)**
· follows the medial aspect of the big toe and foot (1st metatarsal)	(Sp-1–4)
· sweeps upward to the ankle flowing anterior to the medial malleolus	(Sp-5)
· then up the leg, just posterior to the tibia, to the knee	(Sp-6–9)
· it passes along the medial border of the patella into the vastus medialis	(Sp-10)
· then more or less follows the sartorius to the groin	(Sp-11–13)
· ascends the abdomen along the lateral edge of the rectus abdominus to the ribs	(Sp-13–16)
· it shifts laterally & proceeds upward onto the chest midway between the nipple and the mid-axillary line up to the 2nd ICS (almost to Lu-1)	(Sp-17–20)
· then drops down to the 7th ICS, on the mid-axillary line to end	**(Sp-21)**

脾 經 Spleen Channel   (21 pts)

Foot

Sp-1   • the medial nail point on the big toe

Sp-2   • on the medial side of the big toe, just **distal to the base** of the proximal phalanx

Sp-3   • on the medial aspect of the foot, just **proximal to the head** of the 1st metatarsal

Sp-4   • on the medial aspect of the foot, just **distal to the base** of the 1st metatarsal
          inferior to the shaft of the bone, but superior to the plantar fascia
          (Sp-3 & Sp-4 are only about 1 cun apart, be careful to distinguish the base from the joint space)

Ankle

Sp-5   • in the depression at the anterior-inferior corner of the medial malleolus,
        anterior/superior to the posterior tibialis tendon
        (midway between the prominences of the medial malleolus and the navicular)

Leg

     ➤ *There are 15 cun between the prominence of the medial malleolus and the popliteal crease*
        The Sp channel follows the groove between the posterior edge of the tibia and the gastrocnemius

Sp-6   • **3 cun superior** to the prominence of the medial malleolus

Sp-7   • **6 cun superior** to the medial malleolus, in the groove between the tibia & gastroc.

Sp-8   • 10 cun superior to the medial malleolus, in the groove between the tibia & gastroc.
         • **5 cun inferior** to the popliteal crease   (1/3 down)   (3 cun below Sp-9)

Sp-9   • **2 cun inferior** to the popliteal crease, between the tibia & the gastrocnemius
         13 cun superior to the medial malleolus (middle of the curvature of the medial condyle of the tibia)

Thigh

     ➤ *18 cun are measured between the medial epicondyle of the femur and the superior edge of the pubis*
        The Sp channel basically follows the sartorius, i.e. a line from the medial aspect of the patella to the midpoint of the inguinal ligament.

Sp-10   *best located with the knee bent:*   • in the bulge of the vastus medialis
         • **2 cun superior** (and slightly medial) to the medio-superior corner of the patella
          ~ level with ST-34   * note: the patella is considered to be 2 cun in height

Sp-11   • ~ mid thigh, **8 cun superior** to the (superior border of the) patella,   (6 cun above Sp-10)
        at the superior end of the vastus medialis, where the sartorius and rectus femoris cross.
        (9 cun above medial epicondyle = midpoint of thigh)

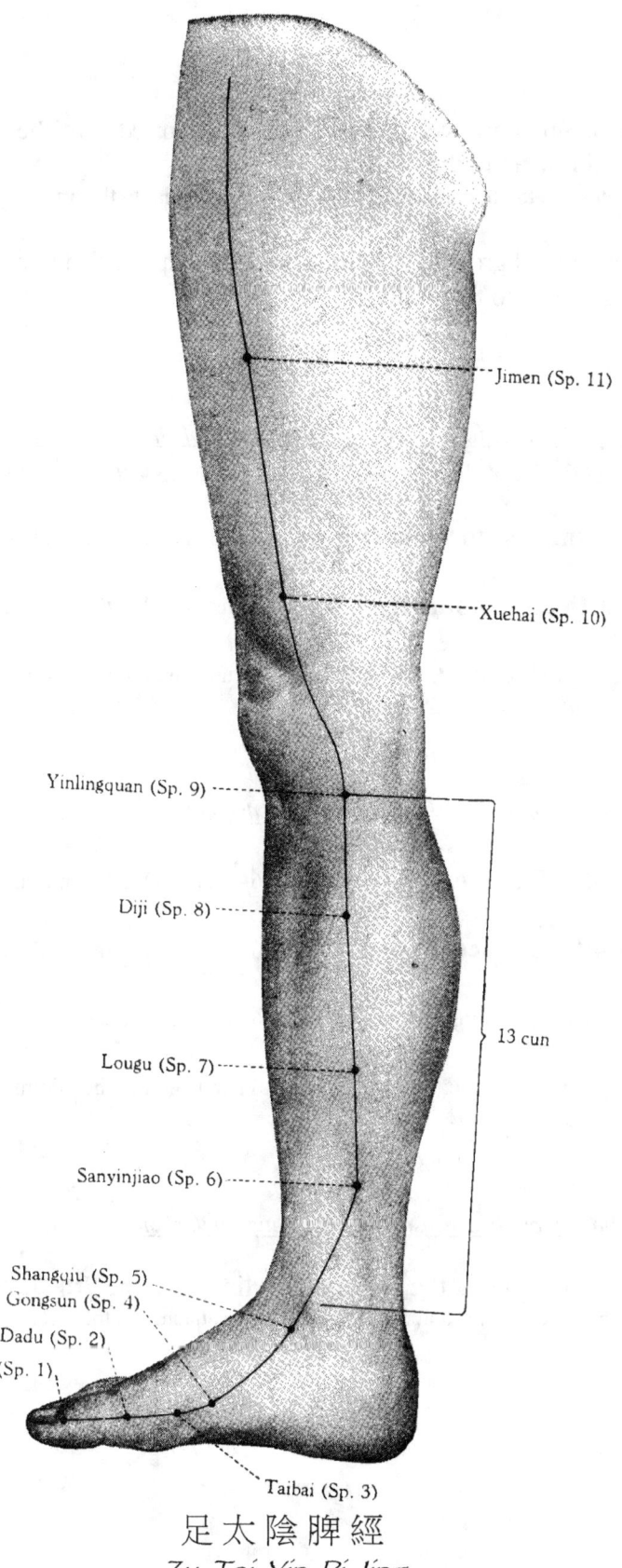

Jimen (Sp. 11)

Xuehai (Sp. 10)

Yinlingquan (Sp. 9)

Diji (Sp. 8)

13 cun

Lougu (Sp. 7)

Sanyinjiao (Sp. 6)

Shangqiu (Sp. 5)
Gongsun (Sp. 4)
Dadu (Sp. 2)
Yinbai (Sp. 1)

Taibai (Sp. 3)

足 太 陰 脾 經
Zu Tai-Yin Pi Jing
Leg Greater-Yin Spleen Channel

Groin

Sp-12   • in the inguinal groove, level with the superior edge of the pubis   <u>level with</u>
             3.5 cun lateral to the midline,   (CV-2 & ST-30)
                just lateral to the femoral artery (ST-30 is just medial to the artery)

Sp-13   • in the inguinal groove, **0.7 cun above** the superior edge of the pubis,
             4 cun lateral to the midline.

Abdomen

➤ *The Sp channel follows the lateral edge of the rectus abdominus from the groin*
to the costal margin. The lateral edge of the rectus is 4 cun lateral to the midline.

Sp-14   • **1.3 cun inferior** to the umbilicus,   4 cun lateral to the midline   (~CV-6)

Sp-15   • **level with the umbilicus,**   4 cun lateral to the midline   (CV-8 & ST-25)

Sp-16   • **3 cun superior** to the umbilicus,   4 cun lateral to the midline   (ST-22)

Chest

➤ *The Spleen channel runs midway between the mid-clavicular and mid-axillary lines (i.e. 6 cun)*

Sp-17   • in the **5th IC space,**   6 cun lateral to the midline   (ST-18)

Sp-18   • in the **4th IC space,**   6 cun lateral to the midline   (ST-17)

Sp-19   • in the **3rd IC space,**   6 cun lateral to the midline   (ST-16)

Sp-20   • in the **2nd IC space,**   6 cun lateral to the midline   (below Lu-1)   (ST-15)

Side

➤ *The mid-axillary line measures 12 cun between the bottom of the axilla and the tip of the 11th rib*

Sp-21   • the mid-point along the mid-axillary line, usu. the **7th IC space,**   (6 cun below the axilla)
             (inferior to the serratus anterior, the lowest slip attaches to the 8th rib)   (~ level with Lr-14)

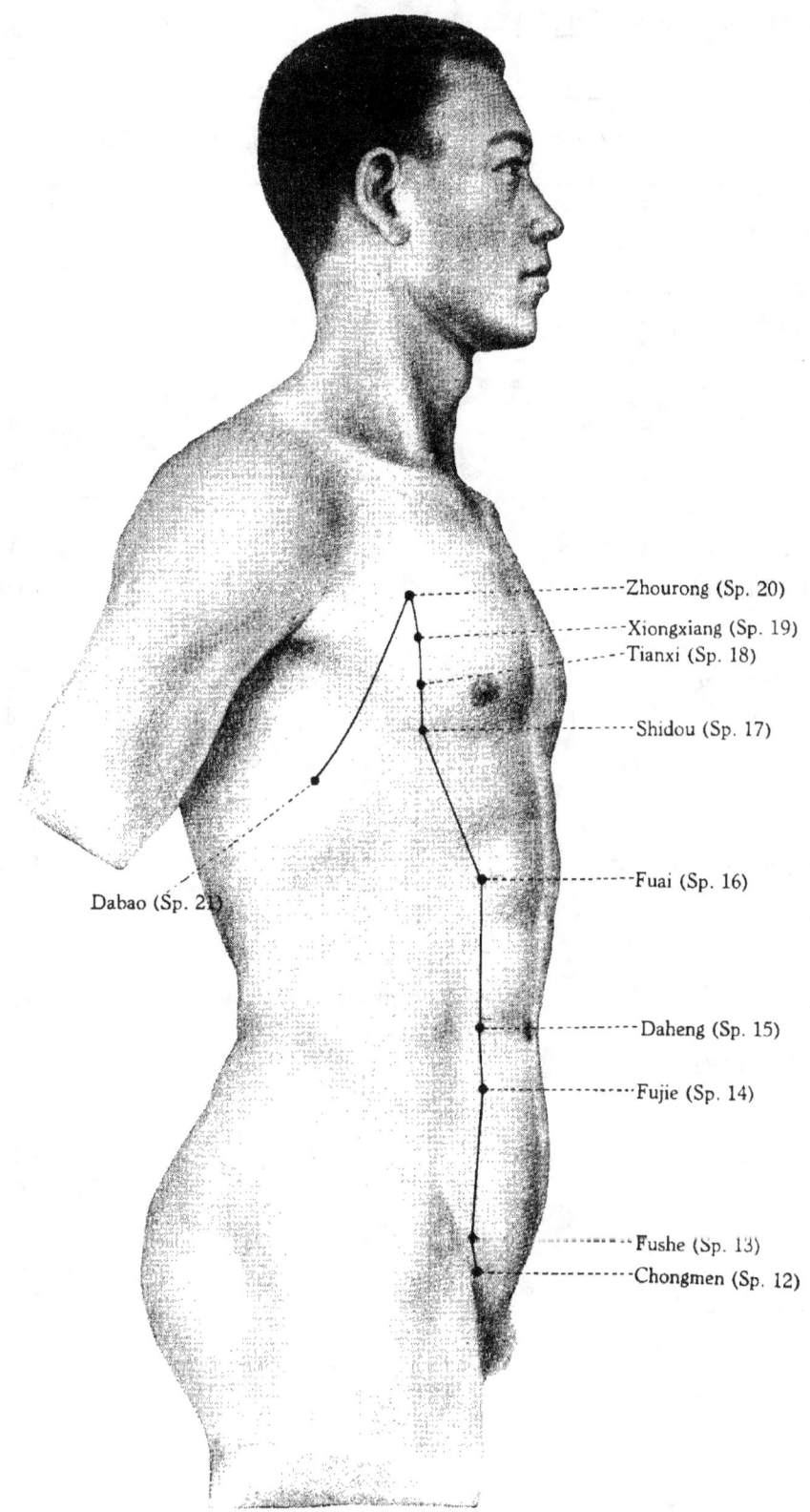

Zhourong (Sp. 20)
Xiongxiang (Sp. 19)
Tianxi (Sp. 18)

Shidou (Sp. 17)

Fuai (Sp. 16)

Daheng (Sp. 15)

Fujie (Sp. 14)

Fushe (Sp. 13)
Chongmen (Sp. 12)

Dabao (Sp. 21)

足 太 陰 脾 經
Zu Tai-Yin Pi Jing
Leg Greater-Yin Spleen Channel

Spleen Channel = Zú **Tài-Yīn** Pí Jīng	**Earth**	**9–11 am**
paired channels } Lu	ST	TB

Mu pt = Lr-13	**Shu pt** = BL-20

	• Main Categories (on every channel)	• Misc. Categories	Pt Name & Translation
Sp-1	• entry pt: *from ST-42* • jing/well–wood–Control pt.	• (3rd) Ghost pt	Yĭn Bái 隱白 Concealed/Hidden White
Sp-2	• ying/brook–fire–Tonif. pt.		Dà Dū 大都 Big City
Sp-3	• shu/stream–earth–Phase pt. • **yuan/source**		**Tài Bái** 太白 Great White
Sp-4	• **luo/connecting**	• **Master pt**: Chong mai	**Gōng Sūn** 公孫 Duke's Grandson/Heir Grandfather & Grandson Ancestor & Descendant
Sp-5	• jing/river–metal–Disp. pt.		Shāng Qiū 商丘 Metal (Note) Hill
Sp-6	• *Cx: pregnancy*	• **Ruler**: (pelvis / LJiao) • **Group Luo**: (3 leg yin) • **9N** (to Rescue Yang)	**Sān Yīn Jiāo** 三陰交 3 Yin Junction
Sp-8	• **xi/cleft**		**Dì Jī** 地機 Terrestrial Machine(ry) Earth Mechanism / Mobilize Earth
Sp-9	• he/sea–water		**Yīn Líng Quán** 陰陵泉 Yin Mound Spring
Sp-10			**Xuè Hăi** 血海 Sea of Blood
Sp-21	• exit pt: *to Ht-1*	• **Great Luo** (of Sp)	**Dà Bāo** 大包 Big Wrap-around Big Embrace

The 2 Wood Channels (58 pts)

Gall Bladder = Zu Shao-Yang Dan Jing

- The **Gall Bladder** flows downward
- from head to toes

(centrifugal / outward flow of yang)

(44 pts)

Liver = Zu Jue-Yin Gan Jing

- The **Liver** flows upward
- from toes to torso

(centripetal / inward flow of yin)

(14 pts)

Fill in the 3 pairings of each channel:

Channel	compartment	Phase	Division	Time
Gall Baldder	*lateral*	yang Wood	zu Shao Yang	11 pm–1 am
	3 pairings }			
Liver	*medial*	yin Wood	zu Jue Yin	1–3 am
	3 pairings }			

膽 經 Dǎn Jīng = Gall Bladder Channel

- **Division:** (Leg) **Shao Yang**
- **Phase/Element:** (Yang) **Wood**
- **High Tide: 11 pm – 1 am**

begins: **on the temple just lateral to the eye** (outer canthus)
ends: **on the lateral side the 4th toe**

❖ *The Gall Bladder Channel external pathway:*

· begins lateral to and level with the outer canthus of the eye	(inferior to TB-23)	**(GB-1)**
· runs across the side of the face toward the lower part of the ear	(level with the infra-tragic notch) (inferior to SI-19)	(GB-2)
· up the side of the face into the temporal hair	(inferior to ST-8)	(GB-3-4)
· then down again toward the upper attachment of the ear		(GB-5-7)
· arcs posteriorly above and behind the ear to the mastoid process		(GB-8-12)
· then arcs anteriorly (higher on the side of the head) all the way to the forehead		(GB-13-14)
· then arcs back again, now on top of the head (slightly lateral to the BL channel)		(GB-15-18)
· descends the back of the head to the occiput (big hollow between the traps & SCM)		(GB-19-20)
· follows the trapezius to the top of the shoulder (midway between the spine and acromion)		(GB-21)
· from the shoulder, it goes internally, and connects to its paired organs		(Lr & GB)
· then reemerges on the side of the torso, just below the axilla (4th/5th ICS)		(GB-22-23)
· flows anteriorly to the chest (7th ICS)		(GB-24)
· posteriorly to the low back (tip of the 12th rib)		(GB-25)
· anteriorly to the abdomen (just medial to the ASIS)		(GB-26–28)
· posteriorly through the TFL to the gluteal hollow		(GB-29–30)
· then follows the ilio-tibial tract to the knee (lateral side)		(GB-31-33)
· from the knee it follows the fibula & peroneal muscles to the ankle		(GB-34-39)
· flowing just anterior to the lateral malleolus into the sinus tarsii		(GB-40)
· across the dorsum of the foot, between the 4th & 5th metatarsals		(GB-41-43)
· ending at the lateral nail point on the 4th toe		**(GB-44)**

膽 經 **Gall Bladder Channel** (44 pts)

Face
GB-1   • level with & lateral to the outer canthus of the eye (lateral edge of the zygomatic, frontal extension)
GB-2   • anterior to the ear, level with the bottom of the infra-tragic notch, on the anterior ear-line
GB-3   • above the zygomatic arch, directly superior to the mandibular notch   (above ST-7)

Side of Head   *GB pts are within the temporal hairline, on a line connecting ST-8 and GB-7*
GB-4   • **1/4** of the distance from ST-8 to GB-7   midway between ST-8 and GB-5
GB-5   • **1/2** of the distance from ST-8 to GB-7   **midway between ST-8 & GB-7**
GB-6   • **3/4** of the distance from ST-8 to GB-7   midway between GB-5 and GB-7
GB-7   • on the pre-auricular vertical line, level with the **apex** of the ear (~ 1 cun anterior to TB-20)

Above Ear
GB-8   • **1–1.5 cun superior** to the apex of the ear   (~ 1/2 the height of the ear)   (above TB-20)
GB-9   • **0.5 cun posterior** to GB-8

Behind Ear   *GB pts of the post-auricular scalp lie along a (slightly curving) line connecting GB-9 & 12*
GB-10   • **1/3** of the arc distance from GB-9 to GB-12
GB-11   • **2/3** of the arc distance from GB-9 to GB-12
GB-12   • immediately inferior to the tip of the **mastoid** process, in the SCM

Forehead   ➤ *The distance between the midline (GV-24) and ST-8 is 4.5 cun, which divides into halves & thirds*
    the height of the forehead from the eyebrow to the hairline is 3 cun
GB-13   • 0.5 cun within the anterior hairline,   **1/3 the distance** from ST-8 to GV-24   (1.5 cun)
       or   3 cun lateral to the midline (GV-24)
    Locating Tip: extend a line up from the outer canthus (not the orbit/TB-23, that line leads you to ST-8)
GB-14   • on the forehead, **1 cun superior to the eyebrow**
    Locating Tip: extend a line up from the pupil and 1/3 of the distance from eyebrow to hairline
GB-15   • 0.5 cun within the anterior hairline,   **1/2 the distance** between ST-8 and GV-24   (2.25 cun)
    Locating Tip: extend a line up from the pupil & GB-14

Top of Head   ➤ *GB pts on the head lie along a line 2.25 cun lateral to the mid-sagittal line (GV)*
    along the line connecting the pupil and GB-20
GB-16   • **2 cun** posterior to the anterior hairline,   (1.5 cun behind GB-15)   (level w/ GV-22)
GB-17   • **3.5 cun** posterior to the anterior hairline,   (1.5 cun behind GB-16)   (level w/ GV-21)
GB-18   • **5 cun** posterior to the anterior hairline,   (1.5 cun behind GB-17)   (level w/ GV-20)
Alt Loc: In 2008 W.H.O. adopted the following: GB-16 is **1.5**, 17 is **2.5**, & 18 is **4.0** cun posterior to the anterior hairline.
    That makes these 3 points level with: ☐   BL-6   BL-7

Back of the Head   *still 2.25 cun lateral to the midline (GV)*
GB-19   • in the large depression level with the EOP, and superior to GB-20   (level w/ GV-17)

Neck/Occiput
GB-20   • immediately inferior to the occiput, in the large depression between the SCM
    and the trapezius muscles.   (level w/ GV-16)

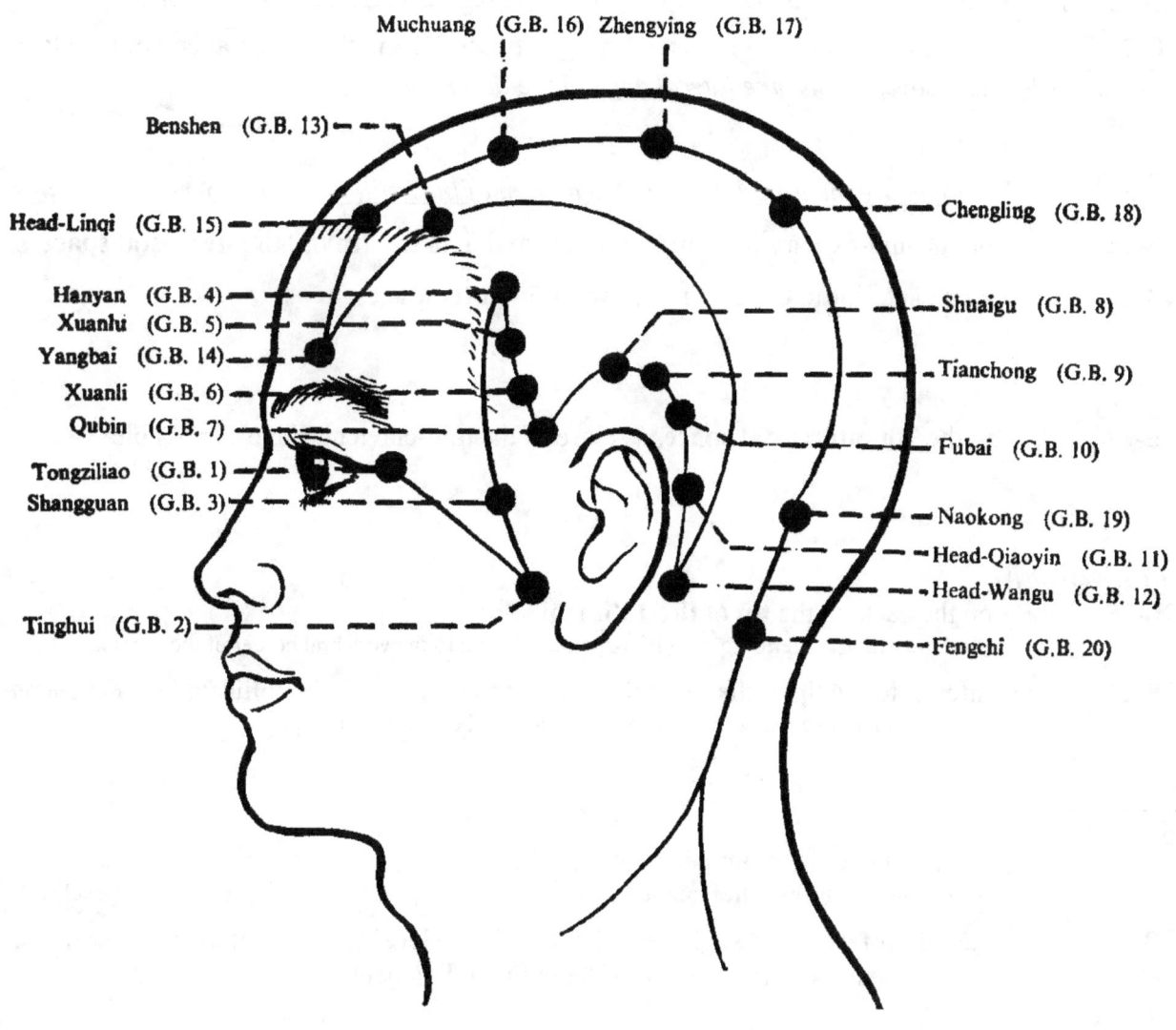

Muchuang (G.B. 16) Zhengying (G.B. 17)

Benshen (G.B. 13)

Head-Linqi (G.B. 15)

Chengling (G.B. 18)

Hanyan (G.B. 4)
Xuanlu (G.B. 5)
Yangbai (G.B. 14)
Xuanli (G.B. 6)
Qubin (G.B. 7)

Shuaigu (G.B. 8)

Tianchong (G.B. 9)

Fubai (G.B. 10)

Tongziliao (G.B. 1)
Shangguan (G.B. 3)

Naokong (G.B. 19)
Head-Qiaoyin (G.B. 11)
Head-Wangu (G.B. 12)

Tinghui (G.B. 2)

Fengchi (G.B. 20)

足少陽膽經
Zu Shao-Yang Dan Jing
Leg Lesser-Yang Gall Bladder Channel

GB points 1–20 are shown
(Nearly half of the GB channel points are on the head)

* Draw in the landmark points ST-8, TB-20, & GV-20. Notice that GB-16, 17, & 18 are all too posterior.
Use a straight-edge to draw a line from the center of the ear lobe to the apex, then extend it to the top of the head.
That line should connect TB-20, GB-8, GB-18 and GV-20.
In the drawing GB-18 should be approx. where they show GB-17.

| Shoulder | ➤ *There are 8 cun between the posterior midline (C7) and the acromio-clavicular prominence* |

GB-21   • on the crest of the trapezius, midway between C$_7$ and the acromial end of the clavicle

variation }   *as above, but use the lateral edge of the acromion*

| Axilla | ➤ *12 cun are measured between the bottom of the axilla to the bottom of the ribcage* |

GB-22   • on the mid-axillary line, inferior to the axilla, in the **4th** or 5th **intercostal space**

GB-23   • 1 cun anterior to GB-22, in the **4th** or 5th **interspace**

| Chest |
GB-24   • in the **7th intercostal space**, as close to the mid-clavicular line as possible   (~ CV-12)

| Back & Waist |
GB-25   • on the back, at the **tip of the 12th rib**
      (find the 12th rib inferior to the 11th & slightly lateral to the vertebral border of the scapula)

GB-26   • inferior to the tip of the 11th rib/Lr-13, at the level of the umbilical plane (~ 1 cun inferior)
      (roughly at the junction of the mid-axillary line and the umbilical plane)

| Abdomen |
GB-27   • just medial to the prominence of the ASIS
      ~ 3 cun below the umbilical plane   (level with CV-4)

GB-28   • **0.5 cun inferior** and slightly medial to GB-27, level with the inferior border of the ASIS
      on the medio-superior border of the inguinal ligament

| Hip & Buttocks | *These two GB pts are best located in the lateral recumbent position* |

GB-29   • in the tensor fascia lata muscle, midway between the ASIS and the greater trochanter*

GB-30   • in the gluteal hollow, **1/3** of the distance between the gr trochanter and the sacral hiatus*

    Tip: * to locate the trochanter – esp. if partner is lying in prone or supine position.
           Place your open hand on the lateral hip region and have partner rotate their leg,
           (wag the foot back & forth), you can easily feel the trochanter moving under your hand.

    Tip: * to find the sacral hiatus (which can extend from the 3rd to below the 4th foramen)
           simply use the top of the natal cleft (~ sacro-coccygeal joint)

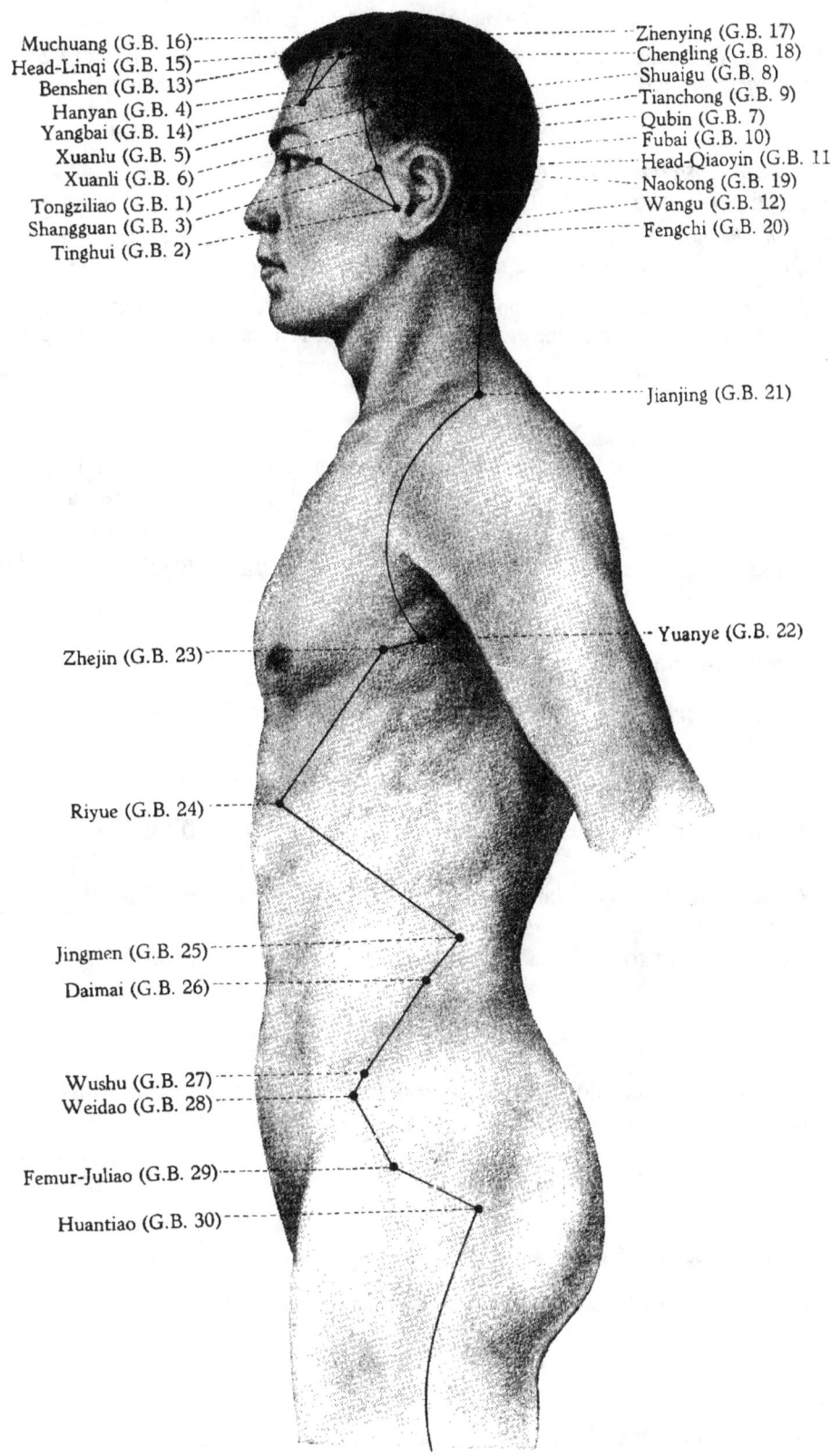

Muchuang (G.B. 16)
Head-Linqi (G.B. 15)
Benshen (G.B. 13)
Hanyan (G.B. 4)
Yangbai (G.B. 14)
Xuanlu (G.B. 5)
Xuanli (G.B. 6)
Tongziliao (G.B. 1)
Shangguan (G.B. 3)
Tinghui (G.B. 2)

Zhenying (G.B. 17)
Chengling (G.B. 18)
Shuaigu (G.B. 8)
Tianchong (G.B. 9)
Qubin (G.B. 7)
Fubai (G.B. 10)
Head-Qiaoyin (G.B. 11)
Naokong (G.B. 19)
Wangu (G.B. 12)
Fengchi (G.B. 20)

Jianjing (G.B. 21)

Yuanye (G.B. 22)

Zhejin (G.B. 23)

Riyue (G.B. 24)

Jingmen (G.B. 25)

Daimai (G.B. 26)

Wushu (G.B. 27)

Weidao (G.B. 28)

Femur-Juliao (G.B. 29)

Huantiao (G.B. 30)

足 少 陽 膽 經
Zu Shao-Yang Dan Jing
Leg Lesser-Yang Gall Bladder Channel

On the thigh, the GB channel follows the ilio-tibial tract, usually along its anterior edge
> *19 cun are measured from the superior border of the greater trochanter to the popliteal crease*
(lateral projection of trochanter is ~1 cun inferior, thus, the midpoint of thigh is 9 cun; 1/3 = 6 cun)

Thigh

GB-31   · **7 cun** above the popliteal crease, in the vastus lateralis along the **anterior edge** of the ITT
    variation }   *along the **posterior edge** of the ITT*
GB-32   · **5 cun** above the popliteal crease, in the vastus lateralis along the **anterior edge** of the ITT
    variation }   *along the **posterior edge** of the ITT, between it and the biceps femoris*
    * *(given 1/3 = 6 cun, GB-31 & 32 are 1 cun above & below the mark 1/3 up from the knee)*

    * 2008 WHO has moved these 2 upward: GB-32 is now 7.0, GB-31 is where the middle finger rests
    They have also decided on the **posterior** border of the IT band, and show 31 being 3 cun above 32.

Knee
GB-33   *lateral aspect of the thigh/knee*
   when the knee is bent 90°: in the large depression between the biceps femoris tendon and the ITT
       (proximal to the lateral epicondyle of the femur)

Leg
> *There are 16 cun between the popliteal crease and the protuberance of the lateral malleolus*
GB-34   · anterior and inferior to the head of the fibula (on the anterior edge of the peroneus/fibularis longus)

GB-35   · **7 cun superior** to the lateral malleolus, **posterior to the fibula** (level w/ ST-39 & BL-58)

GB-36   · **7 cun superior** to the lateral malleolus, anterior to the fibula (just under midway)

GB-37   · **5 cun superior** to the lateral malleolus, anterior to the fibula

GB-38   · **4 cun superior** to the lateral malleolus, anterior to the fibula (1/4 of the distance)

GB-39   · **3 cun superior** to the lateral malleolus, **posterior to the fibula**
    (between the fibula & the peroneal/fibularis tendons) (level w/ BL-59)
    alt. loc. } · 3 cun superior to the lateral malleolus, *anterior* to the fibula

Ankle
GB-40   · in the large depression anterior and inferior to the lateral malleolus (the sinus tarsii)
    (lateral to the extensor digitorum tendon)

Foot
GB-41   · between the 4th and 5th metatarsals, distal to their bases, but proximal to the extensor tendon to the little toe

GB-42   · between the 4th and 5th metatarsals, proximal to their heads, but distal to the extensor tendon

Toes
GB-43   · between the 4th and 5th toes, proximal to the web margin, distal to the MP joint

GB-44   · the lateral nail point on the 4th toe

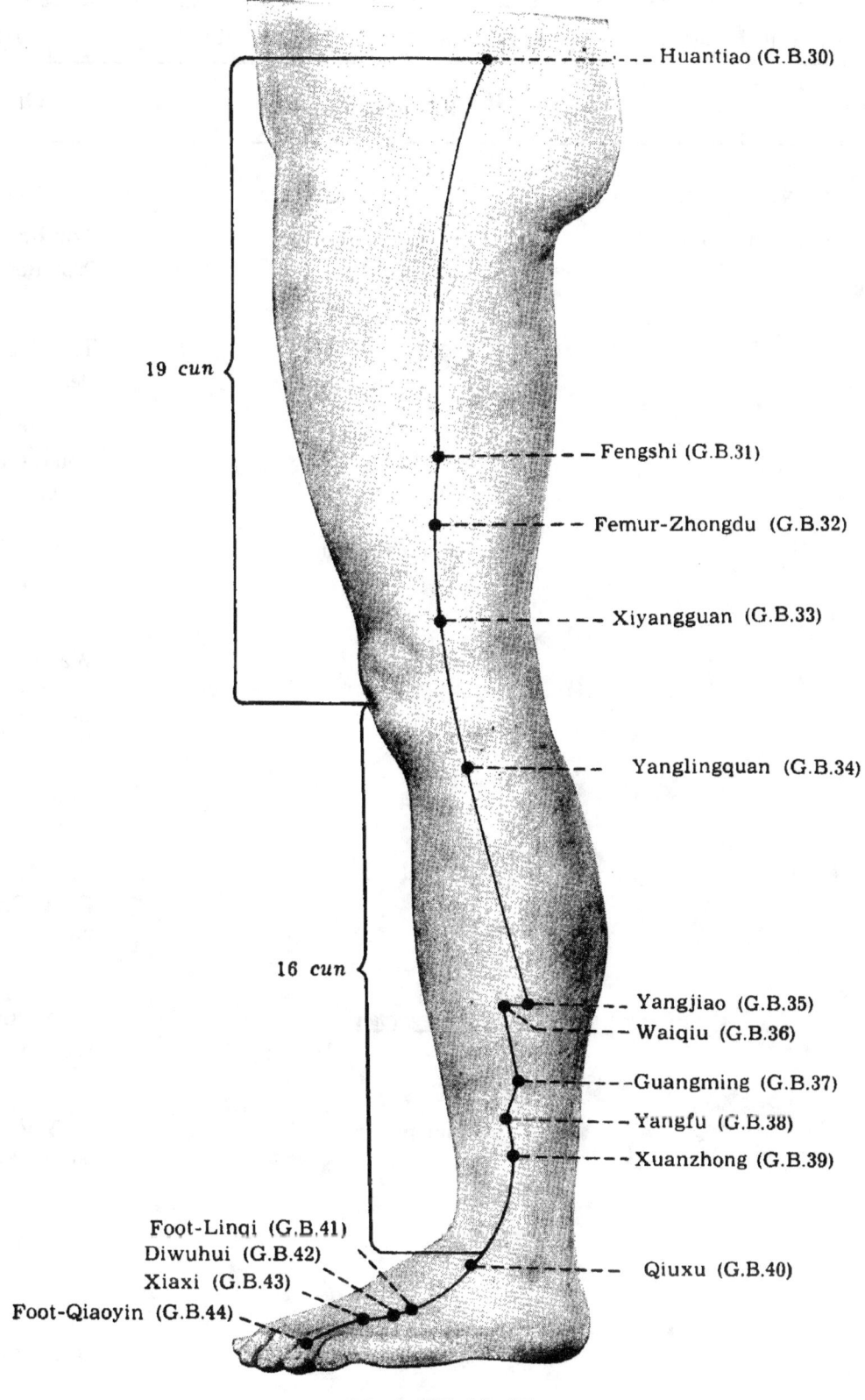

- - - - Huantiao (G.B.30)

19 *cun*

- - - Fengshi (G.B.31)

- - - Femur-Zhongdu (G.B.32)

- - - Xiyangguan (G.B.33)

- - - Yanglingquan (G.B.34)

16 *cun*

- - Yangjiao (G.B.35)
- - Waiqiu (G.B.36)

- - Guangming (G.B.37)

- - - Yangfu (G.B.38)

- - - Xuanzhong (G.B.39)

Foot-Linqi (G.B.41)
Diwuhui (G.B.42)
Xiaxi (G.B.43)
Foot-Qiaoyin (G.B.44)

- - Qiuxu (G.B.40)

足少陽膽經
Zu Shao-Yang Dan Jing
Leg Lesser-Yang Gall Bladder Channel

© 1990–2016   *Jim Cleaver LAc.*

Gall Bladder Channel = Zú **Shǎo-Yáng** Dǎn Jīng		**Wood**	**11 pm–1 am**
paired channels }	TB	Lr	Ht

Mu pt = GB-24	**Shu pt** = BL-19	**Xia-he pt** = GB-34

	• Main Categories _{on every channel}	• Misc. Categories	Pt Name & Translation
GB-1	• entry pt: *from TB-23*		Tóng-zǐ Liáo 瞳子髎 Pupil Bone-hole
GB-2			Tīng Huì 聽會 Hearing Convergence
GB-8			Shuài Gǔ 率谷 Commander of the Valley
GB-9		• alt. Celestial Window	Tiān Chōng 天衝 Celestial Thoroughfare
GB-12			Wán Gǔ 完骨 Complete/Finished/Perfect Bone Ending Bone / End of the Bone Terminus of Bone (mastoid)
GB-14			Yáng Bái 陽白 Yang Clear/White
GB-20			**Fēng Chí** 風池 Wind Pond
GB-21		• *Cx: pregnancy*	**Jiān Jǐng** 肩井 Shoulder Well
GB-24		• GB mu pt	**Rì Yuè** 日月 Sun & Moon
GB-25		• Kidney mu pt	**Jīng Mén** 京門 Capitol Gate
GB-26		• Dai mai: 1st pt	**Dài Mài** 帶脈 Belt Vessel
GB-30		• 9N (to Rescue Yang)	**Huán Tiào** 環跳 Jump/Leap Circle/Ring

	• Main Categories	• Misc. Categories	Pt Name & Translation
GB-31			**Fēng Shì** 風市 Wind Marketplace
GB-34	• he/sea–earth	• **Influential pt**: sinews • **lower uniting pt: GB**	**Yáng Líng Quán** 陽陵泉 Yang Mound Spring
GB-35		• Yang Wei: xi/cleft	Yáng Jiāo 陽交 Yang Junction
GB-36	• GB **xi/cleft**		Wài Qiū 外丘 Outer Hill
GB-37	• **luo/connecting**		**Guāng Míng** 光明 Bright & Clear Bright Light
GB-38	• jing/river–fire–Disp. pt.		Yáng Fǔ 陽輔 Yang Assistant Yang Stabilizing Bar
GB-39		• **Group Luo**: (3 leg yang) • **Influential pt**: marrow	**Xuán Zhōng** 懸鐘 Hanging Bell aka **Jué Gǔ** 絕骨 Disappearing/Vanishing Bone
GB-40	• **yuan/source**		Qiū Xū 丘墟 Hill Burial Grounds/Ruins (Cemetary Hill)
GB-41	• shu/stream–wood–Phase pt. • **exit pt**: *to Lr-1*	• **Master pt**: Dai mai	**Zú Lín Qì** 足臨泣 (Ft) Oversee Tears (Eyes) (see GB-15)
(GB-42)	• *exception to transport pt rule*		Dì Wǔ Huì 地五會 Earth Five Meet
GB-43	• ying/brook–water–Tonif. pt.		Xiá Xī 俠谿 Guard the Stream(bed) Narrow Ravine
GB-44	• jing/well–metal–Control pt.		Zú Qiào Yīn 足竅陰 (Ft) Yin Orifices/Portals (see GB-11)

肝 經 Gān Jīng = Liver Channel

- **Division:** (Leg) **Jue Yin**
- **Phase/Element:** (Yin) **Wood**
- **High Tide: 1–3 am**

---

begins: **on the big toe, lateral side**

ends: **in the 6th ICS, mid-clavicular line**

❖ *The Liver Channel external pathway:*

· begins at the lateral nail point on the big toe   **(Lr-1)**

· proceeds along the inside of the big toe, to the space between the 1st & 2nd toes   (Lr-2)

· continues proximally between the 1st & 2nd metatarsals   (Lr-3)

· and across the dorsum of the foot to the ankle   (Lr-4)
  stays anterior to the medial malleolus (alongside the tibialis anterior tendon)

· follows the shaft of the tibia on the lower leg   (Lr-5–6)

· around mid leg it crosses behind the Spleen channel, i.e. posterior to the tibia,
    and proceeds upward to the medial aspect of the knee   (Lr-7–8)

· ascends the medial thigh following the adductor longus   (between Sp & Kd channels)

· passing through the femoral triangle to the groin   (Lr-10–12)

· it rises obliquely across the abdomen to the side, tip of the 11th rib (~ mid-axillary line)   (Lr-13)

· then anterior & up to end in the 6th ICS, on the mid-clavicular line   **(Lr-14)**

肝經 **Liver Channel**   (14 pts)

Toe
Lr-1   • The lateral nail point on the big toe
    alt loc. 1   *midway between the lateral nail pt and the knuckle*
    alt loc. 2   *at the base of the nail, midway between the med. & lat. nail pts*
    alt loc. 3   *midway between the base of the nail and the knuckle* (hairy area of the toe)

Foot
Lr-2   • between the 1st & 2nd toes (midway between the web margin and the prominence of the knuckle)
Lr-3   • between the 1st & 2nd metatarsals, ~ midway between their heads & bases

Ankle
Lr-4   • medial to the tibialis anterior tendon, level with the prominence of the medial malleolus
old description } • between the tibialis anterior and the extensor hallucis longus tendons, i.e. lateral to the tibialis tendon

Leg
Lr-5   • **5 cun proximal** to the medial malleolus,
        in a small vertical groove in the middle of the shaft of the tibia

Lr-6   • **7 cun proximal** to the medial malleolus,
        in a small depression in the middle of the shaft of the tibia

Knee
Lr-7   • **1 cun posterior** to Sp-9, in the medial head of the gastrocnemius

Lr-8   • the medial aspect of the knee, at the end of the crease formed when the leg is fully flexed,
    (between the tendons of the sartorius/gracilis and semimembranosus)   (anterior to Kd-10)

    alt loc. }   • in the center of the big depression superior to the medial condyle of the femur
    (posterior to the shaft of the femur and anterior to the sartorius)

Thigh
Lr-9   • **4 cun proximal** to the medial epicondyle of the femur
        in the depression between the vastus medialis and the anterior edge of the sartorius

Lr-10   • in the femoral triangle, **3 cun distal** to the pubic tubercle (ST-30)
        on the anterior edge of the adductor longus

Lr-11   • in the femoral triangle, **2 cun distal** to the pubic tubercle (ST-30)
        on the anterior edge of the adductor longus

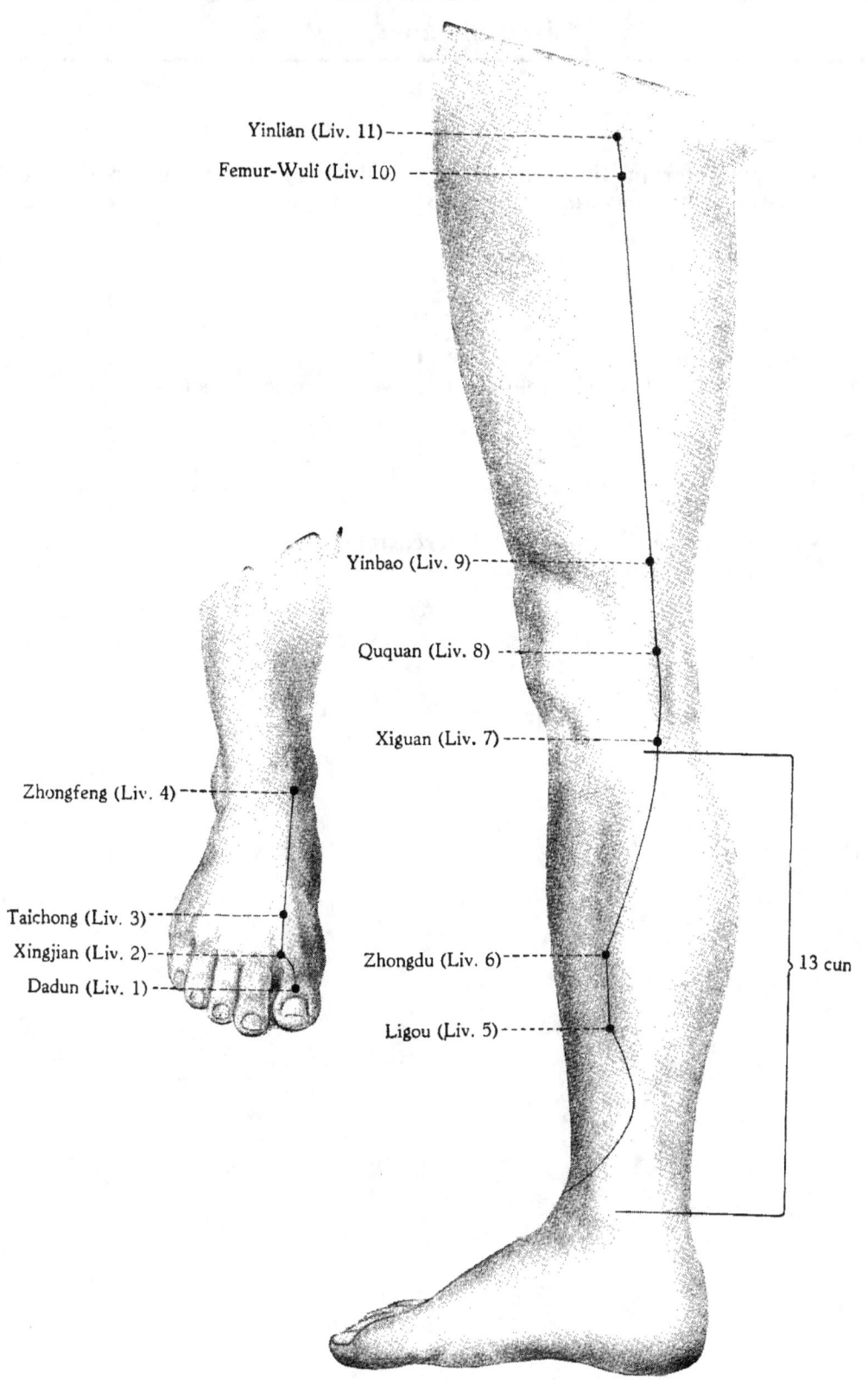

Yinlian (Liv. 11)

Femur-Wuli (Liv. 10)

Yinbao (Liv. 9)

Ququan (Liv. 8)

Xiguan (Liv. 7)

Zhongfeng (Liv. 4)

Taichong (Liv. 3)

Xingjian (Liv. 2)

Dadun (Liv. 1)

Zhongdu (Liv. 6)

Ligou (Liv. 5)

13 cun

足厥陰肝經

Zu Jue-Yin Gan Jing

Leg Faint-Yin Liver Channel

Liver Channel   *(torso)*

Groin
Lr-12   • **2.5 cun lateral** to the midline, just lateral & inferior to the pubic tubercle (ST-30)
             (at the top of the femoral triangle, inferior to the inguinal ligament and medial to the femoral artery)

Side
Lr-13   • at or just inferior to the **tip of the 11th rib**
             (~ the mid-axillary line, usually slightly above the umbilical plane)

Chest
Lr-14   • mid clavicular line, in the **6th intercostal space**   (1 rib space below ST-18)
             (~ level w/ the tip of the xiphoid process or CV-14)

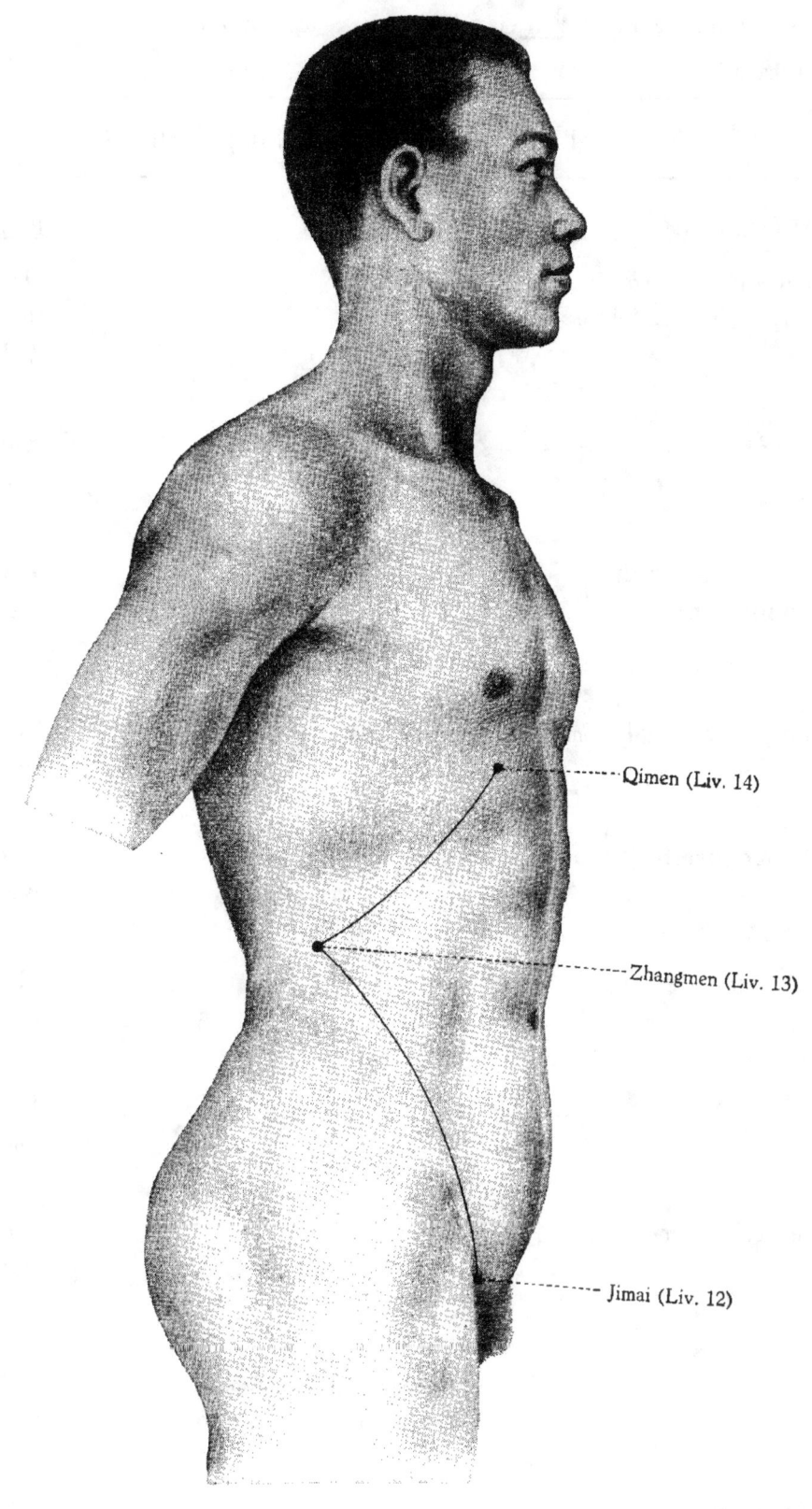

Qimen (Liv. 14)

Zhangmen (Liv. 13)

Jimai (Liv. 12)

足厥陰肝經
Zu Jue-Yin Gan Jing
Leg Faint-Yin Liver Channel

© 1990–2016   Jim Cleaver LAc.

Liver Channel = Zú **Jué-Yīn** Gān Jīng	**Wood**	**1–3 am**
paired channels } Pc	GB	SI

Mu pt = Lr-14	**Shu pt** = BL-18

	• Main Categories _{on every channel}	• Misc. Categories	Pt Name & Translation
Lr-1	• entry pt: *from GB-41* • jing/well–wood–Phase pt.		Dà Dūn 大敦 Big & Important/Esteemed 墩 Block/Post/Stump/Piling
Lr-2	• ying/brook–fire–Disp. pt.		**Xíng Jiān** 行間 Step Between
Lr-3	• shu/stream–earth • **yuan/source**		**Tài Chōng** 太衝 Great Thoroughfare Great Surge
Lr-4	• jing/river–metal–Control pt.		Zhōng Fēng 中封 Sealed in the Middle
Lr-5	• **luo/connecting**		**Lǐ Gōu** 蠡溝 Worm-eaten Groove
Lr-6	• **xi/cleft**		Zhōng Dū 中都 Central City / City Center
Lr-7			Xī Guān 膝關 Knee Gateway
Lr-8	• he/sea–water–Tonif. pt.		Qū Quán 曲泉 Spring at the Bend
Lr-13		• **Influential pt**: zang organs • **Spleen mu**	**Zhāng Mén** 章門 Section Gate
Lr-14	• Liver mu • exit pt: *to Lu-1* (last pt on the 12 regular channels #309)		**Qī Mén** 期門 Gate at Cycle's End Hope Gate / Gate of Hope

奇經八脈   *Qí Jīng Bā Mài = Odd/Unusual/Irregular Channels, 8 Vessels*

Extraordinary Vessels

- *8 Vessels (112 pts)*

- *2 Midline (CV/GV) with their own points (52 pts)*

- *6 other Vessels that share regular channel points (60 pts)*

In the Classics: Su Wen: 17, 21, 41, 44 & 62   Ling Shu: 2, 10, 11, 17, 21, 33, 38, 62, 65   Nan Jing: 27-29 & 37

1. 1295   Zhen Jiu **Zhi Nan** (Acu-Moxa Compass)   author ? early reference
2. 1311   Zhen Jiu **Si Shu** (Acu-Moxa 4 Books)   Dou Jie includes #1 above
3. 1439   Zhen Jiu **Da Quan** (Acu-Moxa Complete)   Xu Feng first correlates trigrams & master points
4. 1529   Zhen Jiu **Ju Ying** (Acu-Moxa Gems)   Gao Wu
5. 1578   Qi Jing **Ba Mai Kao** (Odd Channels, 8 Vessels Investigation) Li Shi Zhen*
6. 1601   Zhen Jiu **Da Cheng** (Great Compendium)   Yang Jizhou

To learn more about Extraordinary Vessels, explore the following books:

1. 1986   Extraordinary Vessels   Matsumoto   history & application
2. 1995   Chasing the Dragons Tail   Manaka   theory & treatment
3. 1996   Meridian Style Acupuncture   Pirog   p. 155–215
4. 1996   Navigating the Channels   Ni   p. 104–134
5. 1997   Eight Extraordinary Meridians   Larre & Rochat   focus on characters & classics
6. 1998   Manual of Acupuncture   Deadman   p. 17–25 (basic description & figures)
7. 2001   Channel Divergences   Shima   uses EV treatments throughout text
8. 2005   Foundations of Chinese M (2nd ed.)   Maciocia   chapters 52 & 53 p. 819–887
9. 2006   The Channels of Acupuncture   Maciocia   Part 7: chapters 24–36 p. 371–648
10. 2008   Applied Channel Theory in CM   Wang/Robertson Chapter 11 p. 273–324
11. 2010   An Exposition on the Eight Extraordinary Vessels   Chace/Shima

---

Recap of the Complete Channel System – Jīng-Luò *or* Jīng-Mài

經 絡 jīng-luò = channels & collaterals   (the main channels (jing) and their network (luo) of vessels/tributaries

經 脈 jīng-mài = channels & vessels   (the main channels (jing) and the extraordinary vessels (mai))

• **Primary/Regular/Ordinary Channels**   (正經 zhèng jīng)   [12]
    a. external pathways: (like rivers)   follow relatively superficial course between muscles & bones
    b. internal pathway: (like ocean currents)   connect to various organs and tissues internally
    • 'homes' to its pertaining organ   circulates qi directly to & from the organ
    • 'nets' i.e. wraps around its yin/yang phase paired organ, connecting them internally

• **Connecting/Network Vessels**   (絡脈 luò mài)   (CV, GV + Great Luo of Sp & ST)   [16]
    Basically there is one luo channel associated with each primary channel,
      but specifically there are several subcategories of luo vessels as follows.

    a. <u>connecting luo</u>: (transverse luo)   A short connecting branch from the luo pt of one channel to the yuan pt on
        the paired channel. Connect the yin/yang (phase paired) channels externally.

    b. <u>reservoir luo</u>: (longitudinal luo)   Run parallel to primary channel pathway.
        Function as reservoirs; storing surplus qi when channel is full, and supply it when channel is low/empty.
        Manifest specific symptoms when xu or shi (see texts for details, from Ling Shu 10)

    c. <u>blood luo</u>: (vascular system)
        1. <u>minute luo</u>:   • the network that delivers qi & blood to every cell in the body (capillary bed)
        2. <u>superficial luo</u>:   • visible veins
        3. <u>blood luo</u>:   • vascular abnormalities (varicosities etc)

• **Channel Divergences**   (經別 jīng bié)   [12]
    * again one is associated with each primary channel
    • they diverge from their primary channel on the upper aspect of the limbs
        (proximal to the knee or elbow) and then proceed internally.
    • they link various tissues and organs and explain how the pertaining organ is related to
        areas its channel does not otherwise seem to traverse.
    • yin divergences connect to their yang counterparts internally, and together rejoin the
        primary yang channel in the vicinity of the neck/throat. (called Reunion Areas/Points)
    • their prime function is to conduct yin energy into the head.

• **Channel Sinews or Muscle-Tendon Channels**   (經筋 jīng jīn)   [12]
    • individual & groups of muscles – connect from joint to joint (結 jié = tie or bind, knot/node)
    • account for both structure and function (anatomy & kinesiology)
    • problems = motor dysfunction, incl stiffness &/or pain (any abnormal sensations or movements)
    • join primary channel at the nail points

• **Cutaneous Regions or Skin Zones**   (皮部 pí bù)   [12]
    • essentially the 6 divisions (analogous to valleys in which the main channel/river flows)
    • anatomically includes the skin and superficial fascia, subcutaneous regions, sweat glands & pores
    • wei qi circulates here   (腠 理 còu lǐ = interstices (sweat glands & pores))

• Curious, Strange, Unusual, **Extraordinary Vessels** (奇 經 八 脈 qí jīng bā mài)   [8]
    • mài = veins (veins & arteries) = vessels (in contrast to jing/channels/rivers), smt. referred to as the 8 lakes

Extraordinary Vessel Characters – Meaning and Translation

任   **Rèn**   = to appoint, employ, esp. in an official position   (Directing) Maciocia
                                                                    (Controlling) Wiseman

壬   Rén   = to carry a load, to bear a burden; 9th stem   工 gōng= work, labor, toil
                  9th stem = yang water = BL (uterus); clock with Lu, Lu-7 is master pt

妊   Rèn   = the load/burden women bear = to be with child, pregnant   (Conception)

督   **Dū**   top L = beans   top R = hand   below = an eye

             = to oversee the picking of the beans = to supervise, superintend   **(Governing)**
             top shū = uncle; a governor (originally one who is related to the ruler);
             to control, watch over, rule;   also to stimulate, to correct

帶   **Dài**   = a belt, ribbon, sash; to girdle   **(Belt)**
               also a zone, region; to wear, or carry; to lead, or bring

沖   **Chōng**   *water radical*   + 中 *zhōng phonetic = central, middle*
                   = to water, rinse, flush; pour boiling water over, make tea   (Penetrating)
                   to clash, collide, rush, dash, charge;   (Thrusting)
      chòng   vigorous, strong, powerful, forceful dynamic   (aterial pulsations)   **(Surging/Pulsing)**
                                       (abd. aorta)   (Vitality Vessel)

衝   chòng   *movement radical* + 重 *zhòng phonetic = heavy, weighty, important, serious*
                    or   + 重 *chóng phonetic = repeatedly, again & again, reiterate*

衝   Chōng   = an open road; public road; highway   **(Thoroughfare)**
             (orig. a stretch of flatland through a hilly region, allowing easy passage)
             [see point names for: ST-30, Sp-12 / ST-42, Lr-3 / Pc-9, Ht-9]
             ST-30 is on the Chòng mài, Sp-12 is on its paired vessel Yin-Wei mài according to some sources;
             the pulse at ST-42 & Lr-3 was traditionally used to assess the Chòng mài.

維   **Wéi**   = to tie down, to fasten, connect, join;   **(Link/Linking)**
               to maintain, safeguard, preserve
                 (wei = tie down, root, ground, connect, link together)

蹺   **Qiāo**   = to raise up, lift; stand on tiptoe   **(Heel)**
              (qiao = lift, raise mobilize, energize)   **(Motility)**
                                                      (Springing) Wiseman
                                                      (Stepping) Maciocia

Vessel	Chong	Yin Wei	Ren	Yin Qiao	Du	Yang Qiao	Dai	Yang Wei
	沖	維	任	蹻	督	蹻	帶	維
transl.	Penetrating, Thoroughfare, Pulsing, Surging	Yin Linking	Conception, Controlling	Yin Heel or Motility	Governing	Yang Heel or Motility	Belt or Girdling	Yang Linking
trigram	Qián	Gèn	Lí	Kūn	Duì	Kǎn	Xùn	Zhèn
trigram	☰	☶	☲	☷	☱	☵	☴	☳
direction	NW	NE	S	SW	W	N	SE	E
relation	father	mother	host	guest	husband	wife	male daughter	female son
luo pt	ø	ø	**CV-15**	ø	**GV-1**	ø	ø	ø
xi pt	ø	**Kd-9**	ø	**Kd-8**	ø	**BL-59**	ø	**GB-35**
master opening pt	**Sp-4**	**Pc-6**	**Lu-7**	**Kd-6**	**SI-3**	**BL-62**	**GB-41**	**TB-5**
# of pts	14 pts	7 pts	24 pts	6 pts	28 pts	13 pts	4 pts	16 pts
pathway begins	kidney / lower jiao	medial leg	kidney / lower jiao	medial heel/ankle	kidney / lower jiao	lateral heel/ankle	ming-men (GV-4)	lateral leg/foot
	CV-1	Kd-9	CV-1	Kd-2	(CV-1)	BL-62	Lr-13	BL-63
	ST-30	(Sp-12)		Kd-6	GV-1	BL-61	GB-26	GB-35
	Kd-11	Sp-13		Kd-8		BL-59	GB-27	GB-29
	Kd-12	Sp-15		ST-12		GB-29	GB-28	SI-10
	Kd-13	Sp-16		ST-9		SI-10	(CV-4) (CV-8)	TB-13
	Kd-14	Lr-14		BL-1		LI-15		LI-14
	Kd-15	CV-22				LI-16		TB-15
	CV-7	CV-23				ST-9		GB-21
	Kd-16					ST-4		GB-20
	Kd-17					ST-3		GB-19
	Kd-18					ST-1		GB-18
	Kd-19				GV-12	BL-1		GB-17
	Kd-20				(BL-12)	thru brain to		GB-16
	Kd-21				GV-13	GB-20		GB-15
	chest							GB-14
	throat							GB-13
	lips		CV-24					(ST-8)
	eyes		(GV-28)					to ear
	(ST-1)		(ST-1)		GV-28			(GV-15) (GV-16)

* In this table I basically follow Li Shi Zhen   (Ch+YnW=21, R+YnQ=30   **Yin = 51 pts**)   (Du+YgQ=41, D+YgW=20   **Yang = 61 pts**)   **Total = 112 pts**

EV – Anatomical and Functional Pairings

- Deeper than the regular channels, they circulate ancestral qi & represent the energetic template around which the physical body organizes: coronal = front/back, sagittal = left/right, umbilical = upper/lower, core = inside/outside (yin/yang)

- 4 are associated with yin, 4 with yang   • 4 on torso, 4 on limbs

- 2 therapeutic pairings result: A. Structural (yin/yang) pairs   B. Functional (same polarity) pairs

I. Structural Pairs   (One Yin – One Yang)   <u>Region</u> (divides into)

A. Core pairs: on Torso   *all 4 begin in lower jiao, but master pts are 2 hand & 2 feet*

Ren mai   = Conception or Controlling vessel (CV)   front   (left/right)
(Jen mo)   controls the yin (storage, nourishment, moistening, cooling, rejuvenation)
    &

Du mai   = Governing vessel (GV)   back   (left/right)
(Tu mo)   controls the yang (function, transformation, warming, drying, activation)

- -

Chong mai   = Penetrating or Thoroughfare vessel   vert. middle (interior/exterior)
(Ch'ong mo)   controls the central core (vertical) axis   (circulation betw core & periphery)
    &

Dai mai   = Belt or Girdling vessel   trans. middle (upper/lower)
(Tai mo)   controls the central (transverse) axis   (circulation betw upper & lower body)

B. Peripheral pairs: *on Limbs*   *all 4 begin on lower limbs, but master pts are 2 arm & 2 leg*

Yin Wei mai   = Yin Linking vessel   medial (anterior/posterior)
       controls the downward movement of Yin
    &

Yang Wei mai   = Yang Linking vessel   lateral (anterior/posterior)
       controls the downward movement of Yang

- -

Yin Qiao mai   = Yin Heel or Motility vessel   medial (anterior/posterior)
(Yin Ch'iao mo)   controls the upward movement of Yin
    &

Yang Qiao mai   = Yang Heel or Motility vessel   lateral (anterior/posterior)
(Yang Ch'iao mo)   controls the upward movement of Yang

II. Functional Pairs (are same Polarity, like Division pairs)

A. **Core/Torso**		B. **Peripheral/Limbs**
Ren	&	Yin Qiao
Du	&	Yang Qiao
Chong	&	Yin Wei
Dai	&	Yang Wei

- **Master Points** (aka Confluent or Coalescent Pts)

Ren	= Lu-7	Yin Qiao	= Kd-6	• one master point for each vessel (opens it)
Du	= SI-3	Yang Qiao	= BL-62	• used in pairs (master + coupled pt)
Chong	= Sp-4	Yin Wei	= Pc-6	• 1 on arm & 1 on leg, both yin or yang channels
Dai	= GB-41	Yang Wei	= TB-5	• analogous to Division pairs
				• 2 pairs are Division pairs (Tai & Shao Yang)

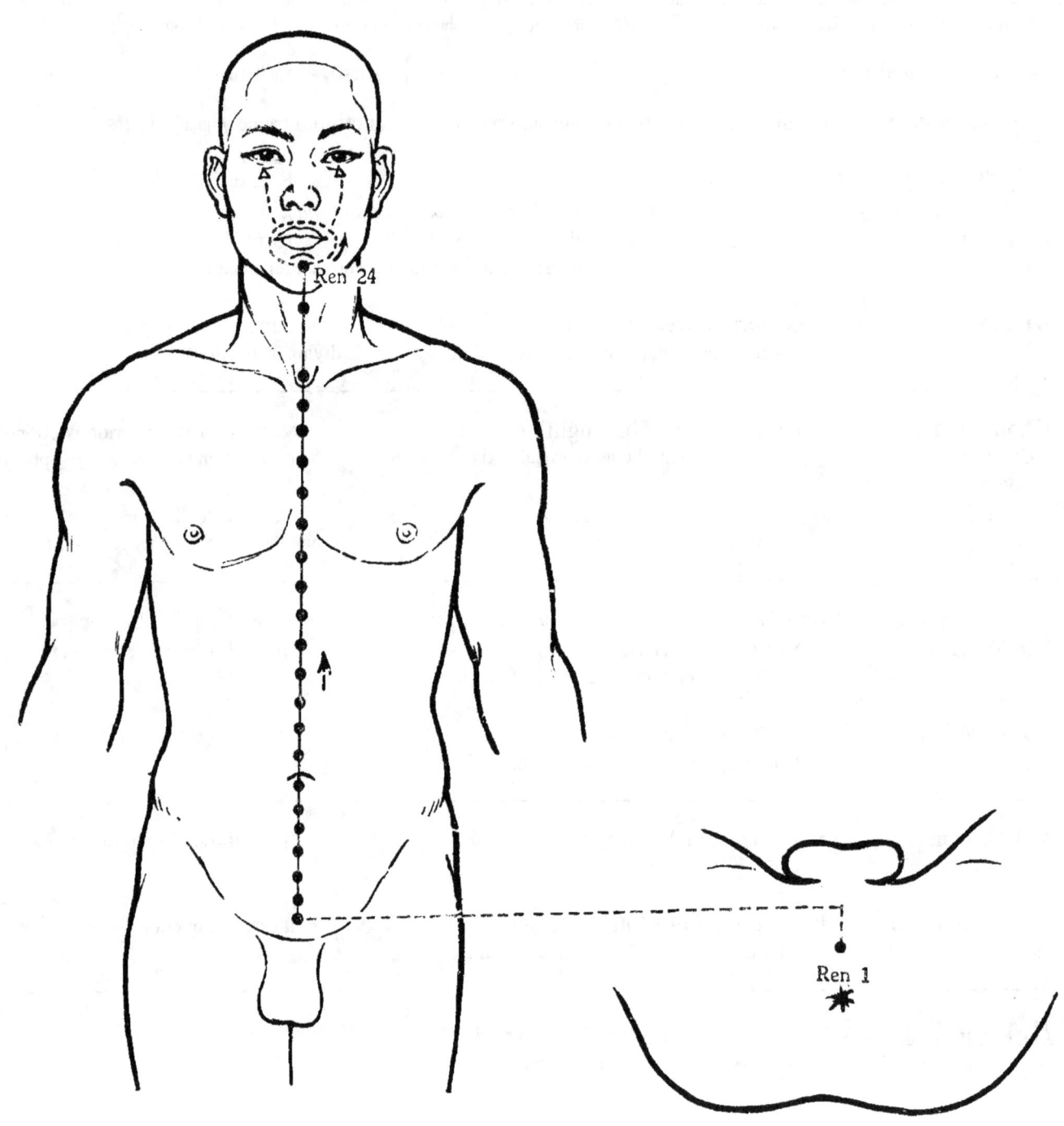

任 脈
Ren Mai
Conception/Controlling Vessel
(24 pts) (+ connection to ST-1)

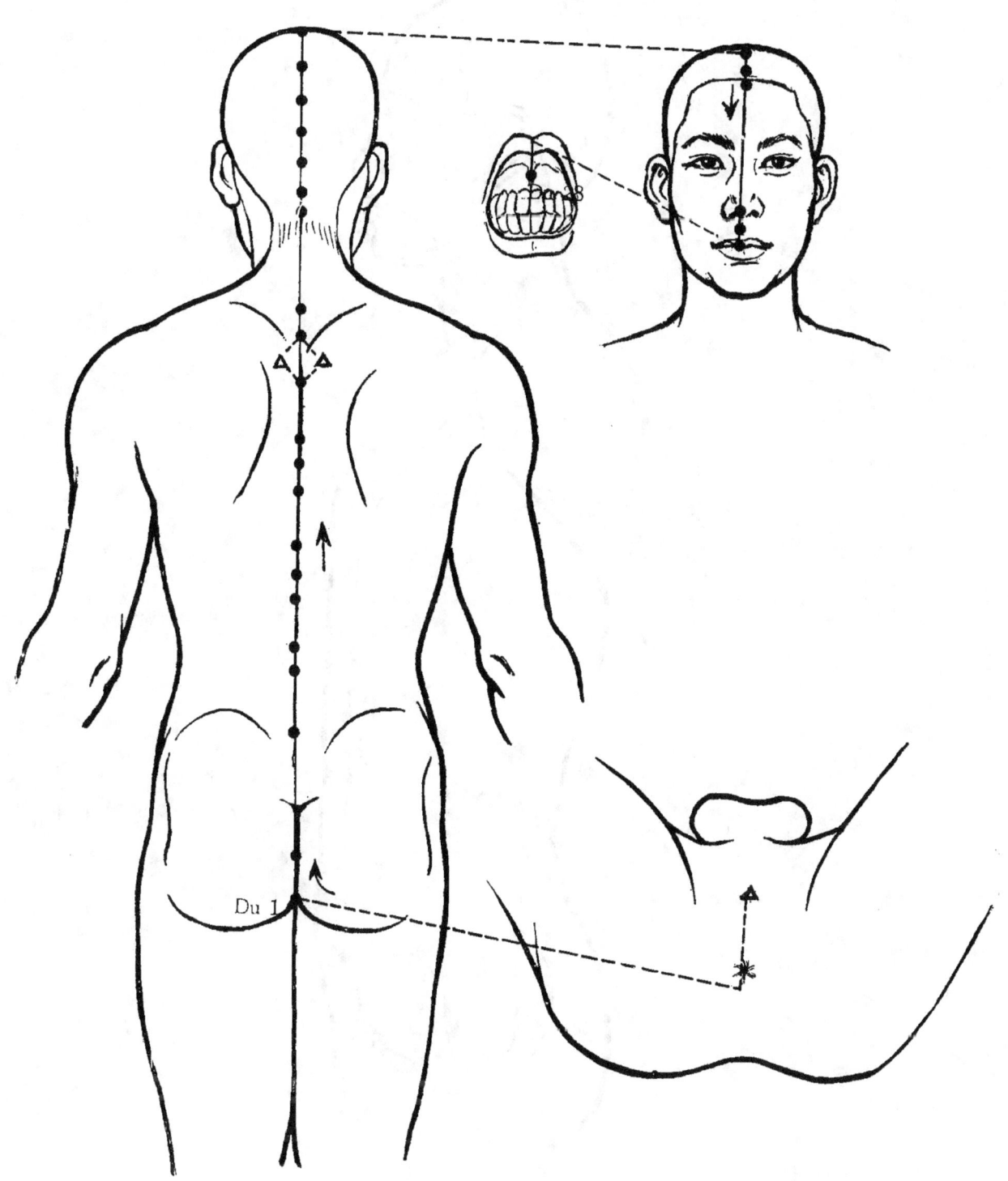

督 脈

Du Mai

Governing Vessel

(28 pts) (+ starts at CV-1 and connects with BL-12)

           © 1990–2016   *Jim Cleaver LAc.*

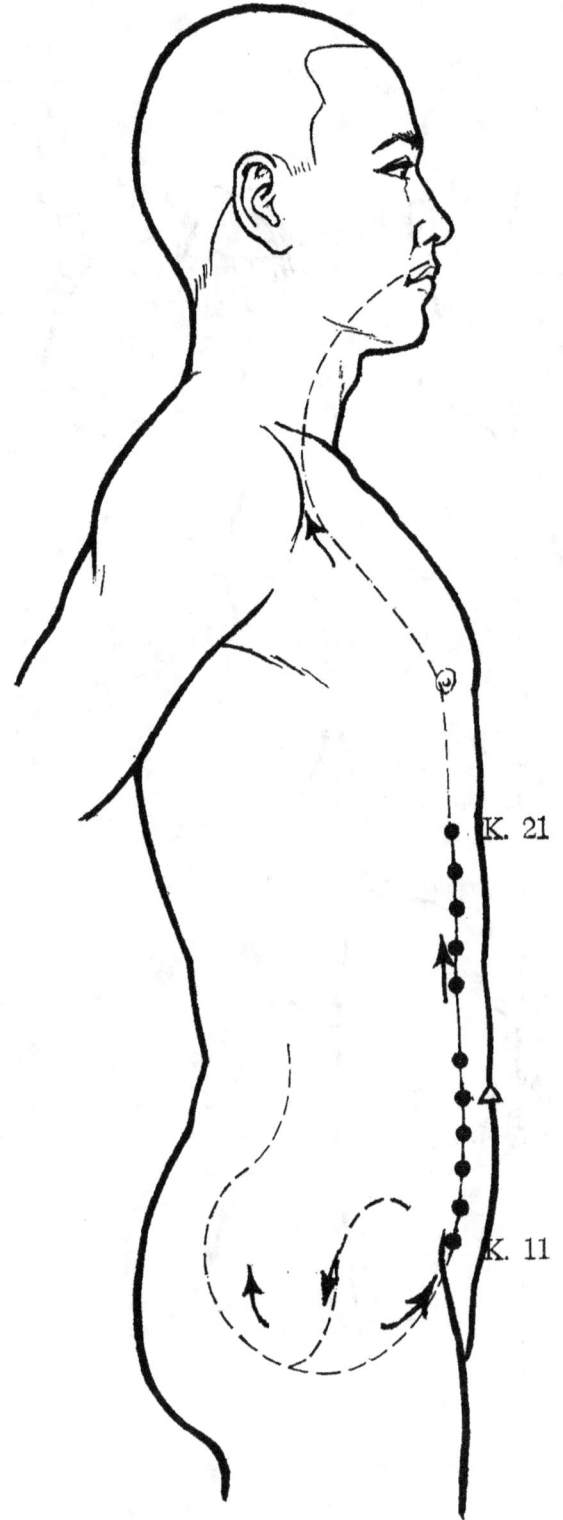

衝／沖 脈
Chong Mai
Surging/Pulsing/Penetrating Vessel
(14 pts)   (11 Kd pts 11-21, CV 1 & 7, & ST-30)

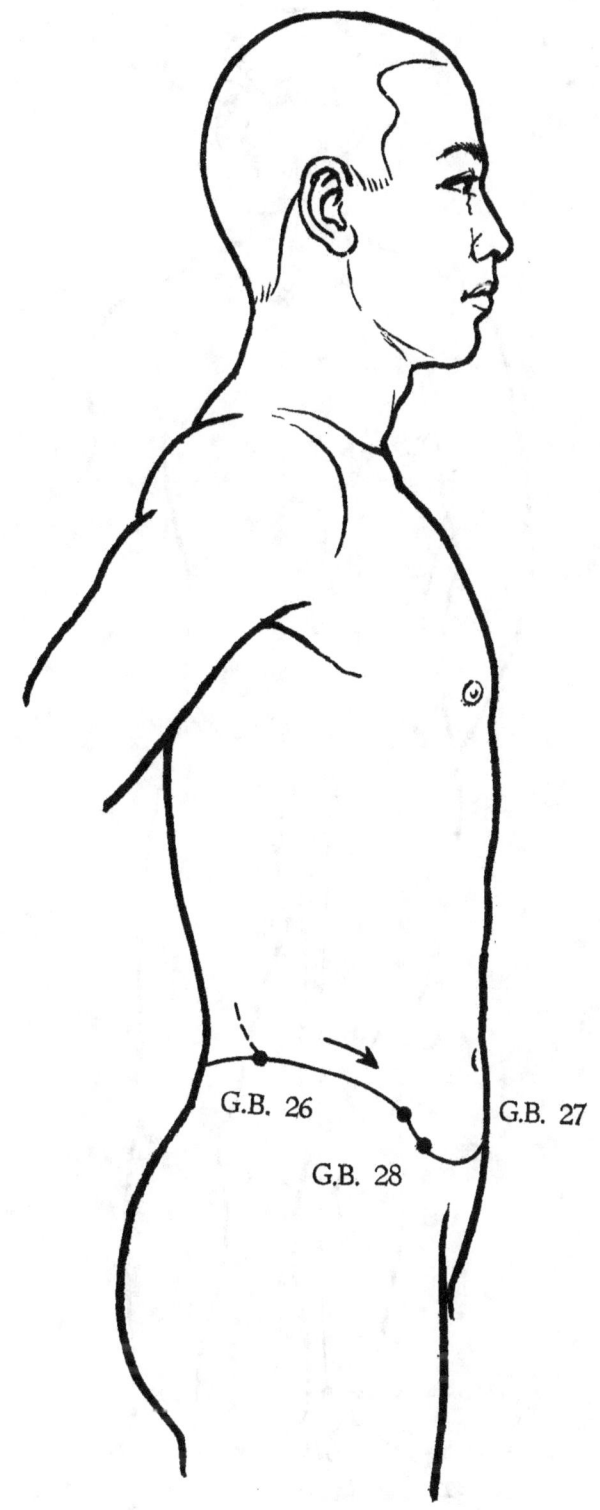

G.B. 26

G.B. 27

G.B. 28

帶 脈
Dai Mai
Belt/Girdling Vessel
(4 pts) (add Lr-13) (+ GV-4 & CV-4 to complete the belt)

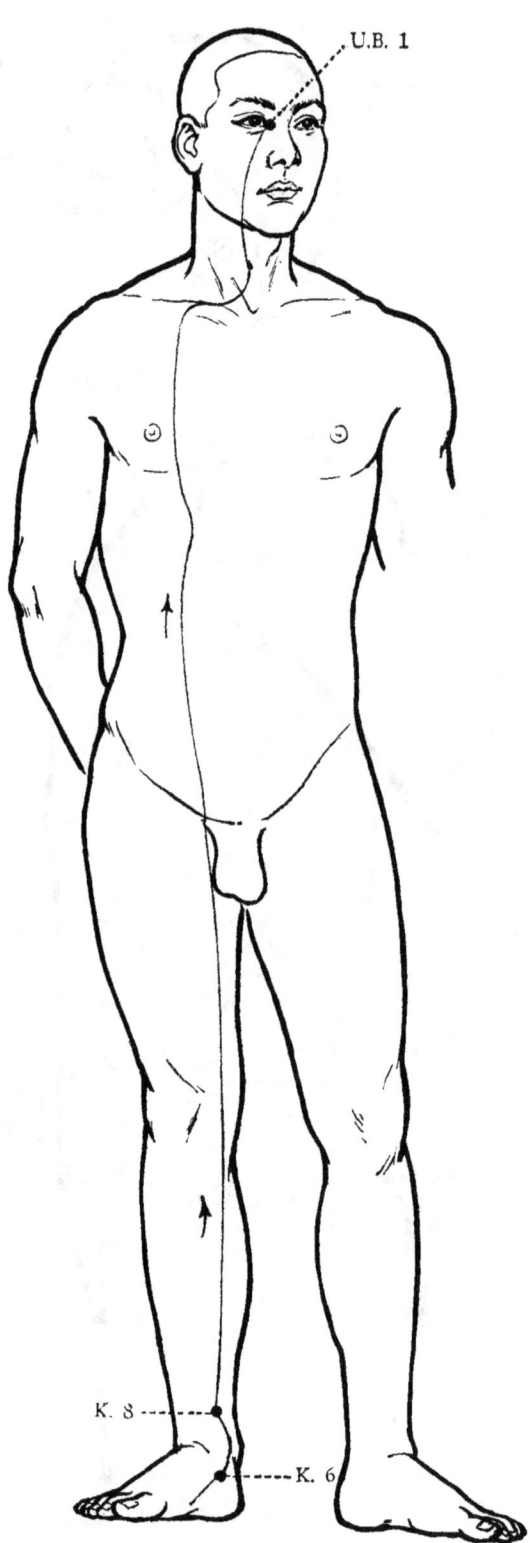

U.B. 1

K. 8

K. 6

陰蹺脈
Yin Qiao Mai

Yin Heel/Motility Vessel

(6 pts) (add Kd-2, ST-12 & St-9)

    © 1990–2016   *Jim Cleaver LAc.*

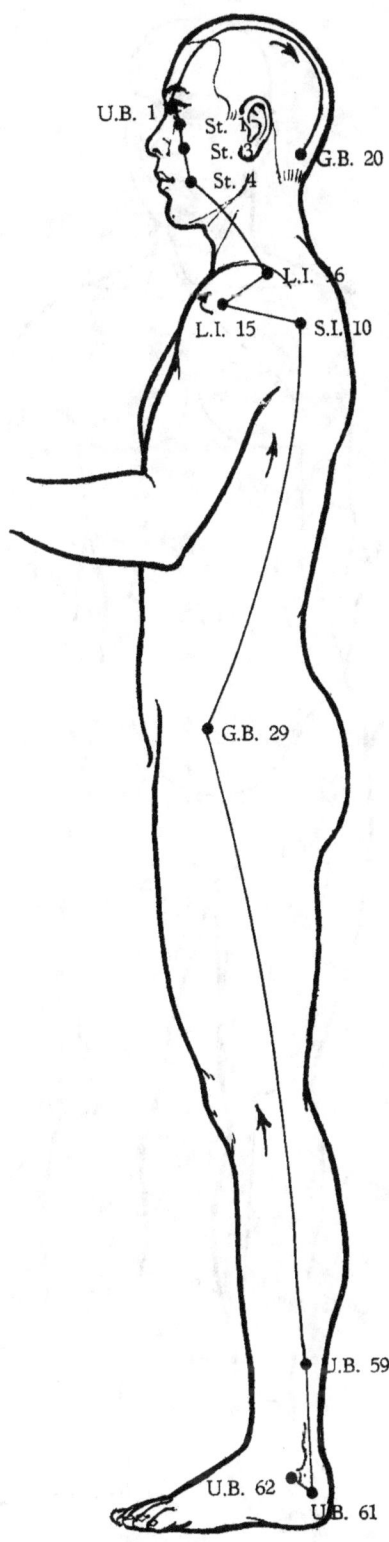

U.B. 1
St. 1
St. 3
St. 4
G.B. 20
L.I. 16
L.I. 15
S.I. 10
G.B. 29
U.B. 59
U.B. 62
U.B. 61

陽 蹻 脈
Yang Qiao Mai
Yang Heel/Motility Vessel
(13 pts) (add ST-9)

© 1990–2016   *Jim Cleaver LAc.*

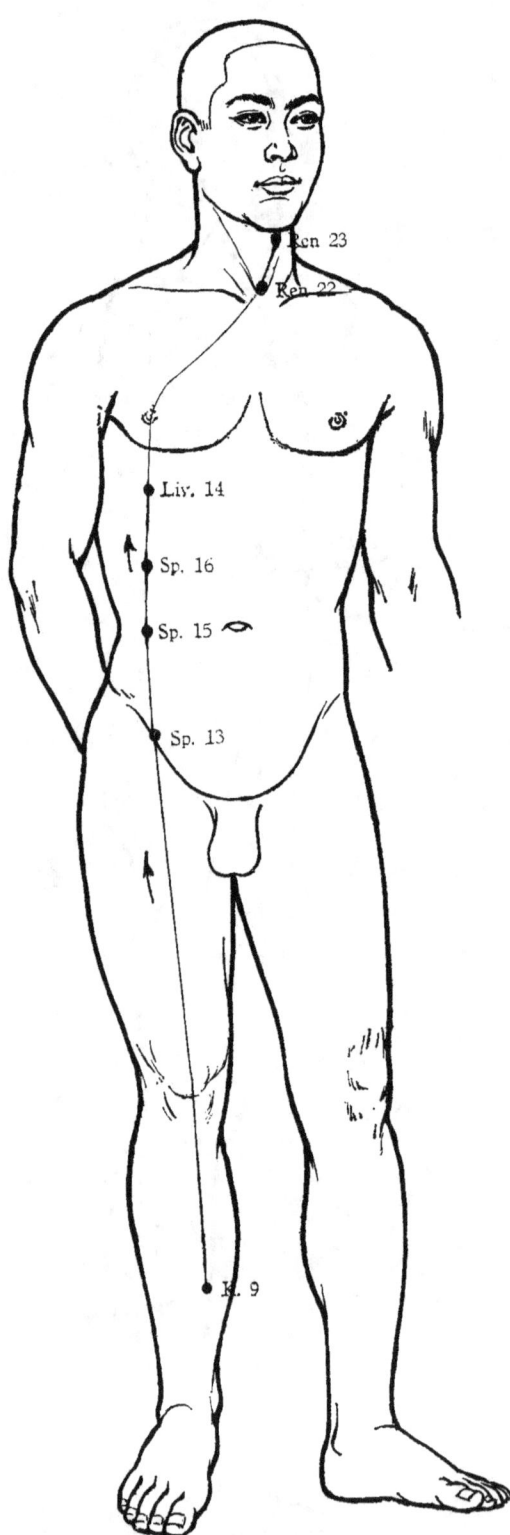

陰 維 脈

Yin Wei Mai

Yin Linking Vessel

(7 pts) (3 Sp pts, 2 CV pts, 1 Kd & 1 Lr pt)

© 1990–2016   Jim Cleaver LAc.

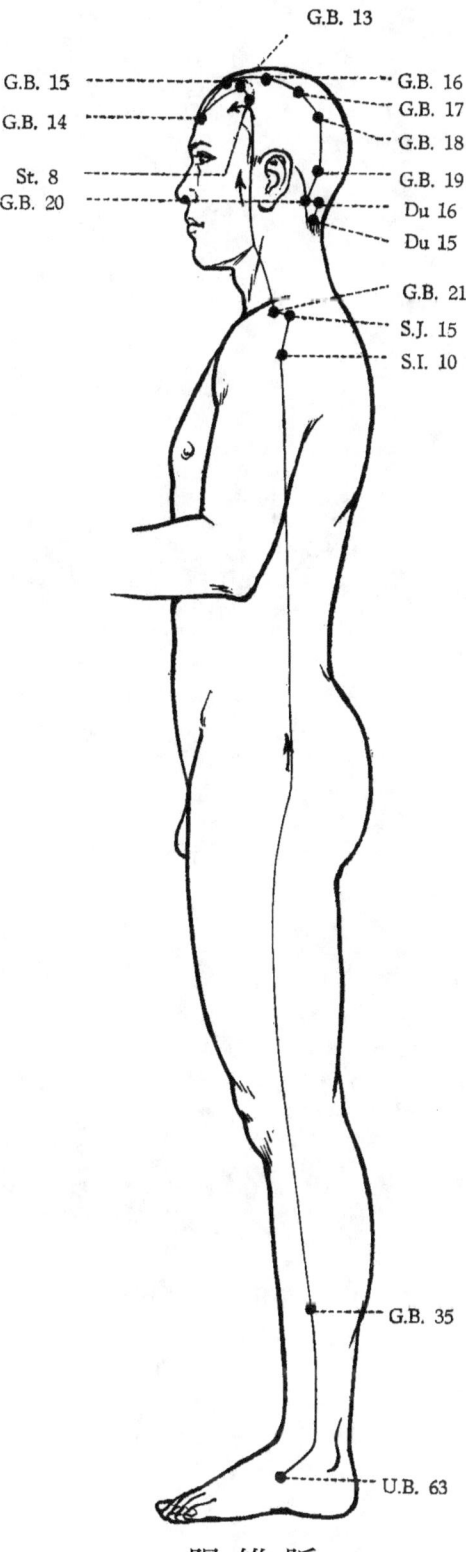

G.B. 13

G.B. 15

G.B. 14

St. 8

G.B. 20

G.B. 16
G.B. 17
G.B. 18
G.B. 19
Du 16
Du 15

G.B. 21
S.J. 15
S.I. 10

G.B. 35

U.B. 63

陽 維 脈

Yang Wei Mai

Yang Linking Vessel

(16 pts)   (add GB-29, TB-13, LI-14   delete Du-15 & 16 & ST-8)

Extra Points

經 外 穴

Jīng Wài Xué

Channel   Outside Acu-Points

Points Outside the Channel System

經外穴 *Jīng Wài Xué = Extra Points*

經外穴 *Jīng Wài Xué = Extra Points*

These are the 54 Extra points NCCAOM expects you to know: (Bold = New)

1) Anmian
2) Bafeng   8 points – 4 per foot
3) Baichongwo
4) Bailao   aka Jing Bai Lao (see #20)
5) Baxie   8 points – 4 per hand
6) Bitong   aka Shang Ying Xiang (see #35)
7) **Bizhong**
8) **Dagukong**   see also #45 Xiao Gu Kong & #52 Zhong Kui
9) **Dangyang**
10) Dannangxue
11) Dingchuan
12) Erbai   2 points on each forearm
13) Erjian
14) **Haiquan**
15) Heding   see also #46
16) **Huanzhong**
17) Huatuojiaji   17 pts on both sides at each vertebral level T1 to L5 (some include the 7 cervicals, making 24)
18) Jiachengjiang
19) Jianqian/**Jianneiling**   actually these are two different points, but they are often considered interchangeable / alt. names
20) **Jingbailao**   aka Bai Lao (see #4)
21) Jinjin & Yuye   JJ is the left side, YY is on the right – referring to the patient's L&R, not the observer's
22) **Juquan**
23) **Kuangu**
24) Lanweixue
25) Luozhen   aka Wai Lao Gong (see #43)
26) **Neihuaijian**   see also #42 Wai Huai Jian
27) **Neiyingxiang**
28) **Pigen**
29) **Qianzheng**
30) **Qiduan**   10 points, 1 at the tip of each toe
31) **Qipang**   2 points that form the base of the San Jiao Jiu triangle (see #33)
32) Qiuhou
33) Sanjiaojiu   this is three points forming a triangle (see #31)
34) **Shanglianquan**
35) **Shangyingxiang**   aka Bi Tong (see #6)
36) Shiqizhui**xue**/Shiqizhuixia
37) Shixuan   10 points, 1 at the tip of each finger
38) Sifeng   4 points per side (1 on each finger at the PIP crease on the palmer side)
39) Sishencong   4 points surrounding GV-20
40) Taiyang
41) Tituo
42) **Waihuaijian**   see also #26 Nei Huai Jian
43) **Wailaogong**   aka Luo Zhen (see #25)
44) Weiguanxiashu   aka Yi Shu (not included)
45) **Xiaogukong**   see also #8 Da Gu Kong & #52 Zhong Kui
46) Xiyan/Neixiyan   2 pts – the eyes of the knee (the outer eye is ST-35, so the extra pt is the inner eye Nei)
47) Yaotongxue   this is 2 pts on each hand
48) Yaoyan
49) **Yiming**
50) Yintang
51) Yuyao
52) **Zhongkui**
53) Zhoujian
54) Zigongxue

* As of Feb. 2014 there are 54 points, up from 34 [I numbered their list and made the new points **Bold**]
There are 22 new/**bold** point names, but really only 17 **new** points, (plus 1 new alt name see #19)
because three pairs are alternate names for the same point [4&20, 6&35, 25&43; and #31 is part of #33]

NCCAOM Extra Points by Body Region

Head & Face	(14 Pts = 15)	Pt Actions #	*Comments*
1. Si Shen Cong	(WHO 1)	(EX 1)	
2. Dang Yang	(WIIO 2)	(EX 2)	
3. Yin Tang	(WHO 3)	(EX 3)	
4. Yu Yao	(WHO 4)	(EX 4)	
5. Tai Yang	(WHO 5)	(EX 5)	
6. Er Jian	(WHO 6)	(EX 6)	
7. Qiu Hou	(WHO 7)	(EX 7)	
8. Bi Tong aka Shang Ying Xiang	(WHO 8)	(EX 8)	* NCCAOM includes **both names = 2 pts**
9. Nei Ying Xiang	(WHO 9)	(EX 9)	* see LI-20 (name is Ying Xiang)
10. Ju Quan	(WHO 10)	(EX 10)	
11. Hai Quan	(WHO 11)	(EX 11)	
12. Jin-jin Yu-ye	(WHO 12 & 13)	(EX 12)	* JJ is Left side, YY is Right side (patient's L&R)
13. Jia Cheng Jiang	(X)	(EX 13)	
14. Qian Zheng	(X)	(EX 14)	

Ear & Neck	(4 Pts = 5)		
15. Yi Ming	(WHO 14)	(EX 16)	
16. An Mian	(X)	(EX 17)	* too many locations for WHO to settle on one?
17. Shang Lian Quan	(X)	(EX 18)	
18. (Jing) Bai Lao	(WHO 15)	(EX 21)	* NCCAOM includes **both names = 2 pts**

Back & Sacrum	(6 Pts)		
19. Ding Chuan	(WHO 17)	(EX 23)	
20. Hua Tuo Jia Ji	(WHO 18)	(EX 27)	* can be called Hua Tuo, or Jia Ji pts
21. Wei Guan Xia Shu	(WHO 19)	(EX 30)	* aka Yi Shu, both WHO & NCCAOM use WGXS
22. Pi Gen	(WHO 20)	(EX 31)	
23. Yao Yan	(WHO 22)	(EX 35)	
24. Shi Qi Zhui Xia	(WHO 24)	(EX 37)	* aka Shi-Qi Zhui

Chest & Abdomen	(4 Pts)		
25. San Jiao Jiu	(X)	(EX 41)	* NCCAOM includes **both** this and the next
Qi Pang	(X)	(EX 41)	* these two pts are part of Sanjiaojiu (see previous)
26. Ti Tuo (Xue)	(X)	(EX 43)	
27. Zi Gong (Xue)	(WHO 16)	(EX 45)	

Upper Extremity	**(13 Pts = 14)**	**Pt Actions #**	*Comments*
28. Jian Qian / Jian Nei Ling	(X)	(EX 47)	* NCCAOM includes **both names** as #19 =1 pt
29. Zhou Jian	(WHO 26)	(EX 50)	
30. Bi Zhong	(X)	(EX 51)	
31. Er Bai	(WHO 27)	(EX 52)	
32. Zhong Quan	(X)	(EX 53)	
33. Yao Tong (Dian/Xue)	(WHO 29)	(EX 54)	
34. Luo Zhen aka Wai Lao Gong	(WHO 30)	(EX 56)	* NCCAOM includes **both names** =2 pts
35. Ba Xie	(WHO 31)	(EX 58)	
36. Da Gu Kong	(WHO 32)	(EX 60)	
37. Zhong Kui	(WHO 33)	(EX 61)	
38. Xiao Gu Kong	(WHO 34)	(EX 62)	
39. Si Feng	(WHO 35)	(EX 64)	
40. Shi Xuan	(WHO 36)	(EX 65)	

Lower Extremity	**(11 Pts)**		
41. Huan Zhong	(X)	(EX 66)	
42. Bai Chong Wo	(WHO 37)	(EX 68)	
43. Kuan Gu	(WHO 38)	(EX 70)	
44. He Ding	(WHO 39)	(EX 71)	
45. (Nei) Xi Yan	(WHO 40 & 41)	(EX 72)	*WHO counts Wai Xi Yan & Nei Xi Yan as distinct pts
46. Lan Wei (Xue)	(WHO 42)	(EX 74)	
47. Dan Nang (Xue)	(WHO 43)	(EX 75)	
48. Nei Huai Jian	(WHO 44)	(EX 80)	
49. Wai Huai Jian	(WHO 45)	(EX 81)	
50. Ba Feng	(WHO 46)	(EX 82)	
51. Qi Duan	(WHO 47)	(EX 84)	

* Of the NCCAOM points, most are also W.H.O. points   The 11 which are not, are marked (X).

** All are included in my Point Actions Book which describes 87 pts (more if one counts alt. names).

Head, Face & Neck Points *(14 pts)*

Points on Top of the Head

(NCCAOM 39)

1.　四神聰　　**Sì Shén Cōng = Four (Points for) Mental Clarity**　　(WHO 1)

literally 4 Spirits w/ Sharp Hearing; 4 Intelligent-Astute-Clever Spirits (4 Spirits See, Hear & Think Clearly)

Location:　　• 4 pts on top of the head - 1 cun anterior, posterior, left & right of GV-20 (the 4 directions)

Indications:　　• calm spirit – headache (esp vertex), dizziness, seizures, mania, hydrocephalus

(NCCAOM 9)

2.　當陽　　**Dāng Yáng = Manage Yang**　　(WHO 2)

Location:　　• 1 cun posterior to the anterior hairline, on a line projected upward from the pupil
　　　　　　　(0.5 cun posterior to GB-15)　　(level with BL-5)

Indications:　　• whole body overheated (w/ swollen neck = frog epidemic); dizziness, hypertension
　　　　　　　eye problems, dim vision, nasal congestion, common cold or flu

---

Points on the Forehead & Temple

(NCCAOM 50)

3. 印堂   <u>**Yìn Táng = Seal Hall, Hall of Seals (the glabella)**</u>   (WHO 3)

<u>Location:</u>   • on the GV at the midpoint between the eyebrows (BL-2)

<u>Indications:</u>   • calm spirit – headache, dizziness/vertigo, insomnia; nasal problems, eye problems;
      swelling of the sublingual veins (blood stag) ; convulsions, vomiting;, hypertension, eclampsia
   * [the Ling Shu states this area can be examined to assess the condition of the Lungs]

(NCCAOM 51)

4. 魚腰   <u>**Yú Yāo = Fish's Waist**</u>   (WHO 4)

<u>Location:</u>   • the midpoint of each eyebrow, directly above the pupil (1 unit below GB-14)

<u>Indications:</u>   • eye problems, supraorbital pain, facial paralysis

(NCCAOM 40)

5. 太陽   <u>**Tài Yáng = Very/Great Yang (Abundant Yang)**</u>   (WHO 5)

<u>Location:</u>   • on the temple 1 cun posterior to the midpoint of a line connecting TB-23 & GB-1
<u>alt Location:</u>   • 1 cun posterior to the outer canthus

<u>Indications:</u>   • headaches (esp. unilateral), eye problems, trigeminal neuralgia, facial paralysis, toothache

(NCCAOM 13)

6. 耳尖   <u>**Ěr Jiān = Ear Apex**</u>   (WHO 6)
      aka Er Yong = Ear Bubbling/Gushing

<u>Location:</u>   • at the apex of the ear; fold the ear forward, the crease marks the spot

<u>Indications:</u>   • high fever, furuncles, conjunctivitis, pannus & other opacities of the eye;
      migraines, high BP

Points Around the Eyes	

(NCCAOM 32)

7. 球後   <u>**Qiú Hòu = Behind the (Eye) Ball**</u>   (WHO 7)

Location: • between the eyeball and the infraorbital ridge, midway between the outer canthus & ST-1

Indications: • eye, vision and optic nerve problems such as optic nerve atrophy or neuritis, myopia, glaucoma, opacity of the vitreous body, retinitis pigmentosa, esotropia (convergent squint)

Points In & Around the Nose	

(NCCAOM 6)

8. 鼻通   <u>**Bí Tōng = Nose Open or Unblock the Nose**</u>   (WHO 8)

aka **Shang Ying Xiang** = Upper LI-20 - (Upper/Above Welcome Fragrance)   (NCCAOM 35)

Location: • on the face, at the superior end of the naso-labial groove

Indications: • all nasal problems

(NCCAOM 27)

9. 內迎香   <u>Nèi Yíng Xiāng = Inner LI-20</u>   (WHO 9)

Location: • inside the nose, at the junction of the alar cartilage and the nasal concha

Indications: • heat stroke, syncope, conjunctivitis

Points In & Around the Mouth

(NCCAOM 22)

10. 聚泉   Jù Quán = Gather/Converge/Assemble at the Spring   (WHO 10)

Location: • on the surface of the tongue, at the midpoint

Indications: • paralysis of the tongue, decreased sense of taste; diabetes; asthma

(NCCAOM 14)

11. 海泉   Hǎi Quán = Sea of Saliva   (WHO 11)

aka She Xia or She Xia Zhong Feng = Under the Tongue, Sealed in the Middle

Ghost pt name: • Guǐ Fēng = Ghost/Demon Enclosed

Location: • on the underside of the tongue - superior to the frenulum attachment (betw Jin-jin & Yu-ye)

Indications: • hiccups, glossitis, xiao-ke/diabetes symptoms (ghost pt. indications: psychosis)

(NCCAOM 21)

12. 金津   **Jīn-jīn = Gold Liquid**   (WHO 12)

　　玉液   **Yù-yè = Jade Fluid**   (WHO 13)

Location: • 2 pts under the tongue - at the midpoint of the left & right sublingual veins
         (Jin jin is on the left vein,   Yu ye is on the right vein)

Indications: • dry mouth, extreme thirst (xiao-ke/diabetes);
         tongue & speech problems (stomatitis, glossitis, tonsillitis; aphasia)

(NCCAOM 18)

13. 夾承漿   **Jiā Chéng Jiāng = Pinch CV-24** **(Catch Saliva/Spittle, For Drooling)**   (WHO X)
aka Ke Liao = Chin Bone-Holes

Location: • on the chin, at the mental foramen, ~1.5 cun to either side of CV-24
         (at the ends of the mento-labial groove, usually below the corners of the mouth)

Indications: • excessive salivation/drooling; trigeminal neuralgia, facial tics, spasms or paralysis

(NCCAOM 29)

14. 牽正   **Qiān Zhèng = Pull Correct or Pull Aright**   (WHO X)

Location: • on the side of the face - 1/2 to 1 cun anterior to the attachment of the earlobe.
         (in the masseter muscle midway between ST-6 & 7)

Indications: • facial paralysis (Bell's palsy), TMD; parotitis; mouth ulcers

Points Behind the Ear

(NCCAOM 49)

15. 翳 明 <u>Yì Míng = Screen Brightness</u> (Eye Screens)

(WHO 14)

Location:
• behind the ear - 1 cun posterior to TB-17 (midway between TB-17 & An Mian)

Indications:
• eye problems: esp. screens = cataracts film, opacity, nebulae;
   myopia, night blindness/nyctalopia
   tinnitus, vertigo, insomnia, headache; mental disorders

(NCCAOM 1)

16. 安 眠 <u>Ān Mián = Peaceful/Calm/Tranquil/Quiet Sleep</u>

(WHO X)

Location:
• behind the ear - midway between TB-17 & GB-20
(posterior edge of mastoid, slightly above & behind GB-12)

Indications:
• insomnia; palpitations, hysteria, mental illness; headache, vertigo

Points on the Front of Neck

(NCCAOM 34)

17. 上 廉 泉 <u>Shàng Lián Quán = Upper CV-23</u> (Upper Pure Spring / Above Ridge Spring) (WHO X)

Location:
• under the chin - on the midline, midway between the hyoid & the chin,
   1/2 cun superior to CV-23

Indications:
• hypo or hyper salivation, impaired/slurred speech, mutism (paralysis of hypoglossal nerve);
   inflammations of the throat or tongue (tonsillitis, pharyngitis, stomatitis)

Points on the Back of Neck

(NCCAOM 20)

18. 頸 百 勞 <u>Jǐng Bǎi Láo = (Neck) 100 Taxations / Complete Fatique</u>

(WHO 15)

aka **Bai Lao**, but this is an alternate name for GV-14, thus the extra point is designated Jing Bai Lao,

(NCCAOM 4)

Location:
• on the back of the neck - 1 cun inferior to the posterior hairline & 1 cun lateral to the midline

Indications:
• scrofula (cervical TB, consumption), neck pain & stiffness,
   cough (whooping cough); postpartum aching

Back & Lumbo-Sacral Points (6 pts)

Points on the Upper Back

(NCCAOM 11)

19. 定喘   <u>**Dìng Chuǎn = Stabilize Dyspnea (Gasping & Panting)**</u>   (WHO 17)

(哮 xiào = wheeze)

<u>Location:</u>   • 0.5 cun lateral to the midline, level with the space inferior to the spinous process of C_7

<u>Indications:</u>   • asthmatic breathing, all types of dyspnea, cough; stiff neck; urticaria

Mid-Back Points

(NCCAOM 17)

20. 華他夾脊   <u>**(Huá-Tuó) Jiā-Jǐ = (Hua Tuo's) Pinch the Spine / Para-Spinal Pts**</u>

<u>Location:</u>   • 17 bilateral pts – on either side of the spine, ~0.75 cun lateral to the midline,   (WHO 18)
level with the space inferior to each spinous process from T_1 to L_5

<u>alt version</u> =   • 24 bilateral pts – from C_1 to L_5

<u>Indications:</u>   • disorders of the spine & nerves; pain or disease at corresponding level of the body
symptom patterns related to zang or fu organ at same level (actions similar to back shu pts)

21. 胰俞   <u>**Yí Shū = Pancreas Shu/Point**</u>   (WHO 19)

aka 胃管下俞   Wèi Guǎn Xià Shū = Lower Stomach Pipe/Duct/Valve Shu (NCCAOM & WHO use this name) (NCCAOM 44)

aka 胃脘下俞   Wèi Wǎn Xià Shū = Lower Epigastrium Shu (pylorus/duodenum/pancreas assoc pt)

<u>Location:</u>   • 1.5 cun lateral to the midline, level with the space inferior to the spinous process of T_8

<u>Indications:</u>   • dry throat, xiao-ke/diabetes, stomach disorders - intercostal neuralgia

(NCCAOM 28)

22. 痞根   <u>**Pǐ Gēn = Abdominal Swelling/Lump Root**</u>   (WHO 20)

<u>Location:</u>   • on the lower back, 3.5 cun lateral to the space inferior to the spinous process of L_1

<u>Indications:</u>   • enlarged liver or spleen (hepato/splenomegaly), stomach, low back or hernia pain;
kidney prolapse; gastritis, enteritis, diarrhea or constipation
(tumors, endometriosis)

Points in the Lumbar Region

(NCCAOM 48)

23. 腰眼   <u>**Yāo Yǎn = Lumbar Eye-sockets (Eyes of the Waist)**</u>

(WHO 22)

• yan = eyes or eye socket (see xi yan #70)

<u>Location:</u>
• the dimple in the lateral lumbar/iliac crest area, the depression is 3 to 4 cun lateral
  to the midline, level with a lumbar spinous process ranging from L$_3$ to L$_5$
  variability is primarily due to differences between male & female pelvic structure

<u>Indications:</u>
• acute or chronic low back pain, kidney prolapse; orchitis; diabetes;
  GYN problems (esp. dysmenorrhea)

(NCCAOM 36)

24. 十七椎下   <u>**Shí-Qī Zhuī-Xià (10+7 Vertebra-Below) Under the 17th Vertebra**</u>

<u>Location:</u>
• on the posterior midline - below the spinous process of L$_5$ (at the lumbo-sacral jct)   (WHO 24)

<u>Indications:</u>
• lumbar &/or sacral pain; paraplegia due to trauma, sequela of childhood paralysis;
  sciatica; anal diseases - dysmenorrhea, uterine bleeding - malposition of the fetus (moxa)

Chest & Abdomen Points (4 pts)

Points on the Lower Abdomen

(NCCAOM 33)

25. 三角灸　　Sān Jiǎo Jiǔ = Three Horns/Angles Moxa (Moxa Triangle)　(WHO X)

Location:
- 3 points forming an equilateral triangle with the apex at CV-8,
  the base & sides are a mouth width
- aka　　**Qí-Páng** = the 2 points forming the base of the above triangle　(NCCAOM 31)

Indications:
- chronic enteritis, colic, abdominal pain & spasm, umbilical hernia, running piglet

(NCCAOM 41)

26. 提托 (穴)　　Tí Tuō (Xué) = Lift & Support (Point)　　　　(WHO X)

Location:
- on the lower abdomen, 3 cun inferior to the umbilicus and 4 cun lateral to the midline
  i.e. on Sp channel, 4 cun lateral to CV-4   (1.7 cun inferior to Sp-14)

Indications:
- prolapsed uterus; hernia; lower abdominal pain

(NCCAOM 54)

27. 子宫　　Zǐ Gōng (Xué) = Child's Palace (Uterus) (& adnexa)　　(WHO 16)

Location:
- on the lower abdomen, 1 cun superior to the pubic crest and 3 cun lateral to the midline
  i.e. 3 cun lateral to CV-3

Indications:
- infertility, irregular menses, dysmenorrhea, prolapsed uterus; eclampsia
  cystitis, orchitis; appendicitis; pelveo-peritonitis; pyelonephritis

Upper Extremity Points (13 pts)

Points on the Upper Arm & Shoulder

(NCCAOM 19)

28. 肩內陵   Jiān Nèi Líng = Shoulder Inner Mound

(WHO X)

Location: • in the anterior deltoid - midway between the anterior axillary fold and LI-15 (on Lu chan.)

Indications: • problems of the shoulder joint & surrounding soft tissues (+ indications as for LI-15)

(NCCAOM 19)

29. 肩前   Jiān Qián = Front of the Shoulder

(WHO X)

Location 1:   • same as Jian Nei Ling: midway between the axillary fold and LI-15 (ACT)
Location 2:   • 1 cun superior to the anterior axillary fold (Atlas & IDCA)
Location 3:   • 1.5 cun superior to the anterior axillary fold (2001)

Indications: • problems of the shoulder joint & surrounding soft tissues (+ indications as for LI-15)

(NCCAOM 53)

30. 肘尖   Zhǒu Jiān = Elbow Apex / Tip of the Elbow

(WHO 26)

Location: • at the tip of the olecranon (flex the elbow)

Indications: • scrofula, abscess, general inflammation, inflammation of the cecum (appendicitis)

Points on the Anterior Forearm

(NCCAOM 7)

31. 臂中   Bì Zhōng = Middle of the ForeArm

(WHO X)

Location: • on the anterior forearm, between the flexor carpi radialis & palmaris longus tendons,
midway between the wrist & elbow folds - i.e. on the Pericardium channel (6 cun up or down)
approx. where the bodies of these muscles end & their tendons begin

Indications: • pain in the forearm, carpal tunnel syndrome; upper limb paralysis; hysteria

(NCCAOM 12)

32. 二白   Èr Bái = 2 Whites (white refers to the anus)

(WHO 27)

Location: • 2 pts on the anterior forearm, 4 cun proximal to the wrist fold
on either side of the flexor carpi radialis (one pt is on the Pc channel, the other is roughly on the Lu = white

Indications: • hemorrhoids, anal prolapse; neuralgia of the forearm

Points on the Dorsum of the Hand

(NCCAOM 47)

33. 腰 痛 (點)   <u>**Yāo Tòng (Diǎn/Xué) = Lumbar Pain (Points)**</u>   (WHO 29)

Location:
3 pts on the dorsum of the hand between the metacarpal bones
#1 - distal to the junction of the <u>bases</u> of the <u>2nd & 3rd</u> metacarpals (aka Wei Ling)
#2 - distal to the junction of the <u>bases</u> of the <u>3rd & 4th</u> metacarpals
#3 - distal to the junction of the <u>bases</u> of the <u>4th & 5th</u> metacarpals (aka Jing Ling)

Indications:
#1 - pain due to trauma to the head, low back or limbs
#2 - pain due to trauma to the chest or limbs
#3 - pain due to trauma to the low back or limbs

(NCCAOM 25)

34.   落 枕   <u>**Luò Zhěn = Fall (off) Pillow = Crick in the Neck**</u>   (WHO 30)

aka 外勞宮 **Wài Láo Gōng** = Outer Labor Palace (Pc-8)   (NCCAOM 43)

Location:
• on the dorsum of the hand, between the 2nd & 3rd metacarpals, just proximal to their heads

Indications:
• torticollis, stiff neck, arm & shoulder pain, numbness, pain or swelling of the fingers;
  migraine; childhood indigestion, abdominal distention, epigastric pain, diarrhea; sore throat

(NCCAOM 5)

35.   八 邪   <u>**Bā Xié = Eight Evils**</u>   (WHO 31)

Location:
• 4 pts on each hand - with the hand in a fist these points are between the knuckles,
  just distal to the MP joint (includes TB-2 & #54 Hu Kou)

Indications:
• numbness, pain, stiffness, inflammation of the fingers & joints,
  inflammation of the hand & forearm, snakebite;
  headache, stiff neck, sore throat, toothache

Points on the Fingers

36. 大骨空 Dà Gǔ Kōng = Big Bone Hollow

Location:
- on the dorsal aspect of the thumb, at the center of the interphalangeal joint

Indications:
- eye diseases: cataracts, film over eyes, excess tearing, itching, or pain; vomiting and diarrhea

37. 中魁 Zhōng Kuí = Middle Eminence (Knuckle)

Location:
- on the dorsal aspect of the middle finger, in the middle of the middle knuckle (PIP joint)

Indications:
- severe vomiting, hiccups, belching, esophageal spasm; nausea, loss of appetite/anorexia; toothache, nosebleed (moxa only pt) (try for severe morning sickness)

38. 小骨空 Xiǎo Gǔ Kōng = Little Bone Hollow

Location:
- on the dorsal aspect of the little finger, at the center of the PIP joint

Indications:
- eye diseases as for Da Gu Kong, sore throat, arthritis of the fingers

39. 四縫 Sì Fèng = Four Fissures / Cracks (Creases)
* the transverse creases on the palmar surface of each finger (excluding the thumb)

Location 1:
- at the center of the PIP joint creases (4 points on each hand)

Location 2:
- at the center of the DIP joint creases

Location 3
- 2 points per crease - at the medial & the lateral ends of each DIP or PIP transverse crease

Indications:
- infant indigestion or loss of appetite, childhood malnutrition syndrome (gan); intestinal parasites (esp roundworm) - pertussis (whooping cough)

40. 十宣 Shí Xuān = Ten Drains

Location:
- 10 points - one at the center of the tip of each finger (5 points per hand)

Indications:
- loss of consciousness, fainting due to fright, shock, heat exhaustion, high fever, convulsions/seizures or hysteria; numbness of the fingertips; hypertension; sore throat

Lower Extremity Points (11 pts)

Points Around the Hip

(NCCAOM 16)

41. 環中   <u>Huán Zhōng = Circle Center (Center of the Circle)</u>

(~~WHO~~ X)

Location: • (best located in the lateral recumbent position) on the buttocks, 2/3 of the distance
between the greater trochanter and the sacral hiatus (midway betw Huan Tiao GB-30 & GV-2)

Indications: • leg pain, sciatica, low back pain, piriformis spasm   w/ GB-30

Points Around the Knee

(NCCAOM 3)

42. 百蟲窩   <u>Bǎi Chóng Wō = 100 Insects/Worms Nest</u>

(WHO 37)

Location: • on the anterior thigh, in the vastus medialis, 1 cun superior to SP-10

Indications: • pruritis, urticaria, eczema

(NCCAOM 23)

43. 髖骨   <u>Kuān Gǔ = Hip Bone (Femur)</u>

(WHO 38)

Location: • 2 points on the thigh, sl. above the knee; spec. 1.5 cun medial and lateral to ST-34

Indications: • arthritis of the knee, paralysis of the lower limb, problems involving the quadriceps

(NCCAOM 15)

44. 鶴頂   <u>Hè Dǐng = Crane's Crown</u>

(WHO 39)

Location: • above the knee - at the midpoint of the superior border of the patella (when the knee is flexed)

alt Location: • the center of the patella (moxa only)

Indications: • weakness of the knees &/or legs; problems of the knee joint or surrounding soft tissues

(NCCAOM 46)

45. 內膝眼   <u>(Nèi) Xī Yǎn = (Inner/Medial) Knee Eye (Eyes of the Knee)</u>

(WHO 40)

aka   Xi Mu = Knee Eye   • yan = eyes or eye socket (see Yao Yan #35)

Location: • below the kneecap - in the depression on the medial side of the patellar ligament
(the lateral eye is ST-35 and in this context is called Wai Xi Yan)

(WHO 41)

Indications: • problems of the knee & surrounding soft tissues
* Nei Xi Yan & Wai Xi Yan are often used together and simply called Xi Yan,
they are often combined with He Ding (#44)
and are very effective for a wide variety of knee problems

Points on the Lower Leg

(NCCAOM 24)

46. 闌尾 (穴)   **Lán Wěi (Xué) = Appendix (Point)**

(WHO 42)

lit. end of the tail (some sources say this is a Right side only pt)

Location: • below the knee - 1 to <u>2 cun</u> inferior to ST-36 (in the tibialis anterior muscle) (1 cun above ST-37)

Indications: • Dx & Tx of acute or chronic appendicitis, indigestion; lower limb paralysis, foot drop

(NCCAOM 10)

47. 膽囊 (穴)   **Dǎn Náng (Xué/Diǎn) = Gall Bladder (Point)**

(WHO 43)

(some sources say this is a Right side only pt)

Location: • below the head of the fibula, along the anterior edge of the peroneus longus muscle,
     1 to 2 cun inferior to GB-34

Indications: • Dx & Tx of gall bladder & bile duct disorders, pain following GB surgery; leg paralysis

---

Points Around the Ankle

(NCCAOM 26)

48. 內踝尖   **Nèi Huái Jiān = Inner Anklebone Tip**

(WHO 44)

Location: • at the tip (high point) of the medial malleolus

Indications: • gastroc spasm, tonsillitis, toothache, lochiorrhea

(NCCAOM 42)

49. 外踝尖   **Wài Huái Jiān = Outer Anklebone Tip**

(WHO 45)

Location: • at the tip (high point) of the lateral malleolus

Indications: • beriberi, spasm of the peroneals, paralysis of the toes, paraplegia, severe headache
     toothache, sore throat, sublingual veins engorged in infants

Points on the Dorsum of the Foot

(NCCAOM 2)

50. 八 風   **Bā Fēng = 8 Winds**   (WHO 46)

Location:
- 4 points on each foot - between the toes, 1/2 cun proximal to the web margin; at the skin change just distal to the MP joints (includes Lr-2, ST-44 & GB-43)

Indications:
- numbness &/or inflammation of the foot or toes, snakebite, peripheral neuritis; headache, toothache, stomach pain; irregular menses; malaria

(NCCAOM 30)

51. 氣 端   **Qì Duān = Extremity of Qi / Qi to Extremities**   (WHO 47)

Location:
- 5 points on each foot - at the center of the end of each toe (analogous to Shi Xuan)

Indications:
- syncope, apoplectic coma; inflam. of the foot, beriberi, numbness or paralysis of the toes

* Because there are two names for 3 points there are actually only 51 points instead of 54.
   I include Qi Pang under San Jiao Jiu for the purposes of this list/text. (see #25)

NCCAOM Points Not Illustrated

Head, Face & Neck

 # 2 Dang Yang   *is labeled, but has no dot*   • lies betw GB-15 & 16

 # 13 Jia Cheng Jiang = Beside For Sauce/Saliva   • either side of CV-24 (Cheng Jiang)

 # 14 Qian Zheng   = Pull Correct   • side of face in masseter m.

 # 16 An Mian   = Tranquil/Peaceful Sleep   • behind Yi Ming

 # 17 Shang Lian Quan = Upper Ridge Spring   • upper CV-23 (Lian Quan)
                Spring above the Ridge (i.e. hyoid b.)

Abdomen

 # 25 San Jiao Jiu   = 3 Angles = Triangle   • 3 points, forming an equilateral triangle
    NCCAOM 33   for Moxa   with the apex of the triangle at the umbilicus
                  or Moxa Triangle   the base and sides being one mouth width each
    aka **Qi Pang**   = Beside the Navel   • the two points that form the base
    NCCAOM 31

 # 26 Ti Tuo (Xue) = Lift & Support   • 4 cun lateral to CV-4

Upper Extremity

 # 28 Jian Qian   = Shoulder Front   • anterior shoulder ~1 cun above axillary crease

 # 28a Jian Nei Ling = Shoulder Inner Mound   • above Jian Qian (midway between crease & LI-15)

 # 30 Bi Zhong   = (Fore)arm Middle/Center   • midpoint of the anterior forearm (on Pc, prox. to Pc-4)

Lower Extremity

 # 41 Huan Zhong = Circle Middle   • near and named for GB-30 (Huan Tiao)

* On the following pages most of the Extra Pt locations are illustrated.
   You should draw in and label the missing points.

Head & Neck (HN)
(13 pts)

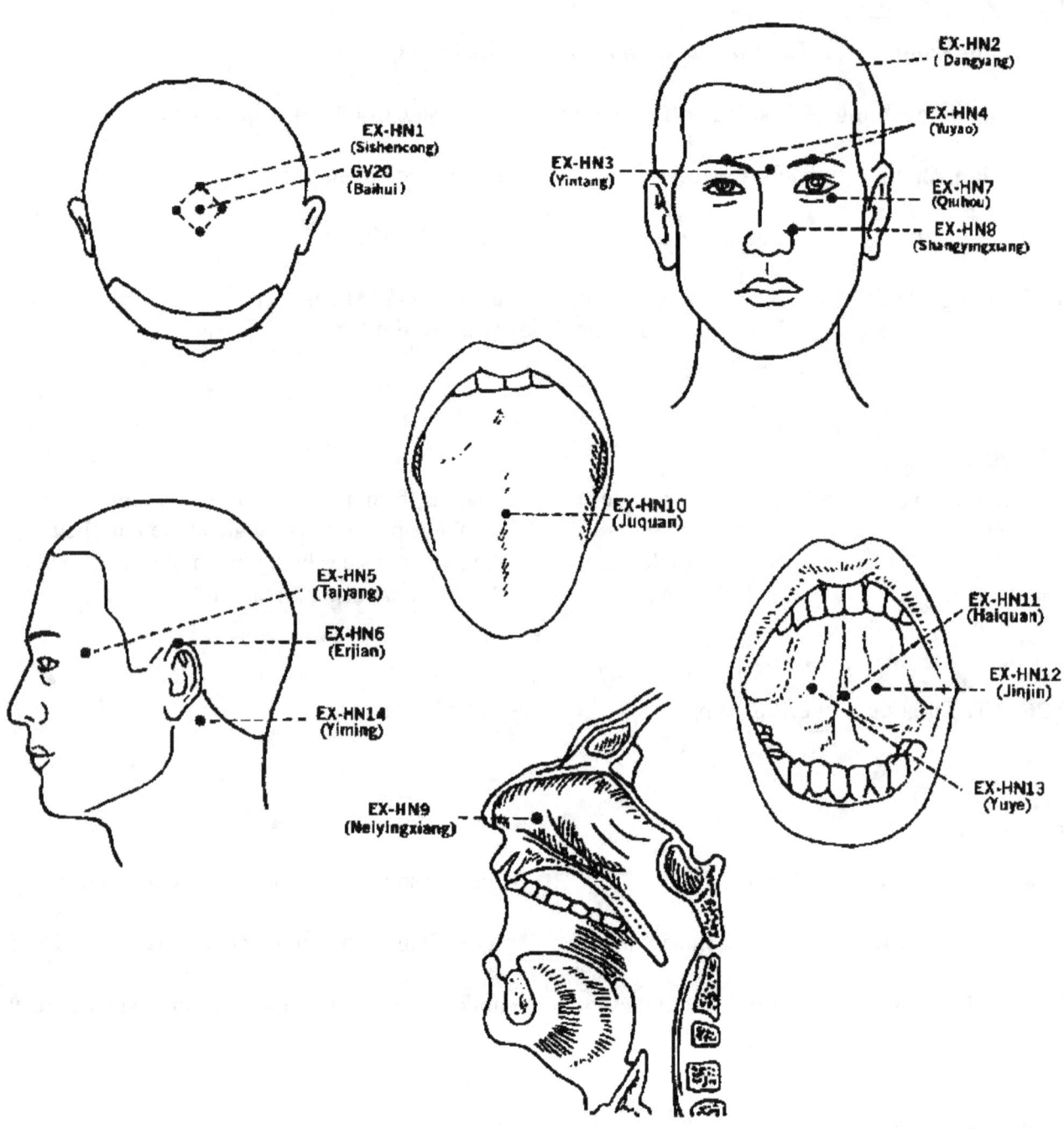

EX-HN1
(Sishencong)

GV20
(Baihui)

EX-HN2
(Dangyang)

EX-HN4
(Yuyao)

EX-HN3
(Yintang)

EX-HN7
(Qiuhou)

EX-HN8
(Shangyingxiang)

EX-HN10
(Juquan)

EX-HN5
(Taiyang)

EX-HN6
(Erjian)

EX-HN11
(Haiquan)

EX-HN12
(Jinjin)

EX-HN14
(Yiming)

EX-HN13
(Yuye)

EX-HN9
(Neiyingxiang)

These numbers ONLY COINCIDENTALLY correspond to the numbers in the text – Use names for ID.

Back & Waist (B or BW)

(9 pts + 1 HN)

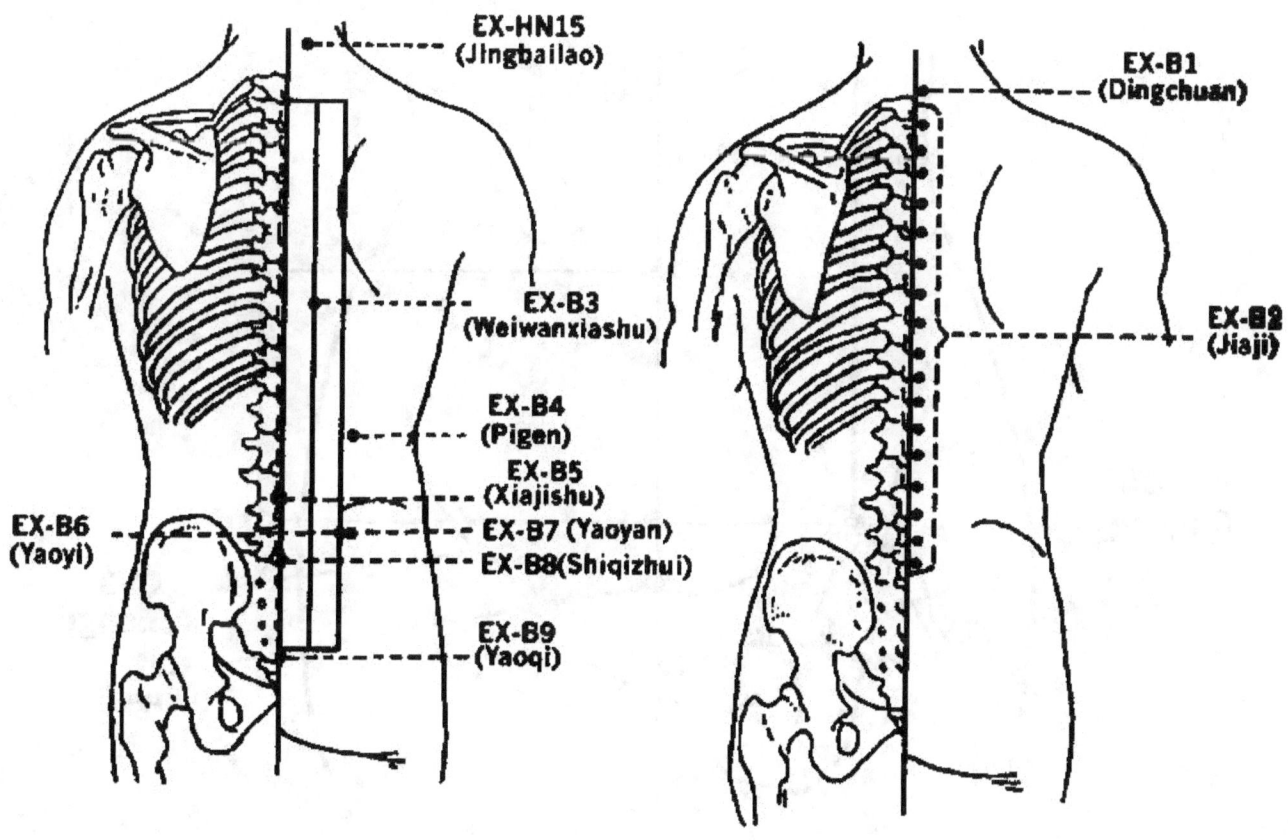

EX-HN15
(Jingbailao)

EX-B1
(Dingchuan)

EX-B3
(Weiwanxiashu)

EX-B2
(Jiaji)

EX-B4
(Pigen)

EX-B5
(Xiajishu)

EX-B6
(Yaoyi)

EX-B7 (Yaoyan)

EX-B8(Shiqizhui)

EX-B9
(Yaoqi)

These numbers DO NOT correspond to the numbers in the text – Use names for ID.

Chest & Abdomen (CA)

(1 pt)

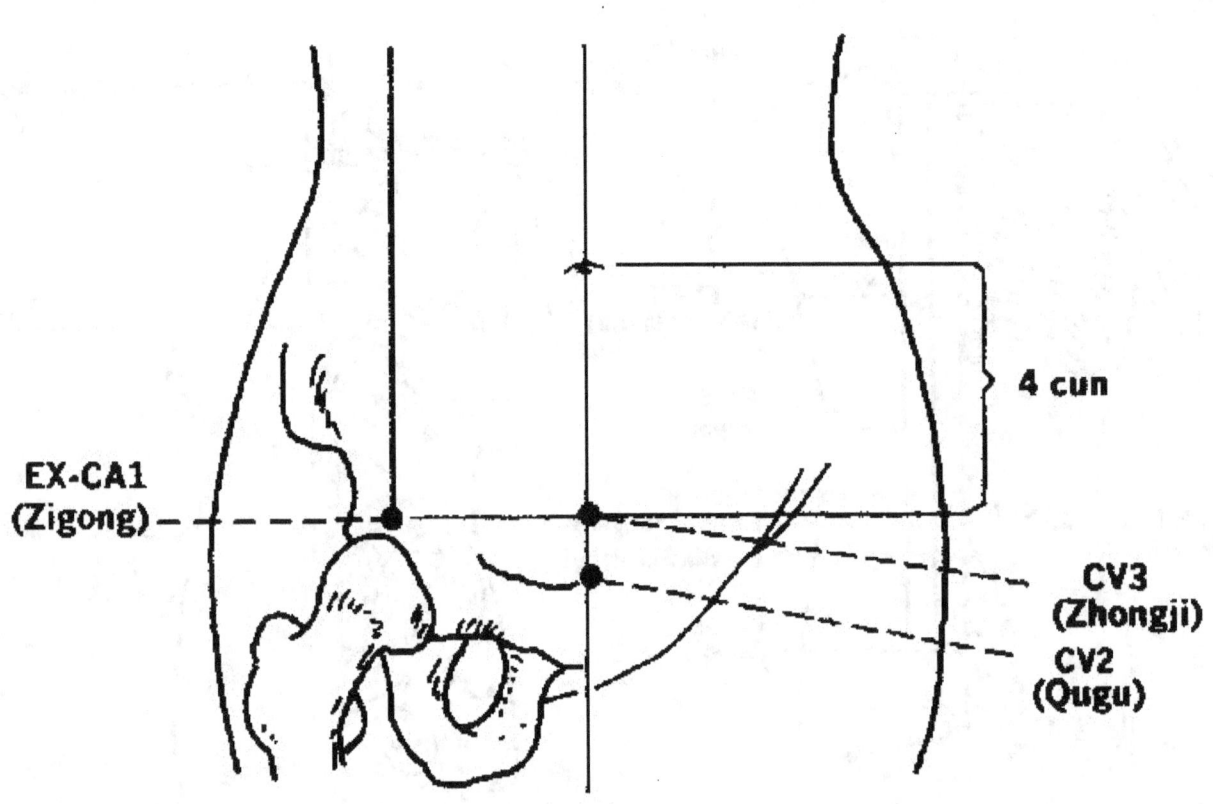

EX-CA1 (Zigong)

4 cun

CV3 (Zhongji)

CV2 (Qugu)

These numbers DO NOT correspond to the numbers in the text – Use names for ID.

Upper Extremity (UE)

(11 pts)

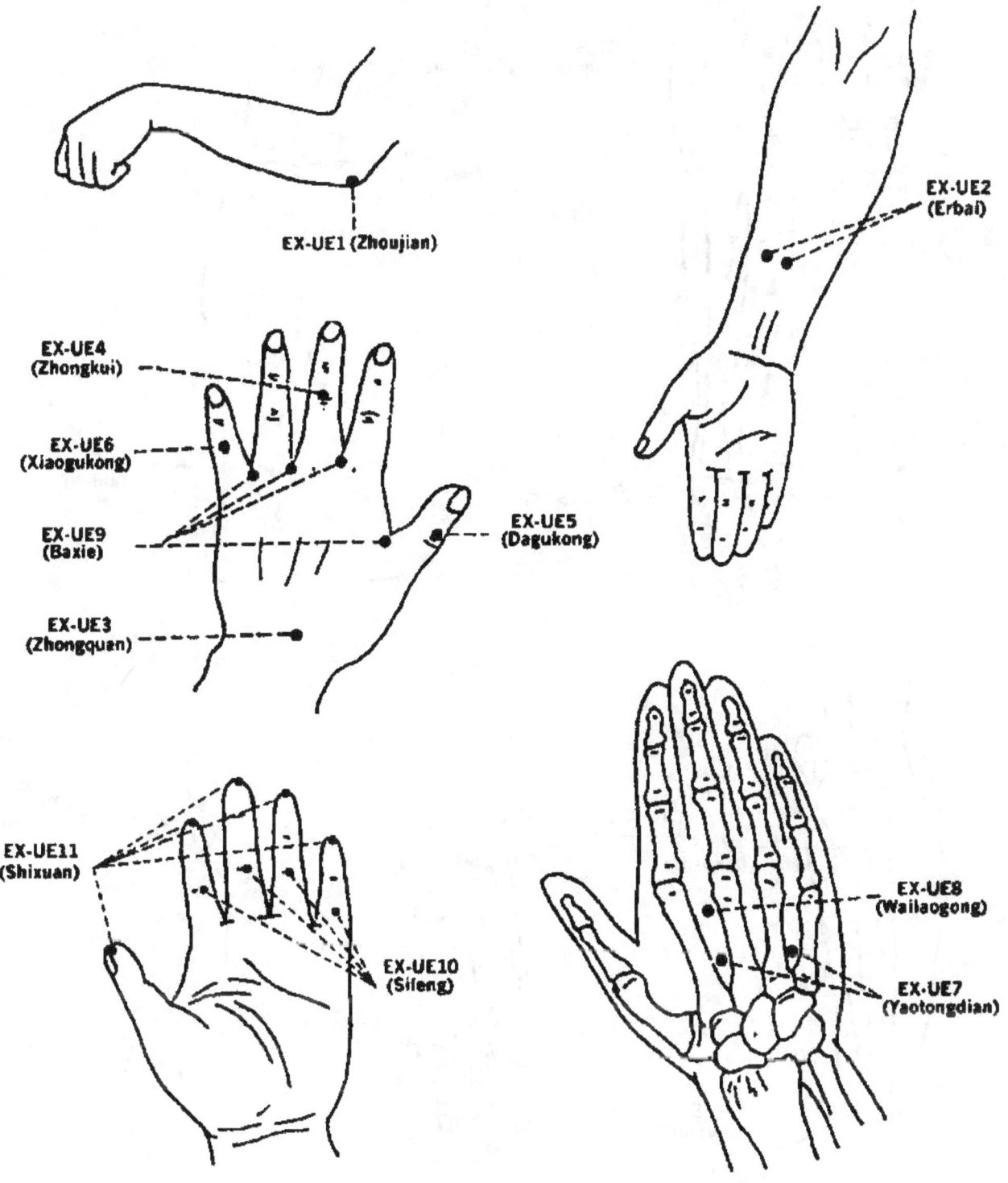

EX-UE1 (Zhoujian)

EX-UE2 (Erbai)

EX-UE4 (Zhongkui)

EX-UE6 (Xiaogukong)

EX-UE9 (Baxie)

EX-UE5 (Dagukong)

EX-UE3 (Zhongquan)

EX-UE11 (Shixuan)

EX-UE10 (Sifeng)

EX-UE8 (Wailaogong)

EX-UE7 (Yaotongdian)

These numbers DO NOT correspond to the numbers in the text – Use names for ID.

Lower Extremity (LE)
(12 pts)

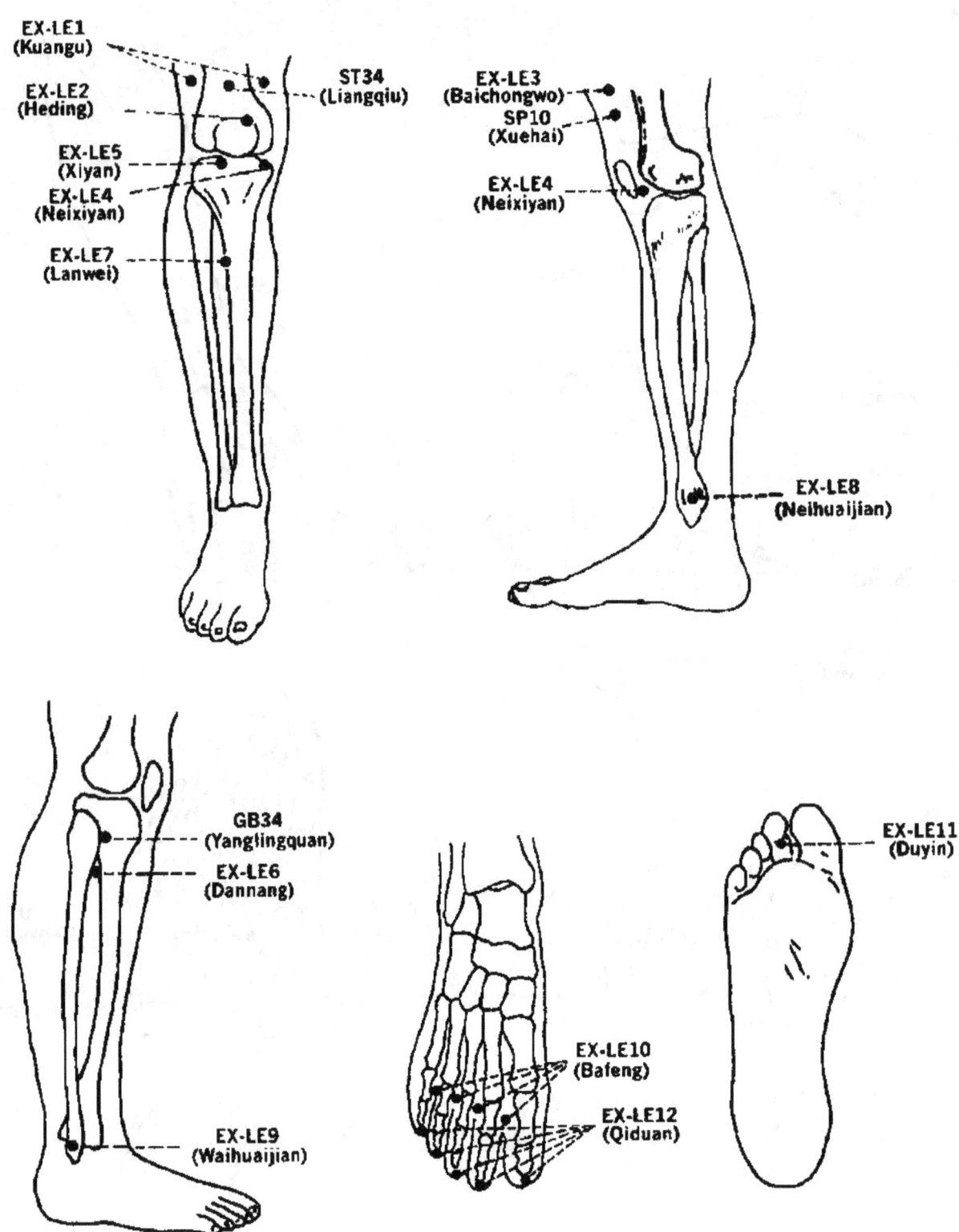

EX-LE1
(Kuangu)

EX-LE2
(Heding)

ST34
(Liangqiu)

EX-LE5
(Xiyan)

EX-LE4
(Neixiyan)

EX-LE7
(Lanwei)

EX-LE3
(Baichongwo)

SP10
(Xuehai)

EX-LE4
(Neixiyan)

EX-LE8
(Neihuaijian)

GB34
(Yanglingquan)

EX-LE6
(Dannang)

EX-LE9
(Waihuaijian)

EX-LE10
(Bafeng)

EX-LE12
(Qiduan)

EX-LE11
(Duyin)

These numbers DO NOT correspond to the numbers in the text – Use names for ID.

Appendix

A

Body Region Tables

These tables show the position of the points relative to one another
(i.e. which points are at the same level)

Arm – Yin Channels (anterior arm)

compartment }	radial	middle	ulnar	{ compartment
Landmarks & Measurements	**LU**	**PC**	**HT**	*Landmarks & Measurements*
chest	**Lu-2** (inf to clavicle) **Lu-1** (level w/ 1st ICS)	**Pc-1** (4th ICS, supralat to nipple)		chest
axillary fold 0 cun			**Ht-1** (armpit)	axillary fold 9 cun
1 cun *distal* ⬇				8 cun
2 cun		Pc-2		7 cun
3 cun	**Lu-3**			6 cun
4 cun	**Lu-4**			5 cun
5 cun				4 cun
6 cun			**Ht-2**	3 cun
7 cun				2 cun
8 cun				⬆ *proximal* 1 cun
9 cun cubital fold 0 cun	**Lu-5** (radial to biceps tendon)	**Pc-3** (ulnar to biceps tendon)	**Ht-3** (radial to med. epicondyle)	0 cun cubital fold 12 cun
1 cun *distal* ⬇				11 cun
2 cun				10 cun
3 cun				9 cun
4 cun				8 cun
5 cun	**Lu-6**			7 cun
6 cun				6 cun
7 cun		**Pc-4**		5 cun
8 cun				4 cun
9 cun		**Pc-5**		3 cun
10 cun		**Pc-6**		2 cun
10.5 cun	**Lu-7**		**Ht-4**	1.5 cun
11 cun	**Lu-8**		**Ht-5**	1 cun
11.5 cun			**Ht-6**	⬆ *proximal* 0.5 c
12 cun wrist fold	**Lu-9**	**Pc-7**	**Ht-7**	0 cun wrist fold
palm	**Lu-10** (mid-pt. 1st metacarpal)	**Pc-8** (betw metacarpals 2 & 3)	**Ht-8** (betw. metacarpals 4 & 5)	palm
nail pt	**Lu-11** (thumb: radial side)	**Pc-9** alt loc: (3rd finger tip)	**Ht-9** (sm. finger: radial side)	nail pt

Arm – Yin Channels (anterior arm)

Lu   Pc   Ht

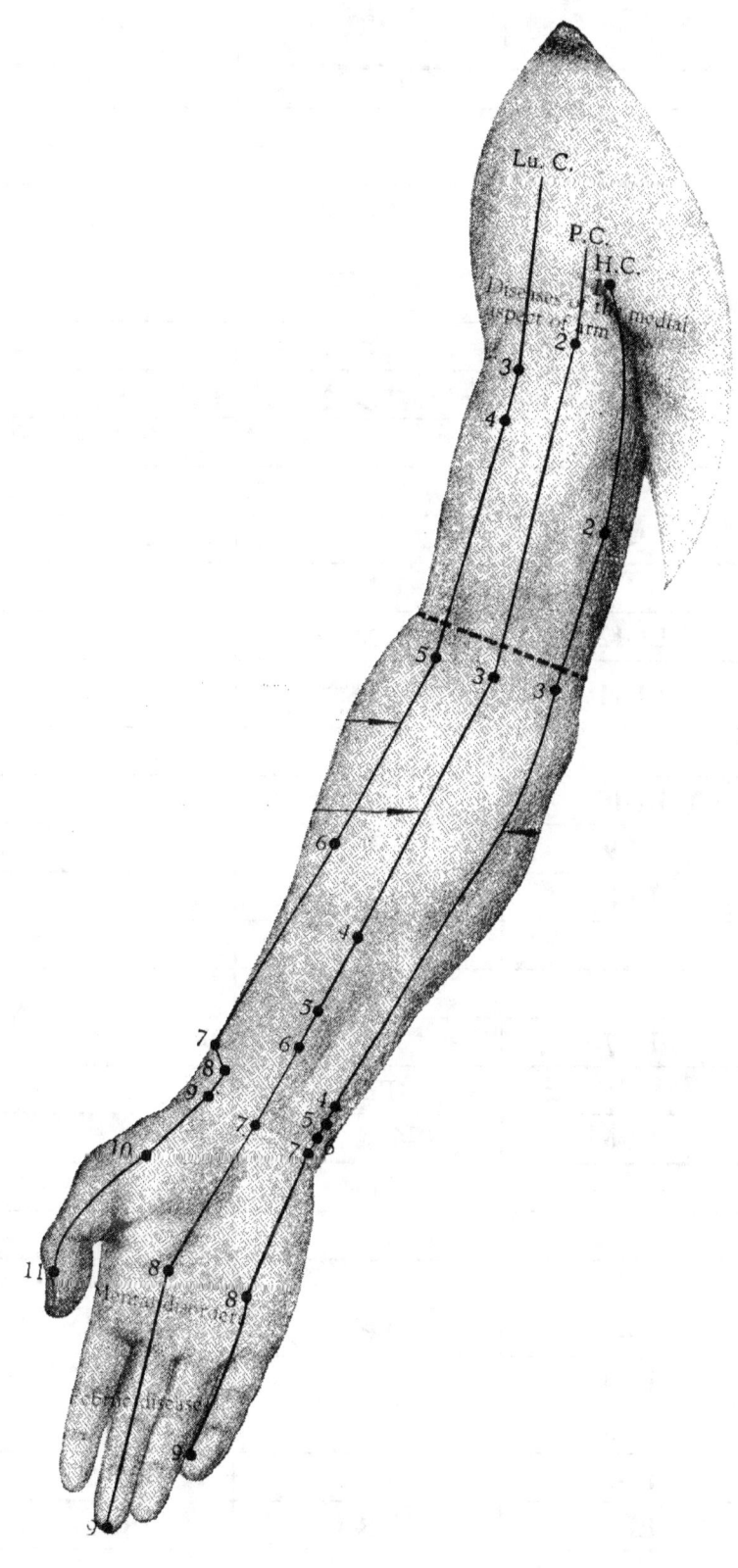

Lu   Pc   Ht

Arm – Yang Channels (posterior arm)

compartment }	radial	middle	ulnar	{ compartment
Landmarks & Measurements	**LI**	**TB**	**SI**	**Landmarks & Measurements**
0 cun = acromion	**LI-15**	**TB-14**	**SI-10**	**acromion** ~ 4 cun
~1 cun				~3 cun
~2 cun				~2 cun
~3 cun		~**TB-13**	**SI-9**	~1 cun
0 c = **axillary fold**				**axillary fold** = 9 c
1 cun *distal* ⬇				8 cun
2 cun	~**LI-14**			7 cun
3 cun		~**TB-12**		6 cun
4 cun				5 cun
5 cun				4 cun
6 cun	**LI-13**			3 cun
7 cun		**TB-11**		2 cun
8 cun	**LI-12**	**TB-10** (90° flexion)		1 cun
9 cun / 0 = **elbow**	**LI-11**	**TB-10** (full extension) tip of olecranon	**SI-8**	**elbow** = 0 / 12 cun
1 cun				11 cun
2 cun	**LI-10**			10 cun
3 cun	**LI-9**			9 cun
4 cun	**LI-8**			8 cun
5 cun		**TB-9**		7 cun
6 cun				6 cun
7 cun	**LI-7**		**SI-7**	5 cun
8 cun		**TB-8**		4 cun
9 cun	**LI-6**	**TB-6 & TB-7**		3 cun
10 cun		**TB-5**		2 cun
10.5 cun			~**SI-6**	1.5 cun
11 cun				⬆ *proximal* 1 cun
12 cun = **wrist**	**LI-5**	**TB-4**	**SI-5**	**wrist** = 0 cun
hand	**LI-4**		**SI-4**	hand
prox. to MP jt	**LI-3**	**TB-3**	**SI-3**	prox. to MP jt
distal to MP jt	**LI-2**	**TB-2**	**SI-2**	distal to MP jt
nail pt	**LI-1**	**TB-1**	**SI-1**	nail pt

Arm – Yang Channels (posterior arm)

SI   TB   LI

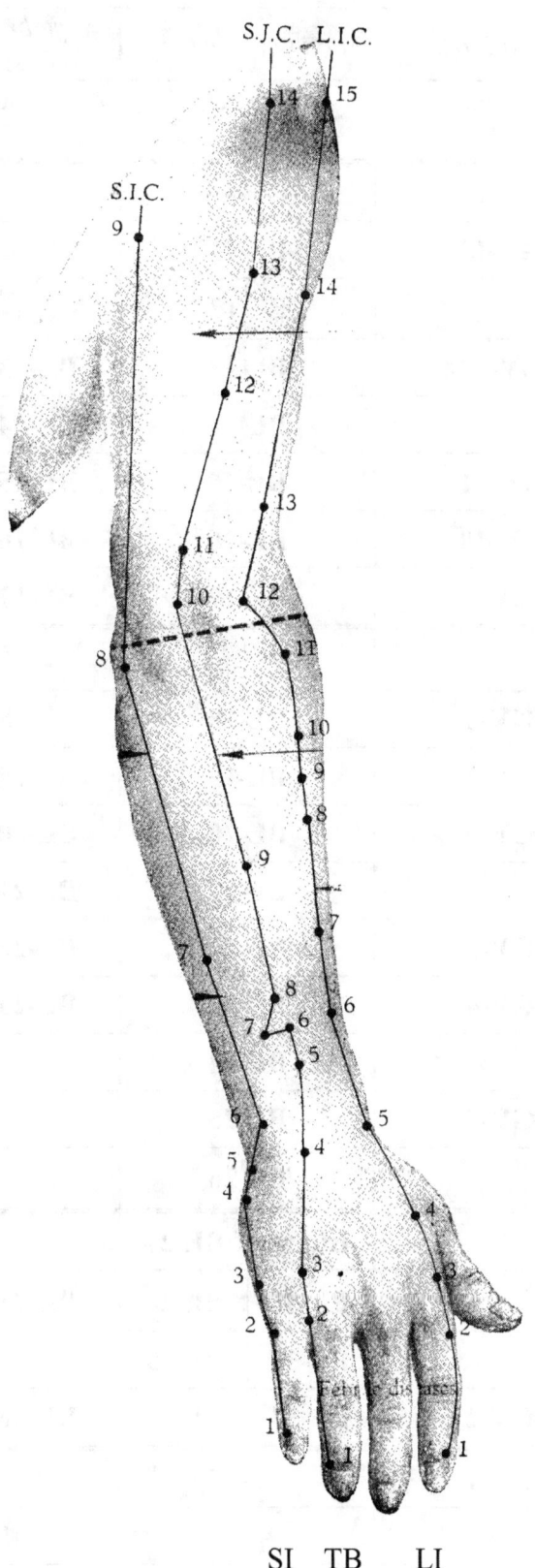

SI   TB   LI

Torso-Back – GV & BL Channels

Measure }	0.0 cun	1.5 cun		3.0 cun	
Vertebral Level	midline	crest of erectors		vertebral border of scapula	
below spinous process of:	Du mai **GV**	inner **BL**		outer **BL**	Shu point Corresponds to:
C7	**GV-14**				
T1	**GV-13**	**BL-11**		**SI-14**	bones
T2		**BL-12**		JC / SH / BJ # **BL-12a**/36/41	wind
T3	**GV-12**	**BL-13**		**BL-13a**/37/42	**Lung**
T4		**BL-14**		**BL-14a**/38/43	**Peric**
T5	**GV-11**	**BL-15**		**BL-15a**/39/44	**Heart**
T6	**GV-10**	**BL-16**		**BL-16a**/40/45	GV
T7	**GV-9**	**BL-17**		**BL-17a**/41/46	diaphragm
T8		**Extra Pt:** Yi Shu			pancreas
T9	**GV-8**	**BL-18**		**BL-18a**/42/47	**Liver**
T10	**GV-7**	**BL-19**		**BL-19a**/43/48	**Gall Bladder**
T11	**GV-6**	**BL-20**		**BL-20a**/44/49	**Spleen**
T12		**BL-21**		**BL-21a**/45/50	**Stomach**
L1	**GV-5**	**BL-22**		**BL-22a**/46/51	**TB** (lower jiao)
L2	**GV-4**	**BL-23**		**BL-23a**/47/52	**Kidney**
L3		**BL-24**			CV-6 shu
L4	**GV-3**	**BL-25**			**Lg. Intestine**
L5	**Extra Pt:** Shi Qi Zhui Xia	**BL-26**			CV-4 shu
S1		**BL-31**	**BL-27**		**Sm. Intestine**
S2	**Extra Pt:** Yao Qi	**BL-32**	**BL-28**	**BL-28a**/48/53	**Bladder**
S3		**BL-33**	**BL-29**		spine & erectors
S4	**GV-2**	**BL-34**	**BL-30**	**BL-30a**/49/54	anus/rectum
tip of coccyx	**GV-1**	**BL-35**			Du mai & yang
perineum	CV-1				Ren mai & yin

Key: JC = Jim / SH = Shanghai / BJ = Beijing

Torso-Back – GV, BL, (& SI) Channels

GV BL TB SI GB   SI LI   TB (ignore arrows)

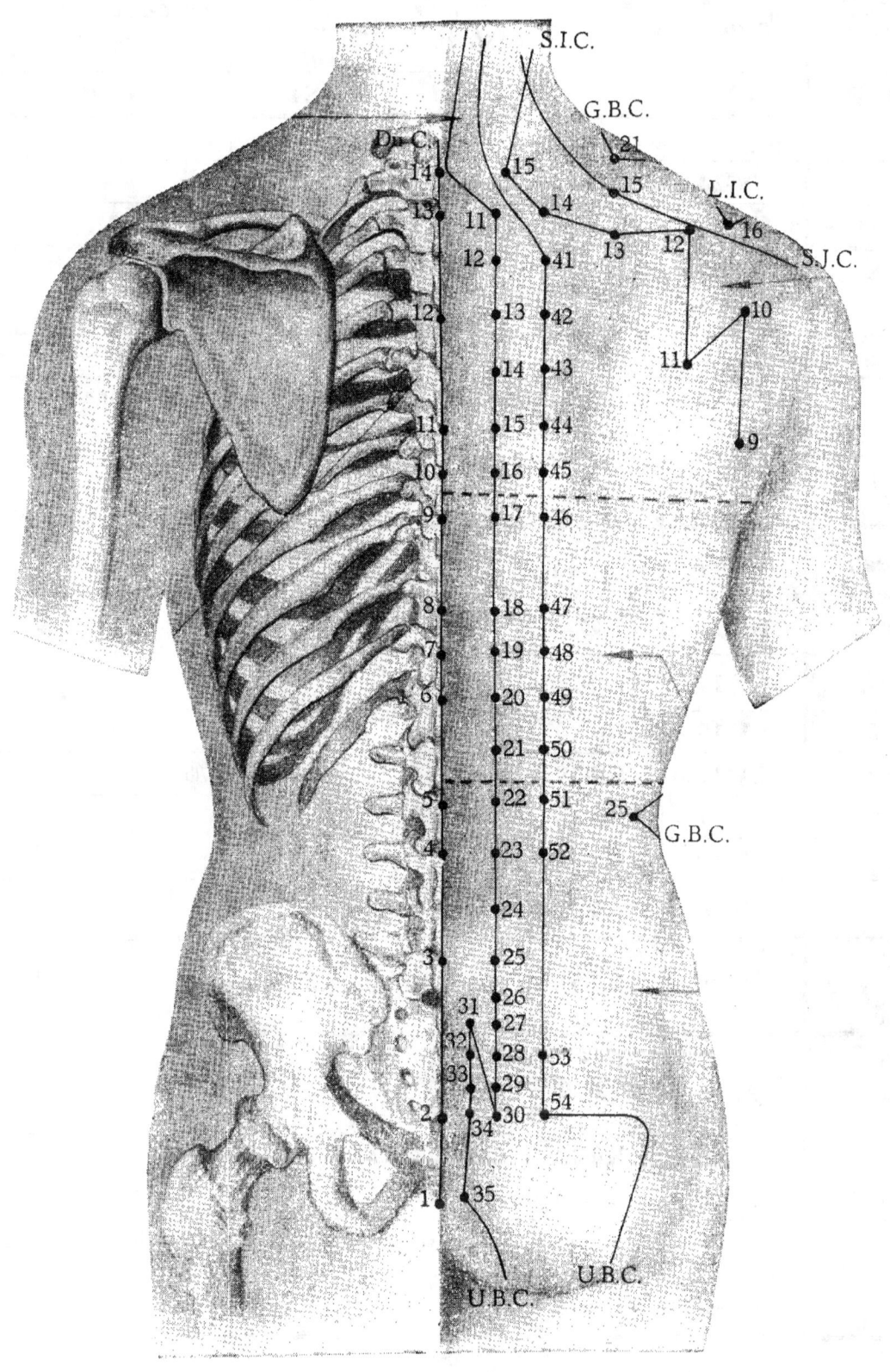

GV   BL   BL GB SI

Torso-Front – Chest & Abdomen

Measure }	0.0 cun	1.0 cun	2.0 cun	4.0 cun	6.0 cun	8.0 cun
Chest	*midline*		*lat. to sternum*	*mid-clavicle line*	*delto-pectoral triangle*	*mid-axillary line*
channel }	**CV**		**Kd**	**ST**	**LU & SP**	
supra-clavicular fossa				**ST-12**		
sternal notch	**CV-22**					
inf. clavicle	**CV-21**		**Kd-27**	**ST-13**	**Lu-2**	
1st ICS	**CV-20**		**Kd-26**	**ST-14**	**Lu-1**	**Ht-1**
2nd ICS	**CV-19**		**Kd-25**	**ST-15**	**Sp-20**	
3rd ICS	**CV-18**		**Kd-24**	**ST-16**	**Sp-19**	
4th ICS	**CV-17**		**Kd-23**	**ST-17** (nipple)	**Pc-1 / Sp-18** (5 cun lat.)	**GB-23 / 22**
5th ICS *xipho-sternal jct* 0 / 8 cun	**CV-16**		**Kd-22**	**ST-18**	**Sp-17**	
Abdomen	*midline*	**Kd** 0.5 – 1.0	**ST** *mid rectus*	**Sp** *lat rectus*		*mid-axillary line*
1 / 7 cun	**CV-15**	Ø				**Sp-21** (7th ICS)
2 / 6 cun	**CV-14**	**Kd-21**	**ST-19**	**Lr-14** (6th ICS)		
3 / 5 cun	**CV-13**	**Kd-20**	**ST-20**			
4 / 4 cun	**CV-12**	**Kd-19**	**ST-21**	**GB-24**	(7th ICS)	
5 / 3 cun	**CV-11**	**Kd-18**	**ST-22**	**Sp-16**		
6 / 2 cun	**CV-10**	**Kd-17**	**ST-23**			
7 / 1 cun	**CV-9**	Ø	**ST-24**			**Lr-13** (11th rib)
8 / 0 cun *umbilicus* 0 / 5 cun	**CV-8**	**Kd-16**	**ST-25**	**Sp-15**		**GB-26**
1 / 4 cun	**CV-7**	**Kd-15**	**ST-26**			
1.5 / 3.5 cun	**CV-6**			**Sp-14** (1.3 ↓)		
2 / 3 cun	**CV-5**	**Kd-14**	**ST-27**			
3 / 2 cun	**CV-4**	**Kd-13**	**ST-28**		**GB-27**	
4 / 1 cun	**CV-3**	**Kd-12**	**ST-29**	**Sp-13** (0.7 ↑)	**GB-28**	
5 / 0 cun *pubic crest*	**CV-2**	**Kd-11**	**ST-30** pubic tubercle	**Sp-12** (3.5 lateral)		
0.5 cun			**Lr-12** (2.5 lat.)			

Torso-Front – Chest & Abdomen

Pc   Lu   ST   Kd   CV

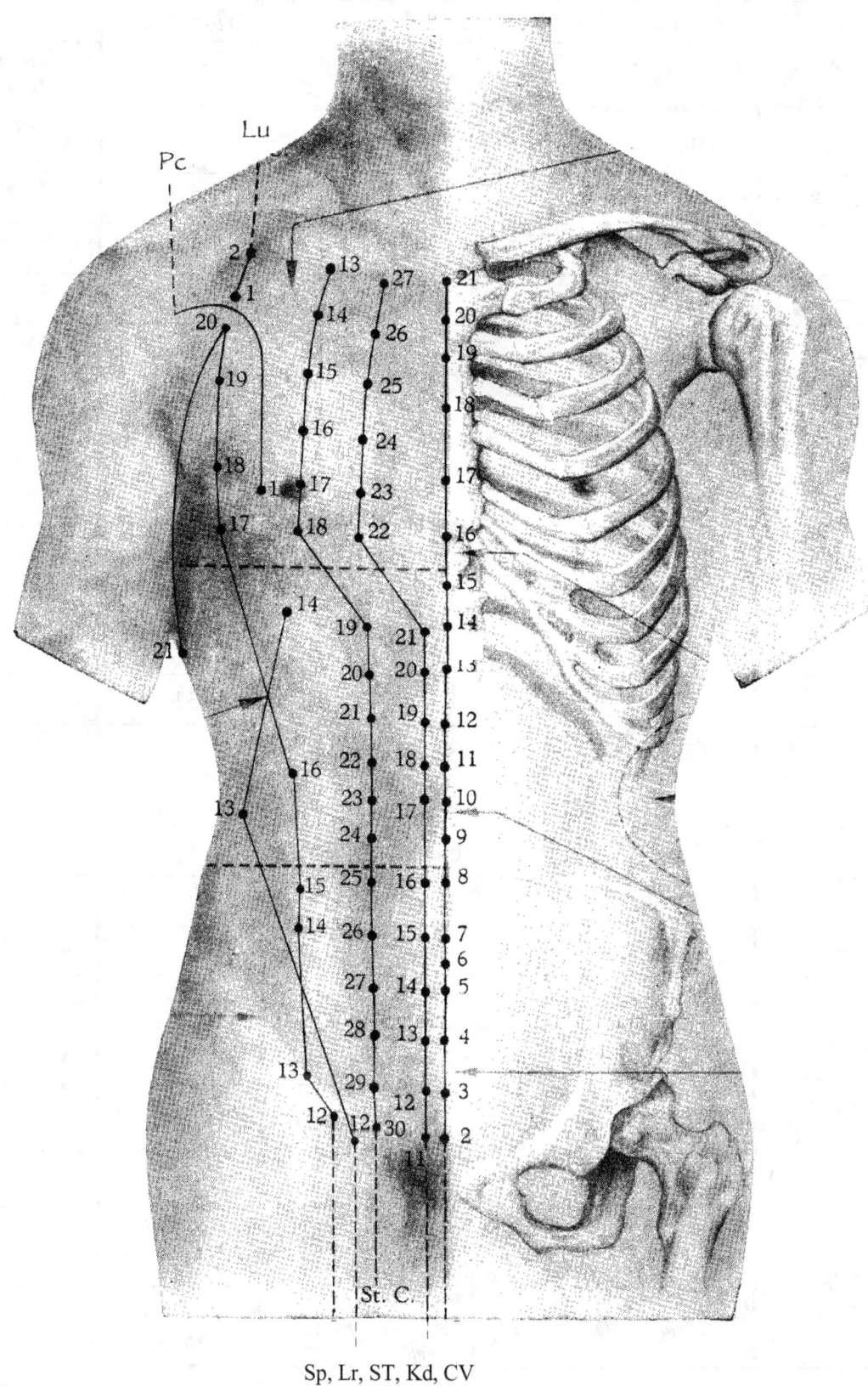

Sp, Lr, ST, Kd, CV

© 1990–2016   *Jim Cleaver LAc.*

Thigh – Yang Channels
(yang aspects – lateral & posterior)

compartment }	anterior thigh	lateral thigh	posterior thigh	{ compartment
Landmarks & Measurements	**ST**	**GB**	**BL**	**Landmarks & Measurements**
sup. **trochanter** 0 cun	ST-30			sup. **trochanter** 19 cun
1 cun *distal* ⬇				18 cun
2 cun				17 cun
3 cun	~ **ST-31**			16 cun
4 cun	~ **ST-31**			15 cun
5 cun	~ **ST-31**		**BL-50**	gluteal fold = 14 cun
6 cun				13 cun
7 cun				12 cun
8 cun				11 cun
9 cun				10 cun
10 cun				9 cun
11 cun			**BL-51**	8 cun
12 cun	**ST-32** (6 cun)	**GB-31**		7 cun
13 cun				6 cun
14 cun		**GB-32**		5 cun
15 cun	**ST-33** (3 cun)			4 cun
16 cun	**ST-34** (2 cun)			3 cun
17 cun				2 cun
18 cun = sup. patella ~ lat. epicond.		~**GB-33**	**BL-52**	⬆ *proximal* 1 cun
19 cun = **popl. cr.** mid patella			**BL-54** / **BL-53**	**popl. cr.** = 0 cun
inf. patella	**ST-35**			
patella is regarded to be 2 cun in height	ST points are measured from the top of patella	GB points are measured from popliteal crease	BL pts are measured betw gluteal fold & popliteal crease	
	on line between ASIS and supra-lateral patella	on line between trochanter and lateral knee	flows between hamstrings	

Thigh – Yang Channels

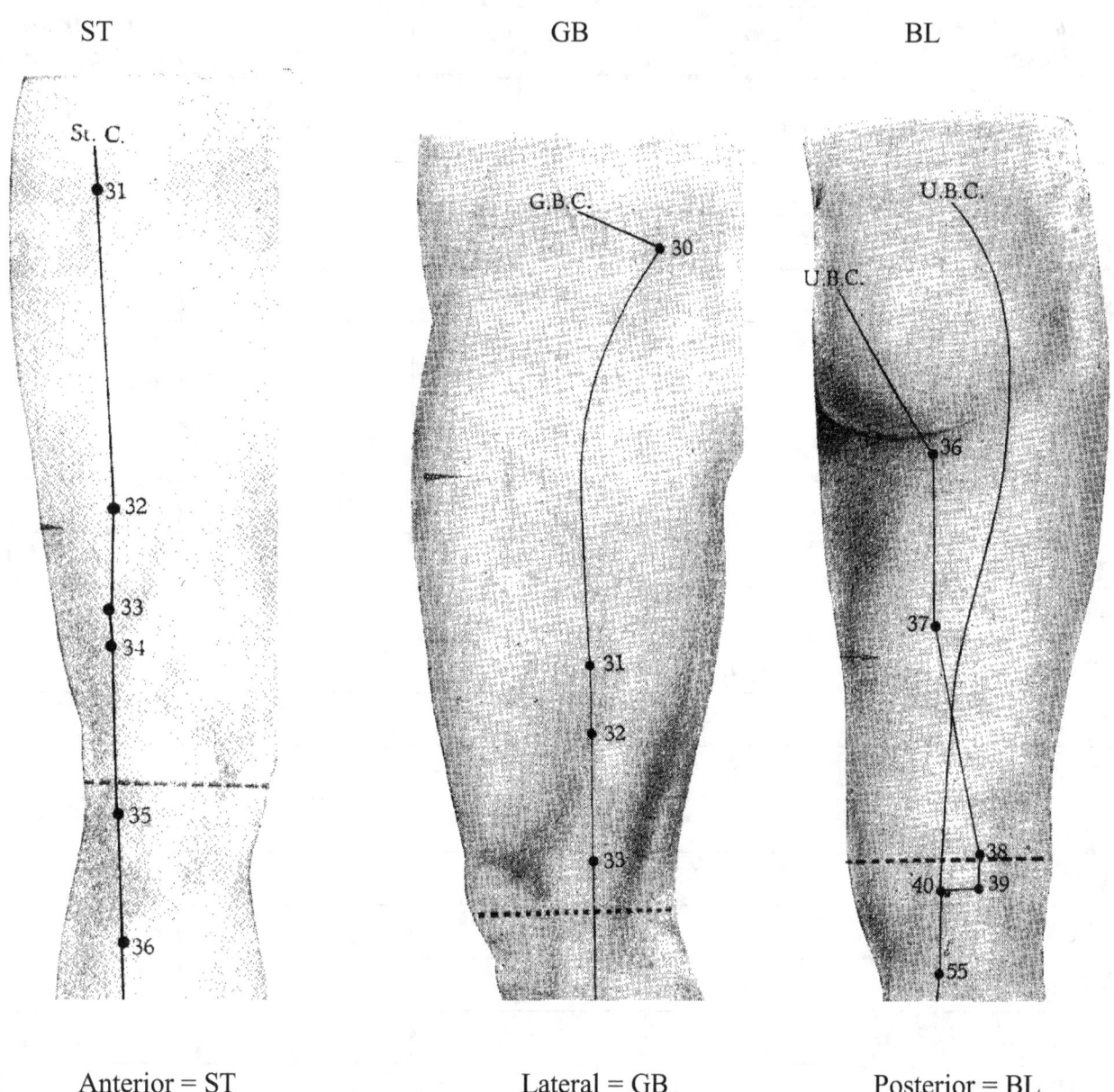

ST   GB   BL

Anterior = ST   Lateral = GB   Posterior = BL

Thigh – Yin Channels (medial aspect)

compartment }	anterior thigh	medial thigh	posterior thigh	{ compartment
Landmarks & Measurements	**SP**	**LR**	**Kd**	**Landmarks & Measurements**
pubic crest 0 cun	Sp-12 (3.5 lateral to midline)	**Lr-12** (0.5 cun inferior) (2.5 lateral to midline)	Kd-11 (0.5 lateral to midline)	**pubic crest** 18 cun
1 cun *distal* ⬇				17 cun
2 cun		**Lr-11**		16 cun
3 cun		**Lr-10**		15 cun
4 cun				14 cun
5 cun				13 cun
6 cun				12 cun
7 cun				11 cun
8 cun				10 cun
9 cun				9 cun
10 cun	**Sp-11**			8 cun
11 cun				7 cun
12 cun				6 cun
13 cun				5 cun
14 cun		**Lr-9**		4 cun
15 cun				3 cun
16 cun	**Sp-10**			2 cun
17 cun				⬆ *proximal* 1 cun
18 cun **medial epicondyle**				0 cun **medial epicondyle**
popliteal crease		Lr-8	Kd-10	popliteal crease

Thigh – Yin Channels (medial aspect)

Sp   Lr   Kd

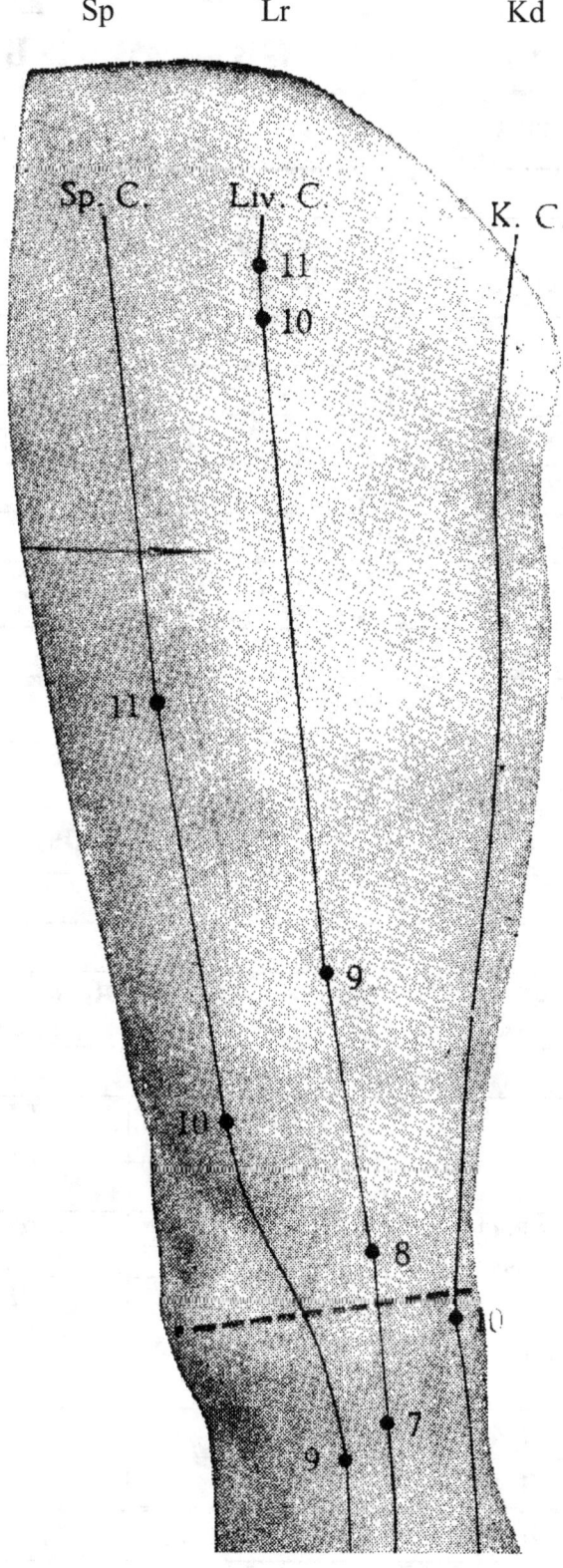

Sp. C.   Liv. C.   K. C.

Sp   Lr   Kd

© 1990–2016   Jim Cleaver LAc.

Leg – Yang Channels
(yang aspects – lateral & posterior)

compartment }	anterior leg	lateral leg	posterior leg	{ compartment
Landmarks & Measurements	**ST**	**GB**	**BL**	**Landmarks & Measurements**
popliteal crease 0 cun = inf patella	**ST-35**		**BL-53 / BL-54**	**popliteal crease** 16 cun
1 cun **distal** ⬇				15 cun
2 cun		**GB-34**	**BL-55**	14 cun
3 cun	**ST-36**			13 cun
4 cun				12 cun
5 cun			**BL-56**	11 cun
6 cun	**ST-37**			10 cun
7 cun				9 cun
8 cun	**ST-38 / ST-40**		**BL-57**	8 cun
9 cun	**ST-39**	**GB-36 / GB-35** (ant. to fib. / post to fib.)	**BL-58**	7 cun
10 cun				6 cun
11 cun		**GB-37** (ant. to fibula)		5 cun
12 cun		**GB-38** (ant. to fibula)		4 cun
13 cun		**GB-39** (ant. or post. to fibula)	**BL-59**	3 cun
14 cun				2 cun
15 cun				⬆ *proximal* 1 cun
16 cun **lateral malleolus**	**ST-41** (midway betw malleolii)		**BL-60** (post. to malleolus)	0 cun **lateral malleolus**

ankle		**GB-40** (sinus tarsi)	**BL-62** (inf. to malleolus)	**ankle**
			BL-61	**heel** 2.0 cun
dorsal foot	**ST-42** (cuneiforms)		**BL-63** (inf. to cuboid)	**lateral foot**
base of metatarsal		**GB-41**	**BL-64** (tuberosity of 5th)	
prox. to MP jt.	**ST-43** (mid shaft)	**GB-42**	**BL-65**	
distal to MP jt.	**ST-44**	**GB-43**	**BL-66**	
nail pt	**ST-45**	**GB-44**	**BL-67**	
	betw 2nd & 3rd	*betw 4th & 5th*	*lateral edge*	

Leg – Yang Channels

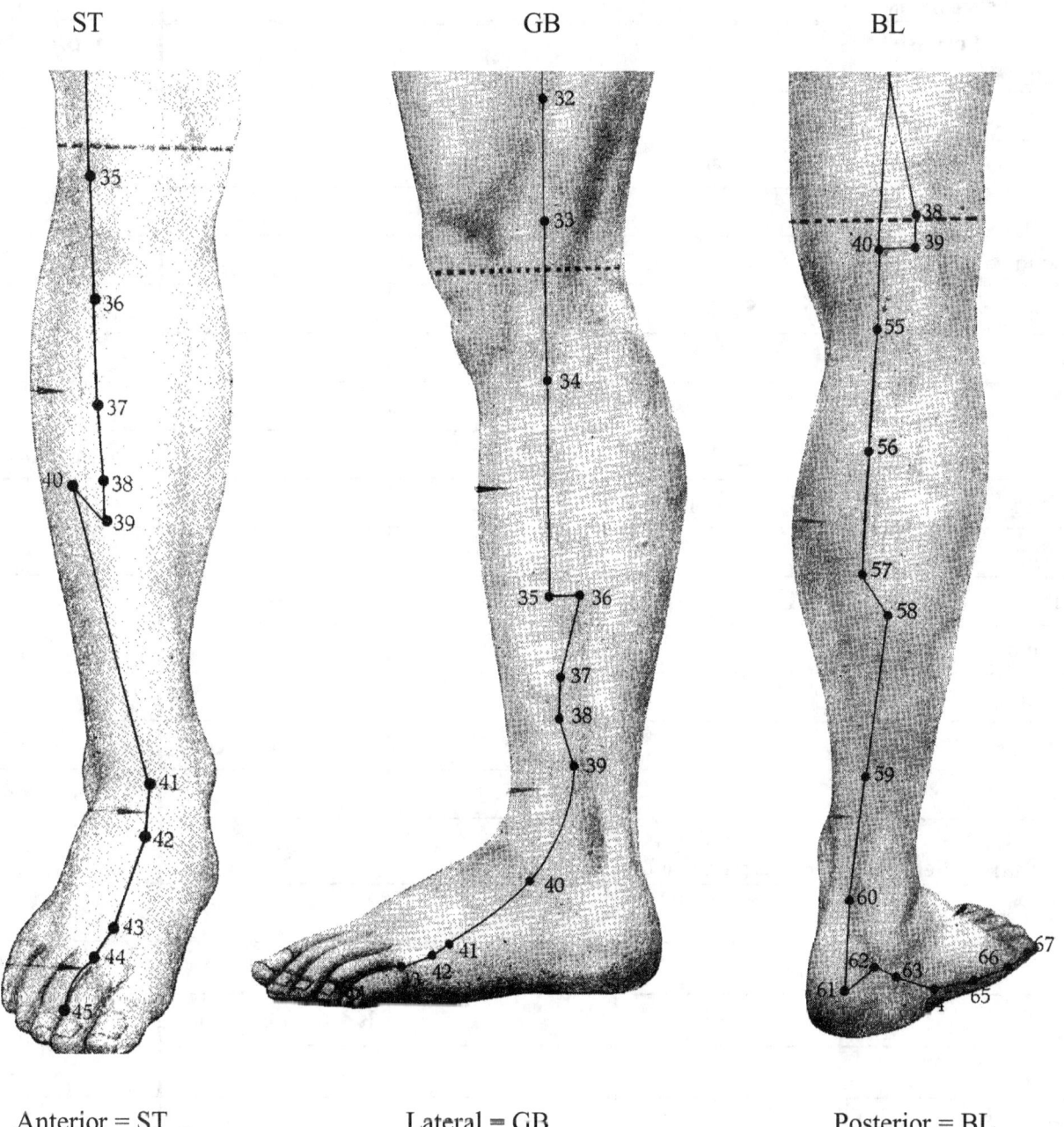

ST   GB   BL

Anterior = ST   Lateral = GB   Posterior = BL

Leg – Yin Channels (medial aspect)

compartment }	anterior leg	medial leg	posterior leg	{ compartment
Landmarks & Measurements	**SP**	**LR**	**Kd**	Landmarks & Measurements
popliteal crease 0 cun		**Lr-8**	**Kd-10**	**popliteal crease** 15 cun
1 cun *distal* ⬇				14 cun
2 cun	**Sp-9**	**Lr-7**		13 cun
3 cun				12 cun
4 cun				11 cun
5 cun	**Sp-8**			10 cun
6 cun				9 cun
7 cun				8 cun
color code }	**LR**	**SP**	**Kd**	{ color code
8 cun	**Lr-6** (on tibia)			7 cun
9 cun		**Sp-7** (post. to tibia)		6 cun
10 cun	**Lr-5** (on tibia)		**Kd-9**	5 cun
11 cun				4 cun
12 cun		**Sp-6** (post. to tibia)		3 cun
13 cun			**Kd-8 / Kd-7**	2 cun
14 cun				⬆ *proximal* 1 cun
15 cun **medial malleolus**	**Lr-4** (med. to ant. tibialis t.)		**Kd-3**	0 cun **medial malleolus**
ankle		**Sp-5** (ant. to post. tibialis t.)	**Kd-4**	0.5 cun
			Kd-5	1.0 cun
			Kd-6 (inf. to sust. tali)	
			Kd-2 (inf. to navicular)	
base of metatarsal		**Sp-4**		
prox. to MP jt.	**Lr-3**	**Sp-3**		
distal to MP jt.	**Lr-2**	**Sp-2**		
nail pt	**Lr-1** (lat. nail big toe)	**Sp-1** (med. nail big toe)	**Kd-0** (med. nail sm. toe)	
			Kd-1 (on the bottom of the foot)	

Leg – Yin Channels (medial aspect)

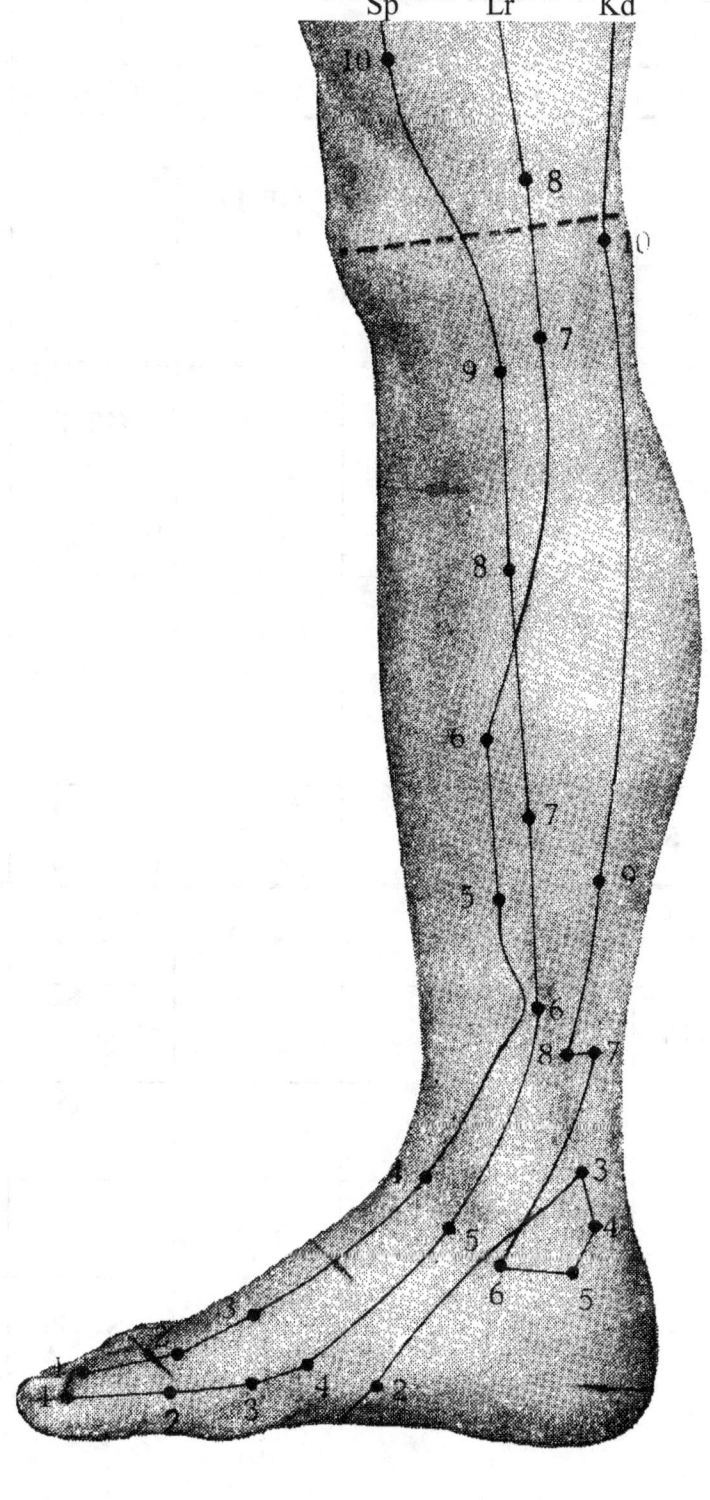

Sp   Lr   Kd

[Lr] / Sp   Kd

© 1990–2016   *Jim Cleaver LAc.*

Face – Anterior View: Front to Side of Face

Measurements }	*0.0 cun*	*0.75 cun*	*1.5 cun*	*2.25 cun*	*3.0 cun*	*4.5 cun*	
scalp divisions }	midline		1/3	1/2	2/3	3/3	
sagittal lines }		*inner canthus*		*pupil line*	*outer canthus*		*anterior ear line*
0.5 cun w/i hair	**GV-24**	**BL-3**	**BL-4**	**GB-15**	**GB-13**	**ST-8**	
anterior hairline							
forehead				**GB-14** (1 cun up)			**~GB-6** (1/4 up)
eyebrow, apex of ear	Yin Tang	**BL-2**		Yu Yao	**TB-23**	Tai Yang	**GB-7**
canthus, superior attachmt of ear		**BL-1**		*pupil*	**GB-1**	**GB-3**	*pre-auricular hairline* **TB-22**
inferior orbit				**ST-1**	Qiu Hou	*zygoma*	
infra-orbital foramen				**ST-2**			**TB-21**
mandibular notch, mid tragus		Bi Tong				**ST-7**	**SI-19**
tip of nose, mid nostril	**GV-25**	**LI-20**					
inferior to maxilla				**ST-3**	**SI-18**	Qian Zheng	**GB-2**
philtrum 1/3 inferior	**GV-26**	**LI-19**					
frenum/gum jct philtrum/lip jct	**GV-28** **GV-27**						
corner of mouth				**ST-4**		**ST-6**	
mento-labial groove	**CV-24**		Jia Cheng Jiang		**ST-5**		

Face – Anterior View

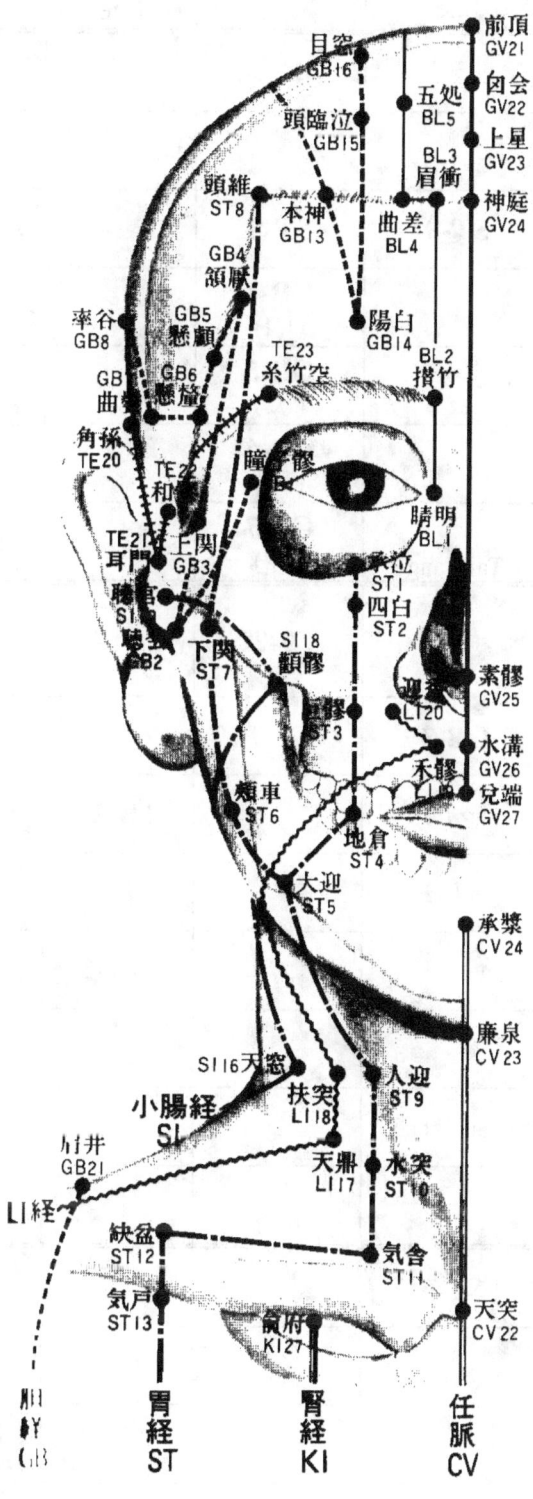

* GB-15 should be between GB-13 and BL-4

© 1990–2016   *Jim Cleaver LAc.*

Head – Lateral View: Side of Face & Head

Sagittal lines }	lateral eyebrow	ST-8 to ST-6 mid-sideburn line	ST-8 to GB-7 line	anterior ear line	apex of ear line	posterior ear line	posterior auricular hairline
scalp					GV-20		
					GB-18		
ant. hairline		ST-8	ST-8				
			GB-4 (1/4)				
side of head, above ear			GB-5 (1/2)		GB-8	GB-9	~ EOP level
			GB-6 (3/4)				
eyebrow, apex of ear	TB-23	Tai Yang	GB-7 (4/4)		TB-20		
outer canthus, superior ear attachment	GB-1		TB-22				GB-10
superior to zygoma		GB-3				TB-19	
supra-tragic notch		zygoma		TB-21			
mid tragus		ST-7		SI-19		TB-18	GB-11
infra-tragic notch	SI-18			GB-2			
earlobe					TB-17		
inferior ear attachment		Qian Zheng					
mastoid						GB-12	
corner of mouth (ST-4)		ST-6					
mento-labial groove	ST-5						
angle of jaw					SI-17 (ant to SCM)	TB-16 (post to SCM)	

Head – Lateral View: Side of Face & Head

GV: 20 21 22 23 24

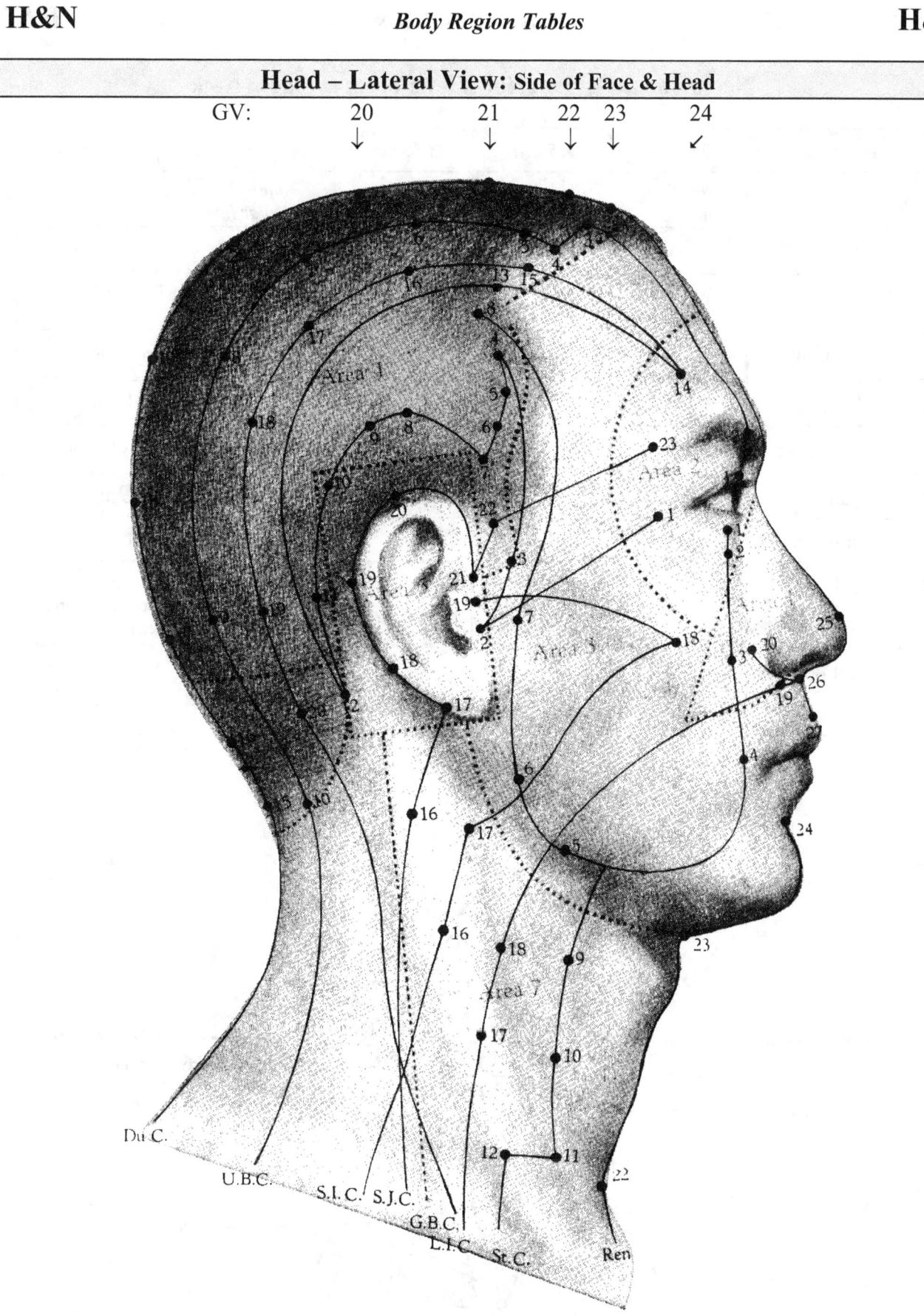

GV   BL   SI   TB   LI ST   CV

Neck/Throat – Anterior View: Front to Side of Neck

Measure }	0.0 cun	1.5 cun	3.0 cun	4.0 cun	{ Measure
	anterior midline	*lat. thyroid cartilage*		*mid-clavicular line*	
channel }	**CV**	**ST**			*{ channel*
mento-labial groove	CV-24	ST-5 (mid mandible)			mento-labial groove
angle of jaw			**SI-17** (ant. to SCM)	**TB-16** (post. to SCM)	angle of jaw
hyoid	**CV-23**				hyoid
laryngeal prom		**ST-9** (ant. to SCM)	**LI-18** (betw. SCM)	**SI-16** (post. to SCM)	laryngeal prom
1 cun inf.			**LI-17**	~ GB-21	1 cun inf.
2 cun inf.		**ST-10**			2 cun inf.
3 cun inf. superior to sternal head of clavicle		**ST-11** (betw heads of SCM)		ST-12 (mid. supra-clavicular fossa)	3 cun inf. superior to sternal head of clavicle
sternal notch	**CV-22**				sternal notch
inf. to clavicle	CV-21	Kd-27		ST-13	inf. to clavicle

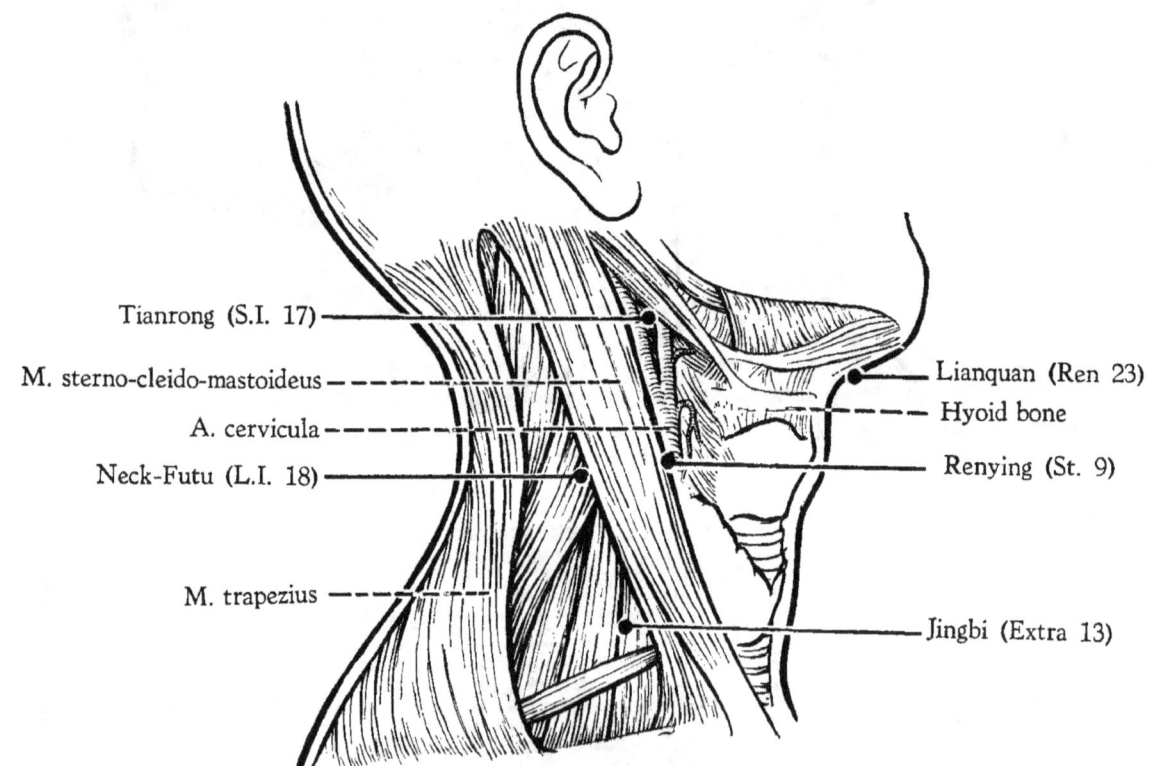

Tianrong (S.I. 17)

M. sterno-cleido-mastoideus

A. cervicula

Neck-Futu (L.I. 18)

M. trapezius

Lianquan (Ren 23)

Hyoid bone

Renying (St. 9)

Jingbi (Extra 13)

Note: LI-18 is too posterior, it should be in the middle of the SCM (as shown it should be labeled SI-16)

Neck/Throat – Lateral View: Front to Side of Neck

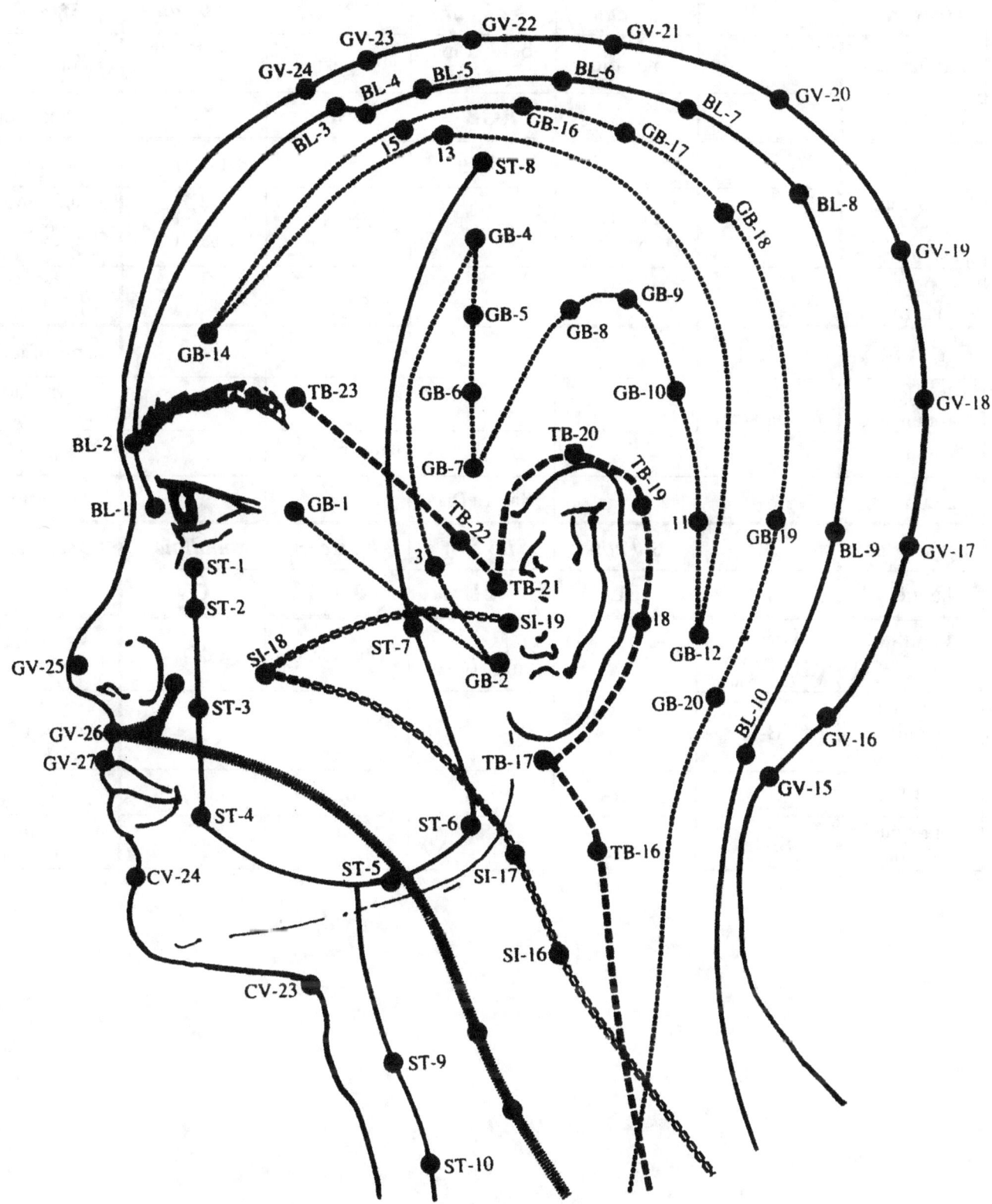

Note: TB-20, GB-8, GB-18, & GV-20 should all be in line, albeit inclined slightly posteriorly. This drawing is slightly off in this regard.
Also you need to label LI-17 and 18.

    © 1990–2016   Jim Cleaver LAc.

Neck – Lateral View: Side & Back of Neck

Measure }		4.5 cun	~2.0 cun	1.3 cun	0.0 cun	{ Measure
Landmarks		mastoid	betw traps & SCM	trapezius	posterior midline	Landmarks
channel }		**GB**	**GB**	**BL**	**GV**	{ channel
occiput			GB-20		GV-16	occiput
0.5 cun above post. hairline		GB-12 (below mastoid)		BL-10	GV-15 (above C2)	0.5 cun above post. hairline
post. hairline						post. hairline
angle of jaw	TB-16 (post. to SCM)					angle of jaw
laryngeal prominence	SI-16 (post. to SCM)					laryngeal prominence
1 cun inf.				Jing Bai Lao		1 cun inf.
2 cun inf.			Xue Ya Dian			2 cun inf.
Upper Back		3.0 cun	1.5 cun	0.75 cun	midline	**Upper Back**
channel }		**BL**	**BL**	**Jia Ji**	**GV**	{ channel
3 cun inf. **C7**	GB-21 mid-way betw C7 & acromion		SI-15 (2.0 cun lateral)	Ding Chuan	GV-14	3 cun inf. **C7**
superior angle of scapula	TB-15					superior angle of scapula
T1		SI-14	BL-11	Jia Ji	GV-13	**T1**
supra-spinous spoon	SI-13					supra-spinous spoon

Neck – Lateral View: Side & Back of Neck

* In this picture GB points 15, 16, 17, & 18 are displaced posteriorly.

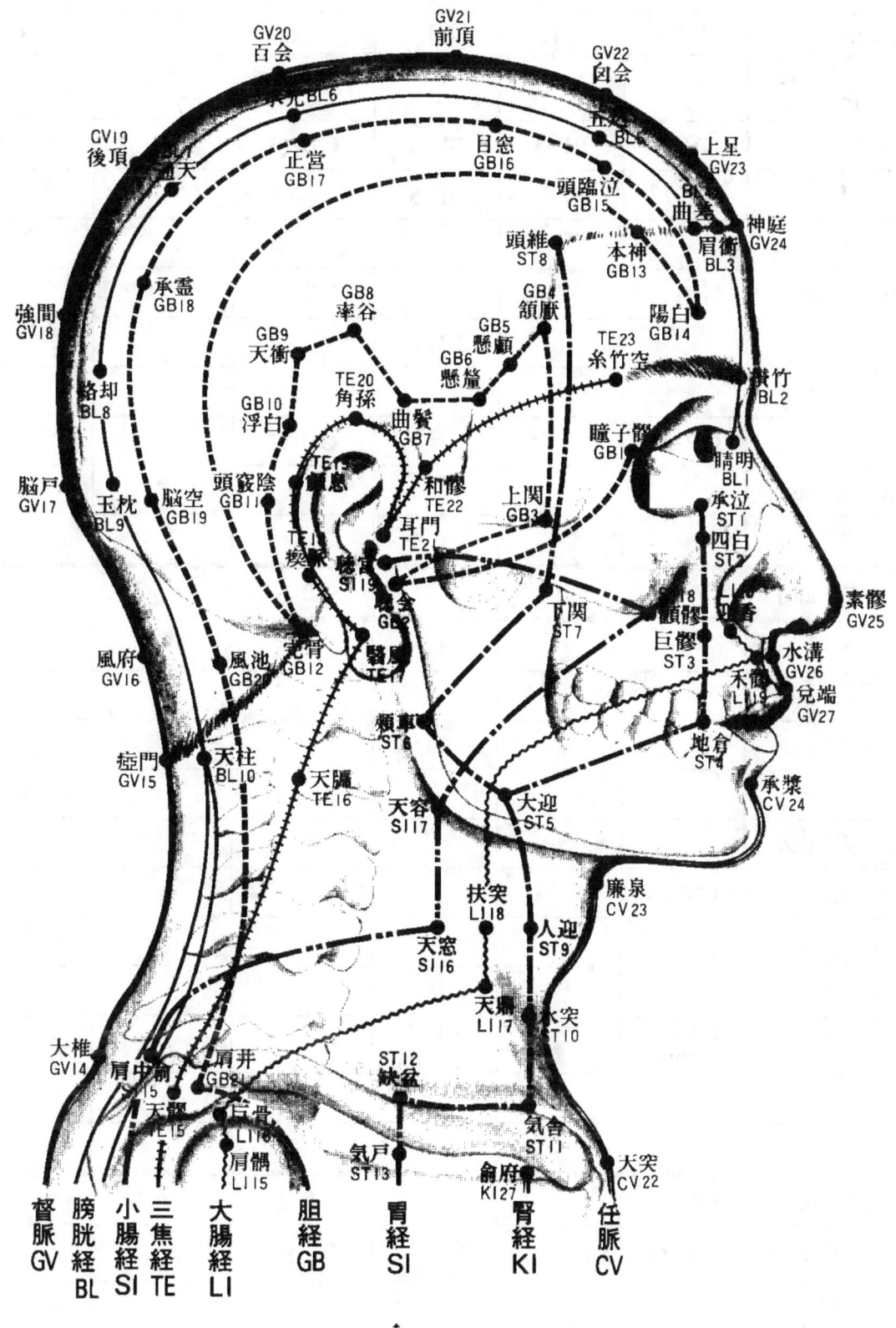

↑
ST is mislabeled as SI

      © 1990–2016   *Jim Cleaver LAc.*

Head – Superior View: Top & Back of Head

Measure }	0.0 cun	0.75 cun	1.5 cun	2.25 cun	3.0 cun	4.5 cun
Head	midline		1/3	1/2	2/3	3/3
channel }	**GV**	**BL**	**BL**	**GB**	**GB**	**ST**
ant. hairline 0.0 / 12.0 cun						head corner
0.5 / 11.5 cun	**GV-24**	**BL-3**	**BL-4**	**GB-15**	**GB-13**	**ST-8**
1.0 / 11.0 cun	**GV-23**		**BL-5**	Dang Yang		
1.5 / 10.5 cun						
2.0 / 10.0 cun	**GV-22**			**GB-16**		
2.5 / 9.5 cun			**BL-6**			
3.0 / 9.0 cun						
3.5 / 8.5 cun	**GV-21**			**GB-17**		
4.0 / 8.0 cun			**BL-7**			
4.5 / 7.5 cun						
5.0 / 7.0 cun	**GV-20**			**GB-18**		
5.5 / 6.5 cun			**BL-8**			
6.0 / 6.0 cun						
6.5 / 5.5 cun	**GV-19**					
7.0 / 5.0 cun						
7.5 / 4.5 cun						
8.0 / 4.0 cun	**GV-18**					
8.5 / 3.5 cun						
9.0 / 3.0 cun						
9.5 / 2.5 cun	**GV-17** (EOP)		**BL-9** (1.3 lat.)	**GB-19**		
10.0 / 2.0 cun						
10.5 / 1.5 cun						
11.0 / 1.0 cun	**GV-16**			**GB-20**		
11.5 / 0.5 cun	**GV-15**		**BL-10** (1.3 lat.)			
12.0 / 0.0 cun **post. hairline**						

Head – Superior View: Top & Back of Head

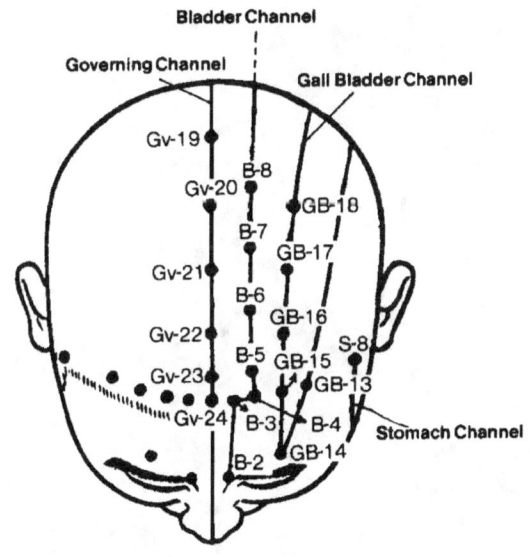

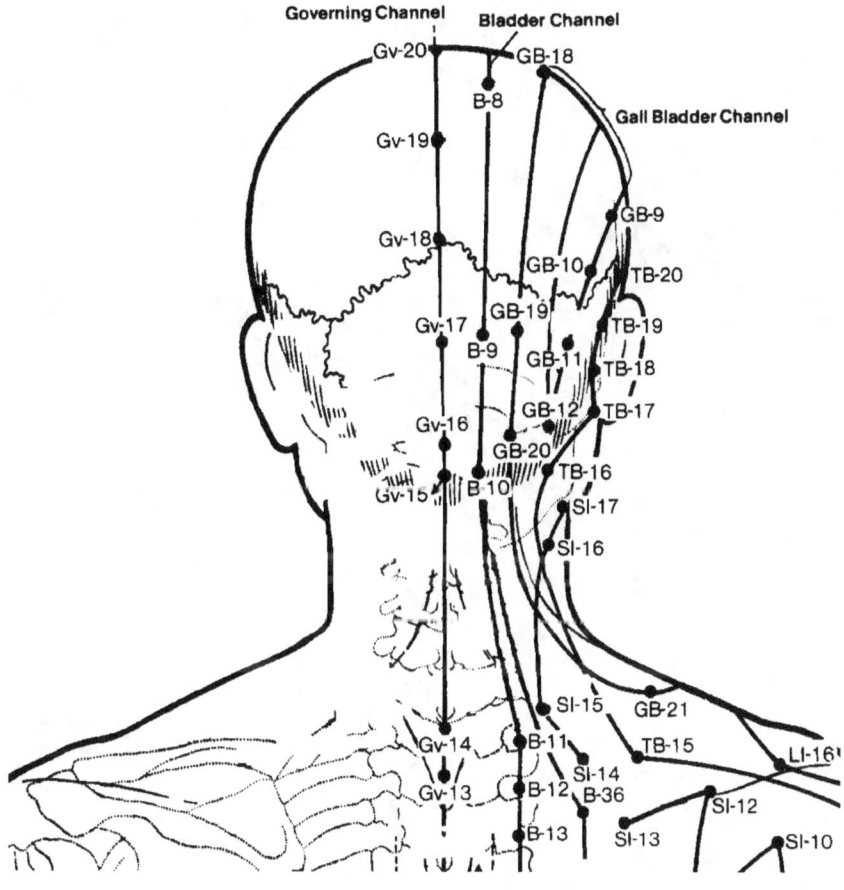

Appendix

B

經 羅

Jīng-Luó

Internal Pathways

A Synopsis: Points III and Board Review Study Guide

Ling Shu 5	根 結	Gēn Jié	= [Channel] Roots & Nodes
Ling Shu 10	經 脈	Jīng Mài	= Channels & Vessels
Ling Shu 11	經 別	Jīng Bié	= Channel Branches/Divergences
Ling Shu 12	經 水	Jīng Shuǐ	= Channels & Rivers
Ling Shu 13	經 筋	Jīng Jīn	= Channels [& their] Sinews
Ling Shu 14	骨 度	Gǔ Dù	= Bone Measurement

Table of Contents

Jing Luo – The Complete Channel System – Synopsis of Pathways

> **Jīng-Luò: Channel & Connecting Vessels, i.e. Channel Network / Network of Channels**
> Limb & Yin-Yang Sub-Division: Phase: polarity & Phase-element   Time: high tide in channel

Think of arrows as the equivalent of 'to' ('goes/proceeds to', 'goes into, through', 'goes out/up/down to')

Int. Path:
(內 經 nèi jīng)

LS:10 the internal pathway & flow – its connections and transitions.
Think of these like currents in the ocean.

wraps *means it surrounds the organ, but remains relatively surface/exterior.*
enters, *means it penetrates and permeates the organ.*
This constitutes a more subtle understanding of what the interior-exterior pairings mean at an anatomical level.

Ext. Path:
(外經 wài jīng)

Branches of the external channel that may not be obvious simply connecting the points.
The primary pathways are assumed to be known and I have dealt with them elsewhere.

Connecting Luo:
(絡 脈 luò mài)

LS:10 aka **Transverse Luo**: generally understood to bridge from the luo pt of one channel
to the yuan/source point on its phase partner

Superficial Luo:
(浮 fú luò/mài)

LS:10 aka **Longitudinal Luo**: generally understood to parallel the external pathway,
alongside or superficial to them
They function as a **reservoir**, *absorbing overflow and replenishing when primary channel is low.*

Symptoms:

LS:10 also provides symptoms associated with **surplus** & **insufficiency** for these channels.
Shi: *Sx of surfeit/surplus*

Xu: *Sx of deficit/insufficiency*

Subsidiary Luo:
(孫 sūn luò/mài)
Venous Luo:

LS:10? (lit. grandchildren) aka Tertiary or Capillary Luo
I suggest these are an attempt to incorporate visible blood vessels (i.e. veins)
within the channel system. Of course a capillary bed is exactly the idea that luo
is designed to communicate.

Divergent:
(經 別 jīng bié)

LS:11 (lit. channel divergences)   離 lí = leave (branch off) – 入 rù = enter (re-connect)
an auxiliary internal flow   出 chū = leave (depart/exit) – 合 hé = re-unite (merge)

Sinew:
(經 筋 jīng jīn)

LS:13 (lit. channel sinews) aka tendon-muscle channels
These account for the muscular system within the channel system
primarily they follow muscles (including their attachments, i.e. tendons)
from joint to joint (and by extrapolation connective tissue in general)

Root:
(根 gēn)

LS:5.2&3   the origination pt of the channel   **Node:** the termination pt of the channel
(結 jié) node, to tie, bind, knot)
ACT: p. 61 Origin & End   p.62 Root & Branch Areas

Jct Pts:

junction pts, traditional **points of intersection** with other channels, aka crossing pts.

Heart Network – Xīn Jīng-Luò
Shǒu Shǎo-Yīn   Yin-I. Fire   11am-1pm

• arrows can be translated in a variety of ways, but simply put: → 'to' or 'goes to', ↑ 'goes up', ↓ 'goes down'

Int. Path: originates within the **heart**   [incl. the coronary arteries & cardiac veins]
                descends: ↓ **diaphragm, ↓ *wraps* SI**   [follows the abdominal aorta & iliac arteries]
                ascends: ↑ **esophagus, ↑ face ↑ eyes**   [follows the carotid artery & jugular vein]
                laterally: → **lungs, → axilla/armpit** (emerging at Ht-1)

Ext. Path: follows ulnar side of the biceps (brachialis) from axilla to medial epicondyle side of the elbow (Ht-3)
                continues along the ulnar aspect of the forearm (flexor carpi ulnaris) to the wrist (pisiform) (Ht-7)
                across the palm between the 4th & 5th metacarpals (Ht-8)
                to the radial nail pt on the 5th digit (small finger) (Ht-9).

Connecting Luo: Ht-5 → SI-4

Reservoir Luo: follows the primary channel back to the **heart → pericardium**
                ↑ up to **root of tongue → eyes**
                ↓ down to **SI** (LJiao/hypogastrium).

Symptoms: ***Shi:***   distention & fullness in the chest and diaphragm area
                Xu: aphasia, disorders of the vocal cords

Venous Luo: follows the axillary-brachial-ulnar nerve; axillary-ulnar artery; basilic vein.

Divergent: departs from the primary channel in the **armpit** → into the **chest** → **heart**
                → **throat** → **face** → converging with SI at the **inner canthus** (BL-1).

Sinew: little finger → wrist/pisiform → flexor carpi ulnaris → medial epicondyle → brachialis → axilla
                joins the Lu sinew → chest/sternum ↓ diaphragm ↓ central tendon → anteriorly to the umbilicus.

Root: Ht-9   **Node:**

Jct Pts: **none**

手少陰心經

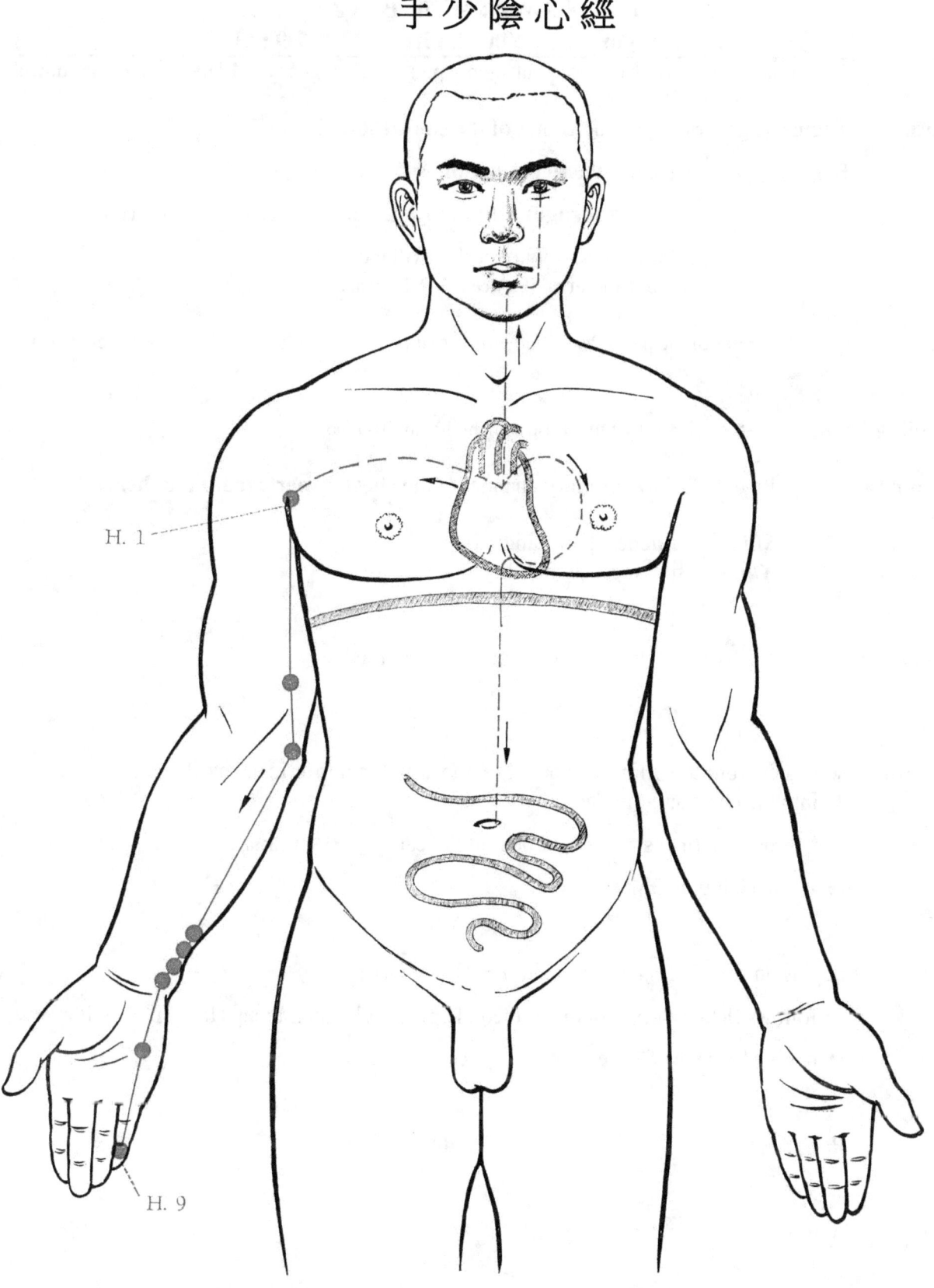

H. 1

H. 9

Shŏu Shăo/Shào Yīn Xīn Jīng
Solid line is the external channel.   Dashed lines show the internal pathway.

Pericardium Network – Xīn-Bāo Jīng-Luò
Shǒu Jué-Yīn   Yin-M. Fire   7-9 pm

• arrows can be translated in a variety of ways, but simply put: ➜ 'to' or 'goes to', ↑ 'goes up', ↓ 'goes down'

Int. Path: originates generically in the center of the **chest/thoracic cavity**

      Branch A.   permeates the **pericardium** & heart

                ↓ thru **diaphragm** ↓ **M.Jiao** ↓ **L.Jiao** (thus connecting all 3 jiao)

      Branch B.   surfaces at Pc-1 ↻ over the axillary fold
                    then out the arm (between Ht & Lu channels) i.e. ext. pathway.

Ext. Path: from the center of the palm/Pc-8 (Lao Gong, exit pt) ➜ tip of the ring finger (TB-1 entry pt).

Connecting Luo: Pc-6 ➜ TB-4 (yuan) (also straight thru to TB-5 luo)

Reservoir Luo: Pc-6 ➜ follows primary channel to the **chest** ➜ **pericardium** & **heart**

Symptoms: *Shi:*   heart/chest pain (angina)
              Xu: restlessness, irritability

Venous Luo: axillary v. ➜ brachial v. ➜ cubital v. ➜ median

Divergent: separates from the primary channel on the arm 3 cun inferior to axilla (just below Pc-2)
      ↻ into the chest and divides:

      1. ↑ throat, continues ↑ mastoid/behind the ear (& joins TB channel)

      2. ↓ connecting all 3 jiao.

Sinew: begins on middle finger (palm side) ➜ ties at wrist

      ➜ follows flexor carpi radialis to medial epicondyle, then biceps brachii ➜ axilla

      ➜ chest/ribs (pects & intercostals) ➜ ties to diaphragm.

Root: Pc-9   **Node:**

Jct Pts: **none**

手厥陰心包經

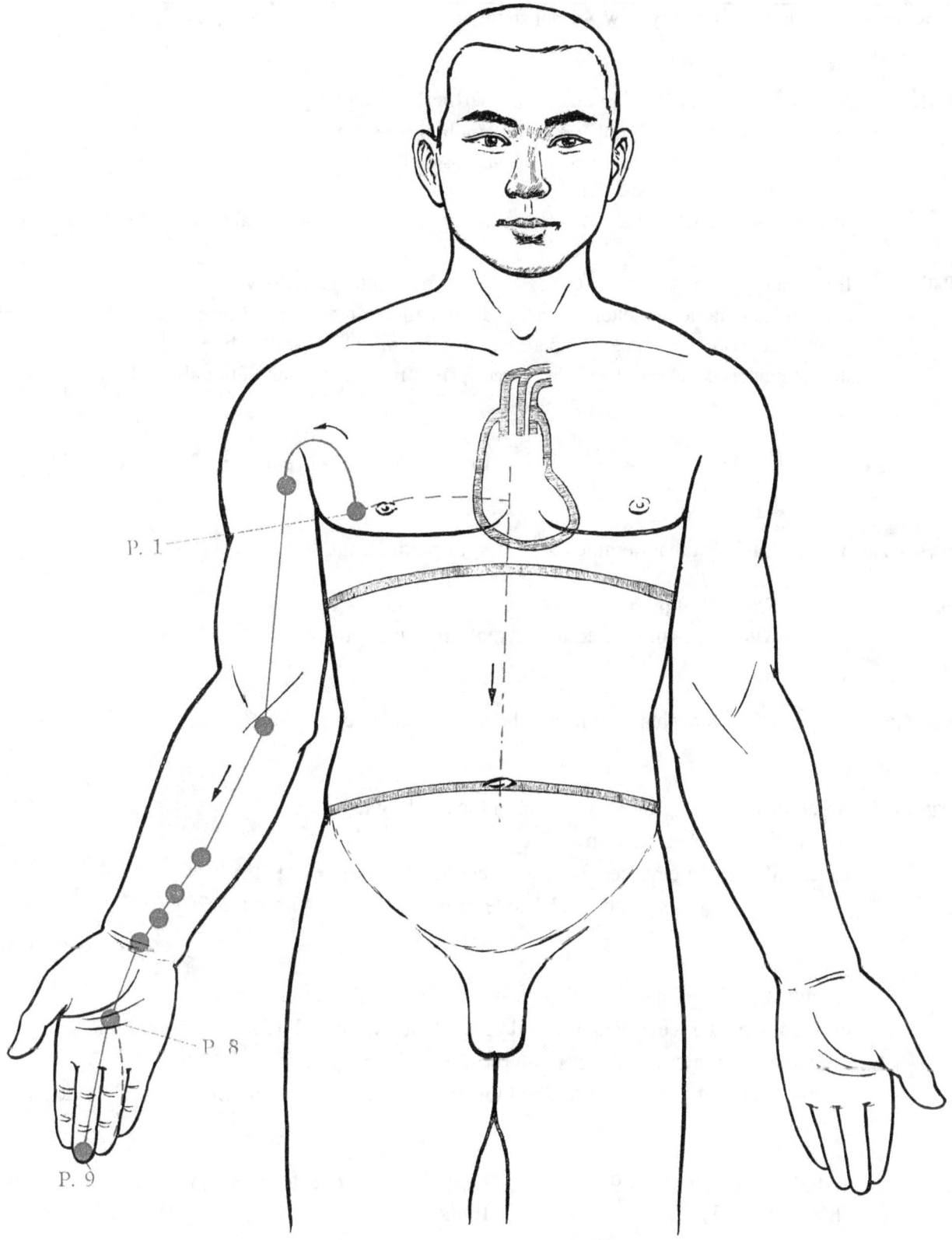

Shǒu Jué Yīn Xīn-Bāo Jīng
Solid line is the external channel.   Dashed lines show the internal pathway.

Lung Network – Fèi Jīng-Luò
Shǒu Tài-Yīn   Yin-Metal   3-5 am

• arrows can be translated in a variety of ways, but simply put: → 'to' or 'goes to', ↑ '(goes) up', ↓ '(goes) down'

Int. Path: (MJ: (Lr-14 or CV-12)

MJiao ↓ *wraps* LI ↑ ST (Yang-ming partner) → diaphragm

→ *permeates* lungs (alveoli) → *out* bronchial tree → throat

[throat = trachea, larynx (vocal cords), pharynx, naso-pharynx, nose, sinuses, cheeks]

[in other words, lungs = the entire airway]

throat → supraclavicular fossa → under clavicle → delto-pectoral triangle (Lu-2 & 1)

Ext. Path: from delto-pectoral triangle (Lu-2 & 1) ⤴ arcs over anterior axillary fold →

ant. deltoid (anterior to deltoid insertion & humerus) → radial side of biceps (cephalic groove) →

cubital fossa (Lu-5) → radial compartment of forearm → base of thumb →

thenar eminence (palmer edge of first metacarpal) → radial nail point of thumb (Lu-11)

Connecting Luo: Lu-7 → LI-4   Lu-7 (exit) → LI-4 (entry) → forefinger → LI-1

Reservoir Luo: Lu-7 → thenar eminence → across palm & out thumb

Symptoms: **Shi:** hot palms
             Xu: yawning, frequent urination or incontinence

Venous Luo: follows cephalic vein → subclavian vein → chest (heart) (coronary & pulmonary vessels)

Divergent: diverges from the primary channel in the axillary region →
        internally: chest → Lung ↓ LI
        externally: re-emerges from supraclavicular fossa (ST-12)
                  joins LI channel ↑ side of neck (LI-18), ↑ nose (LI-20)

Sinew: thumb (Lu-11) → thenar eminence → wrist → brachioradialis → elbow
       → brachialis & biceps → anterior deltoid → acromion (LI-15)
       → pectoralis major & minor → intercostals → floating ribs
       → diaphragm → central tendon → lumbar vertebral bodies (anterior surface) → (kidneys)

Root: radial artery/pulse (Lu-9)   **Node:**   (axillary artery) (Lu-1)
Begins: thumb (Lu-11)   **Ends:**   chest (Lu-1)

Jct Pts: **none** *but* Lu-1 is the jct/intersection of the leg & arm Tai-Yin channels (Sp-20 → Lu-1)

手太陰肺經

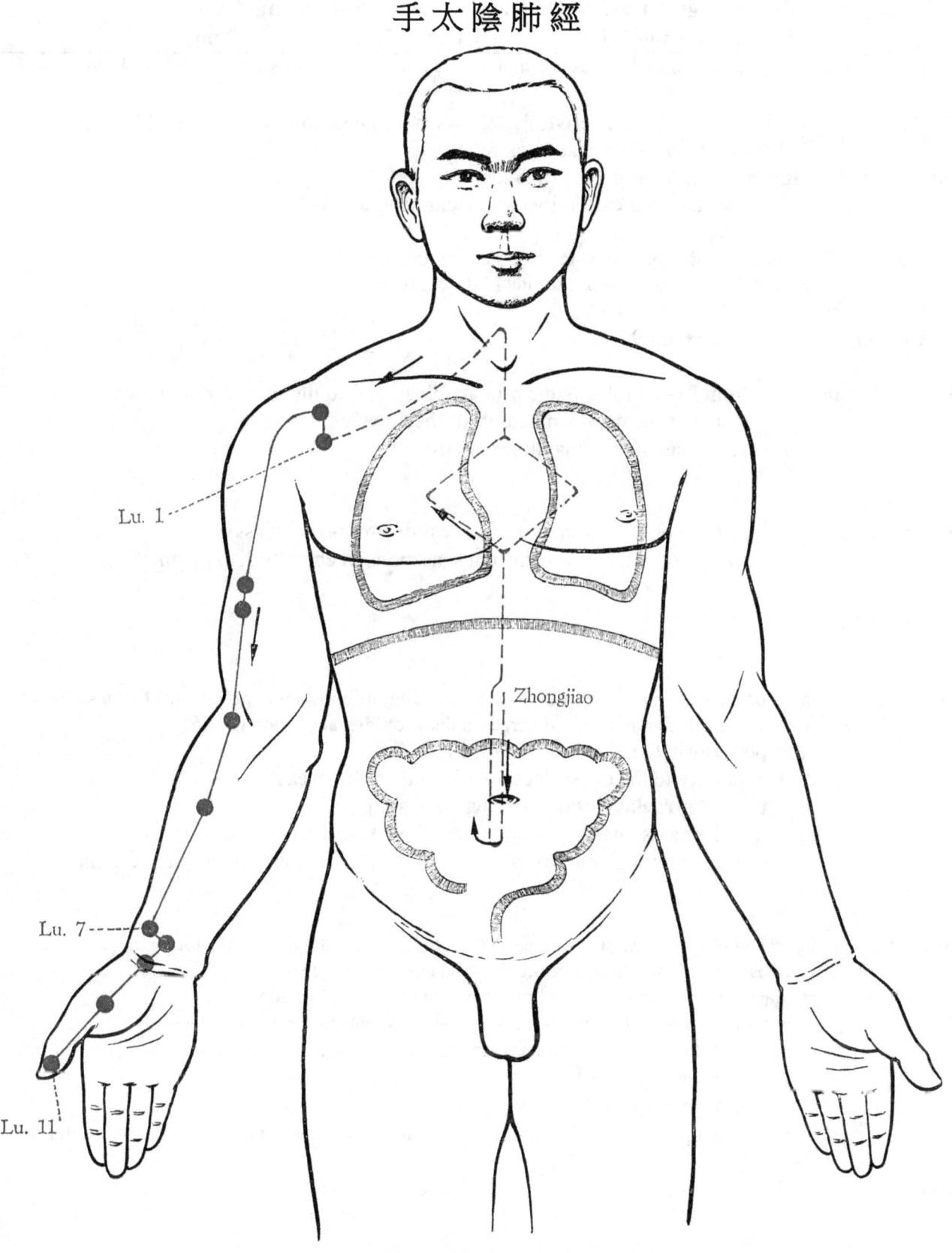

Lu. 1

Zhongjiao

Lu. 7

Lu. 11

Shǒu Tài Yīn Fèi Jīng

Solid line is the external channel.   Dashed lines show the internal pathway.

Large Intestine Network – Dà-Cháng Jīng-Luò
Shǒu Yáng-Míng   Yang-Metal   5-7am

• arrows can be translated in a variety of ways, but simply put: → 'to' or 'goes to', ↑ 'goes up', ↓ 'goes down'

Ext. Path: from LI-16 at the acromio-clavicular 'V' ↘ supra-spinous fossa SI-12 → GV-14
↶ shoulder → supraclavicular fossa (ST-12)

Int. Path: ↓ **lungs** ↓ **diaphragm** ↓ **LI** (ST-25)
a branch ↓ the lower extremity (w/ ST channel) to **ST-37**.

Ext. Path: is now generally considered to cross sides on the upper lip,
running thru GV-26 → opposite side LI-19 & 20.

Connecting Luo: LI-6 → Lu-9

Reservoir Luo: from LI-6 it follows the primary channel ↑ to the shoulder/acromion/LI-15
↑ side of the neck ↑ mandible ↑ cheek where it divides:
1. → mandible & maxilla → **teeth**
2. → enters the **ear**

Symptoms: ***Shi:***   toothache, gum disease; ear disorders (deafness)
Xu: sensitive teeth; stifling sensations in chest & diaphragm

Venous Luo:

Divergent: traditional sources say it separates on the hand, but it follows the reg. channel to the shoulder
so for all intents & purposes it diverges at the **shoulder/acromion** (LI-15)
1. → posteriorly to the **spine**/C7/GV-14
2. → anteriorly to the **chest/pectorals** including the **breasts**
3. → to the **supraclavicular fossa**, where it splits:
   a. descends internally to join both the **LU & LI**,
   b. rises through the **throat** to **LI-18**, where it rejoins the primary channel.

Sinew: index/fore-finger → wrist/snuffbox (ext. pollicis longus, brevis & abductor pollicis)
→ forearm (ext. carpi longus & brevis) → lateral epicondyle
→ brachialis/biceps/humerus/deltoid → acromion where it divides:
1. → spreads across the upper back → spine (scapula to upper thoracic & cervical)
2. ↑ side of the neck (SCM), ↑ jaw/ramus, ↑ TMJ and divides again:
   a. → nose (LI-20)
   b. ↑ up to top of forehead/ST-8
→ over the top of the head to the opposite side (ST-8), ↓ mandible/ramus/masseter.

Root: LI-1   **Node:**   ST-8

Jct Pts: **SI-12, GV-14, ST-4, GV-26**
(4 pts)

手陽明大腸經

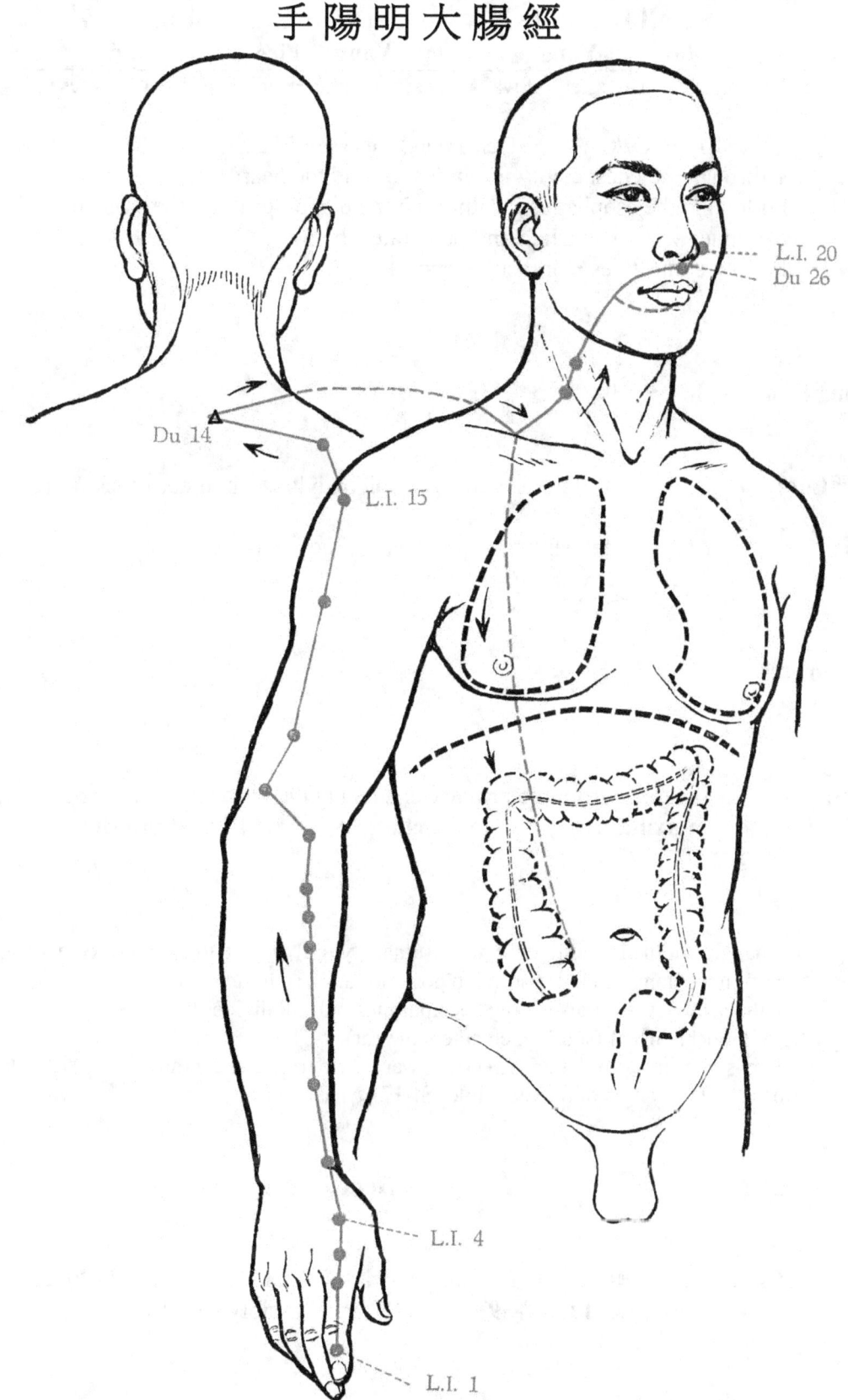

L.I. 20
Du 26

Du 14

L.I. 15

L.I. 4

L.I. 1

Shǒu Yáng Míng Dà Cháng Jīng

Solid line is the external channel.   Dashed lines show the internal pathway.

Small Intestine Network – Xiǎo-Cháng Jīng-Luò
Shǒu Tài-Yáng   Yang-I. Fire   1-3pm

• arrows can be translated in a variety of ways, but simply put: → 'to' or 'goes to', ↑ 'goes up', ↓ 'goes down'

Ext. Path: from SI-15 → C7/GV-14 → then around the base of the neck into the supraclavicular fossa (ST-12)

Int. Path: ↓ through the chest cavity *wrapping* around the heart.
Following the esophagus it ↓ through the diaphragm into the stomach (CV-13 & 12)
continues ↓ into the LJiao and penetrates the SI.
From the intestines a branch extends ↓ to ST-39.

Connecting Luo: SI-7 → Ht-7

Reservoir Luo: SI-7 → Ht channel → medial epicondyle → shoulder (back & front)

Symptoms: *Shi:*   weakness &/or paralysis of the joints (wei/atrophy)
               Xu: flat warts (skin disorders)

Venous Luo:

Divergent: separates from the primary channel at the posterior shoulder (**SI-10**)
               → **axilla** (Ht-1) → into the **chest**, → **heart**, ↓ **small intestine**.

Sinew: ulnar side of the little finger → wrist (ulnar styloid) → ulna to elbow (medial condyle)
               → follows [long head of] triceps to posterior axillary fold → scapula (teres, infraspinatus & subscapularis)
               ↑ the neck (levator/trapezius) → occiput/mastoid and divides?:
               1. posterior branch: GB-11 (sub-branch enters the ear), ↑ TB-20 → TB-22
                  ↓ masseter [insertion], then sweeps upward ↻ to the outer canthus (GB-1) (also Ht rules canthii)
               2. anterior branch: → angle of the mandible (SI-17) ↑ masseter insertion/teeth, ↑ the outer canthus ↑ ST-8.

Root: SI-1   **Node:**   BL-1

Jct Pts: **BL-1, BL-11, BL-41/36** (Fu Fen), **GV-14, ST-12, GB-1 & 11, TB-20&22,**
(13-14 pts)   **CV-17, CV-13 & 12, ST-39**   Possibly: (LI-14)

手太陽小腸經

S.I. 19

S.I. 18

Du 14

S.I. 1

Shǒu Tài Yáng Xiǎo Cháng Jīng
Solid line is the external channel.   Dashed lines show the internal pathway.

© 1990–2016   Jim Cleaver LAc.

Triple Burner Network – Sān-Jiāo Jīng-Luò
Shǒu Shǎo-Yáng   Yang-M. Fire   9-11pm

• arrows can be translated in a variety of ways, but simply put: → 'to' or 'goes to', ↑ 'goes up', ↓ 'goes down'

Ext. Path: from TB-15 → GV-14 → ST-12

Int. Path: separating from the ext. channel it descends ↓ through the **supraclavicular fossa** (ST-12)
permeates the **chest** and connects with the **Pericardium** (& CV-17)
↓ **MJiao** ↓ **LJiao** (thus connecting all three jiao/burners)
From the LJiao (intestines/bladder) there is a branch ↓ to BL-39/53 (Wei Yang).

Connecting Luo: TB-5 → Pc-7 (yuan) (also straight thru to Pc-6 (luo))

Reservoir Luo: from TB-5 it follows the primary channel to the **shoulder** then flows
anteriorly to the **chest** where it connects with the **Pericardium**.

Symptoms: *Shi:*   spasms of the elbow
                Xu: arm muscle flaccidity, difficulty flexing elbow

Venous Luo:

Divergent: starts at the vertex (GV-20) ↓ behind ear ↓ through the supraclavicular fossa (ST-12)
                alt: separates from primary channel behind the ear (TB-17-20)/mastoid
                        1. ↑ **vertex** (GV-20)
                        2. ↓ **supraclavicular fossa** (ST-12) goes internally and continues
                            ↓ permeates the **chest/U.Jiao**, ↓ **M. & L.Jiao** connecting all three jiao.

Sinew: ulnar side of the ring finger → wrist → dorsal forearm → olecranon fossa
            → between triceps to postero-lateral shoulder → neck (trapezius)
            → intersects SI sinew (SI-17) and splits:
            1. goes under the mandible to the root of the tongue.
            2. goes up anterior to the ear (GB-2, SI-19, TB-21) continues ↑ (TB-22 & GB-3)
                → temple → outer canthus (GB-1), ↑ ST-8.

Root: TB-1   **Node:**   SI-19 / ST-8

Jct Pts: **SI-12, BL-11, GV-14, GB-21, ST-12, CV-17 & 12,**
(16-19 pts)   **GB-11, GB-14, GB-6-5-4-3; SI-18 & 19, GB-1**   (+ BL-1, GB-20; Pc-1)

手少陽三焦經

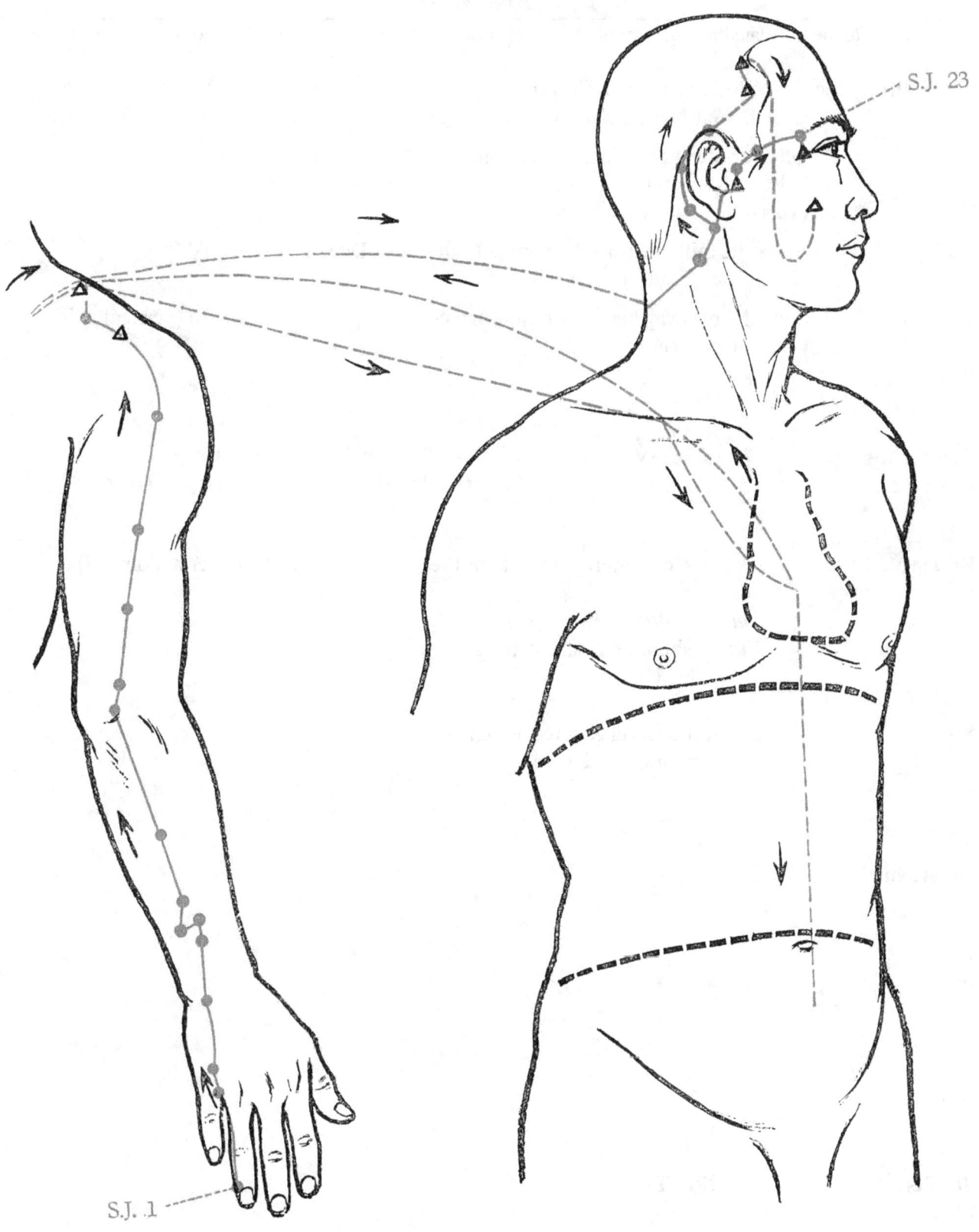

S.J. 23

S.J. 1

Shǒu Shǎo/Shào Yáng Sān Jiāo Jīng

Solid line is the external channel.   Dashed lines show the internal pathway.

© 1990–2016   *Jim Cleaver LAc.*

Conception/Controlling Vessel
Rèn Mài

• arrows can be translated in a variety of ways, but simply put: → 'to' or 'goes to', ↑ 'goes up', ↓ 'goes down'

Int. Path: begins in lower abdomen (lower dan tian) (uterus) ↓ perineum (CV-1).
　　　　　[Ren, Du & Chong, all have the same origin]

　　　1. follows anterior midline from pubic bone ↑ abdomen ↑ thorax
　　　↑ throat ↑ around mouth/lips ↑ GV-28 ↑ eyes (ST-1).
　　　(This is the External pathway)

　　　2. enters the tailbone (GV-1) ↑ spine (anterior to Du?) ↑ vertex (GV-20).
　　　(for all intents and purposes this IS the Du)

　　　3. flows ↑↓ midway between Ren & Du connecting CV-1 & GV-20 (vertical axis).
　　　(This is the Chong mai)

Connecting Luo:　CV-15 → GV-1　　[CV-15 → ST-18 → Sp-21 → BL-15? → GV-9-10-11]
　　　　　　　　　　　　　　　[CV luo → Gr. luo ST → Gr. luo Sp → Ht shu → GV Ht/Pc levels]

Reservoir Luo:　CV-15 ↓ dispersing throughout the upper abdomen (↓ lower abdomen?)

Symptoms:　*Shi:*　abdominal skin pain
　　　　　　Xu:　abdominal skin itching

Venous Luo:　abdominal aorta & inferior vena cava
　　　　　　coronary arteries & veins

Divergent:　n/a

Sinew:　n/a

Root:　n/a　　　　**Node:**　n/a

Jct Pts:　**GV-28, ST-1**
(2 pts)

任脈

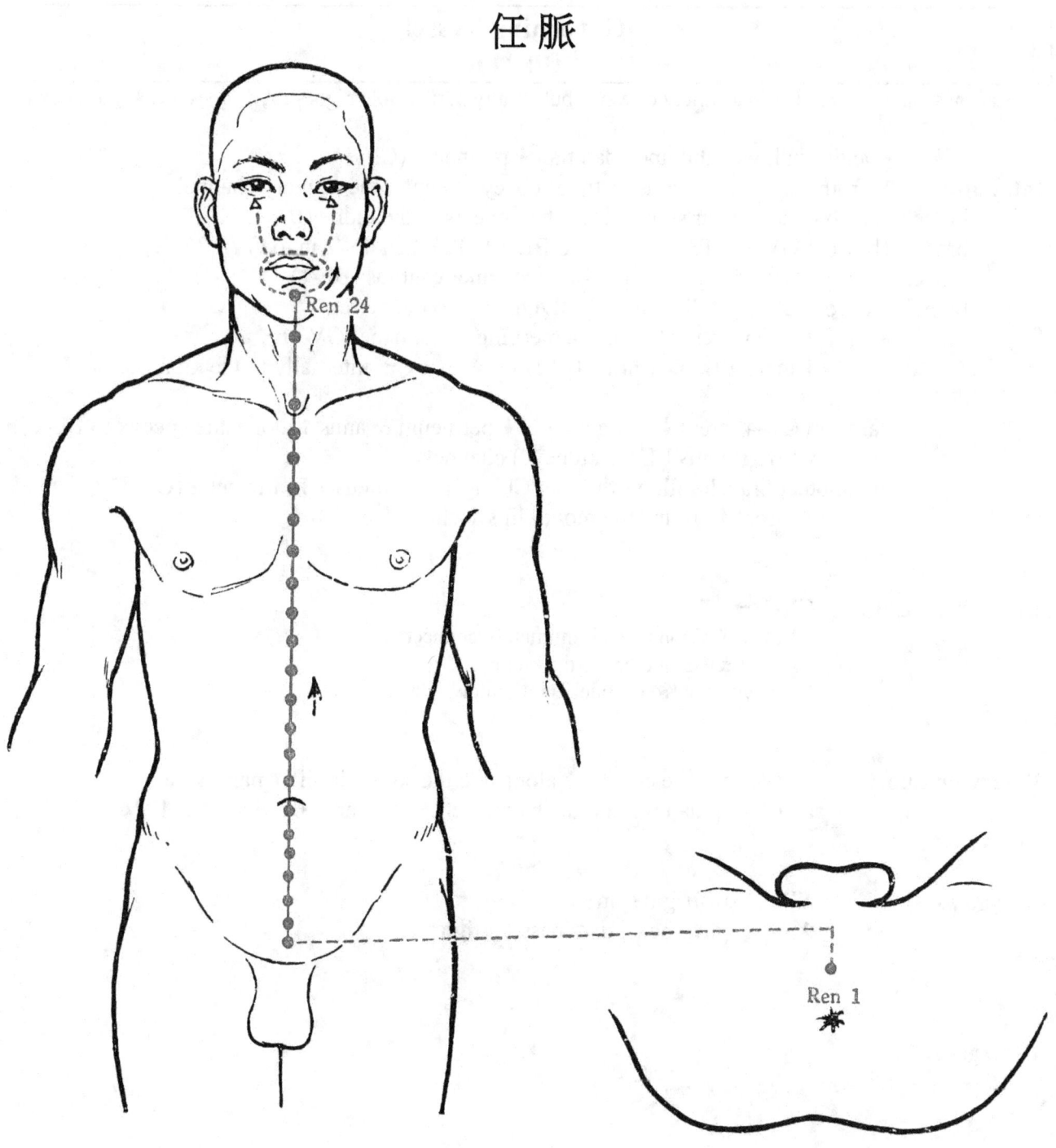

Rèn Mài

Solid line is the external channel.   Dashed lines show the internal pathway.

Governing Vessel
Dū Mài

• arrows can be translated in a variety of ways, but simply put: → 'to' or 'goes to', ↑ 'goes up', ↓ 'goes down'

• begins in lower abdomen/dan tian ↓ perineum (CV-1)

Int. Path: 1. from perineum → anus → tip of coccyx to enter the primary channel.
branch 1a. from the lumbar spine a branch connects to the kidneys.
branch 1b. from GV-12 (T3) up & out to BL-12 (T2) then up & in to GV-13 (T1).
branch 1c. from GV-16 into and thru brain → inner canthus (BL-1).
branch 1d. from BL-1 ↑ following the BL channel to the vertex,
  ↓ re-enters the brain, re-emerging at the nape (GV-16),
  ↓ inner BL line (thru BL-12) ↓ low back → internally to the kidneys.

2a. from CV-4 (area) ↓ ext. genitalia ↓ perineum & anus ↑ alongside coccyx to BL-35, where it joins BL (& kidney?) channels.
2b. another branch follows the Ren/Chong ↑ umbilicus ↑ heart center (CV-17?)
  ↑ throat ↑ around the mouth/lips ↑ cheek ↑ eye.

Connecting Luo: GV-1 → CV-1 or 15.
GV, CV & Chong are all intimately connected.
also GV & BL and hence the kidneys.
Moreover, the Kd channel is intimately related to the Chong.

Reservoir Luo: separates at the coccyx ↑ alongside the spine (jia-ji) ↑ nape ↑ head.
at the scapula level a branch connects to the inner BL line. BL-12?

Symptoms: **Shi:** stiff/rigid spine
  Xu: heavy head, dizziness/vertigo

Divergent: n/a

Sinew: n/a

Root: n/a   **Node:** n/a

Jct Pts: **CV-1, BL-12; CV-4, BL-1, BL-35**
(5 pts)

督脈

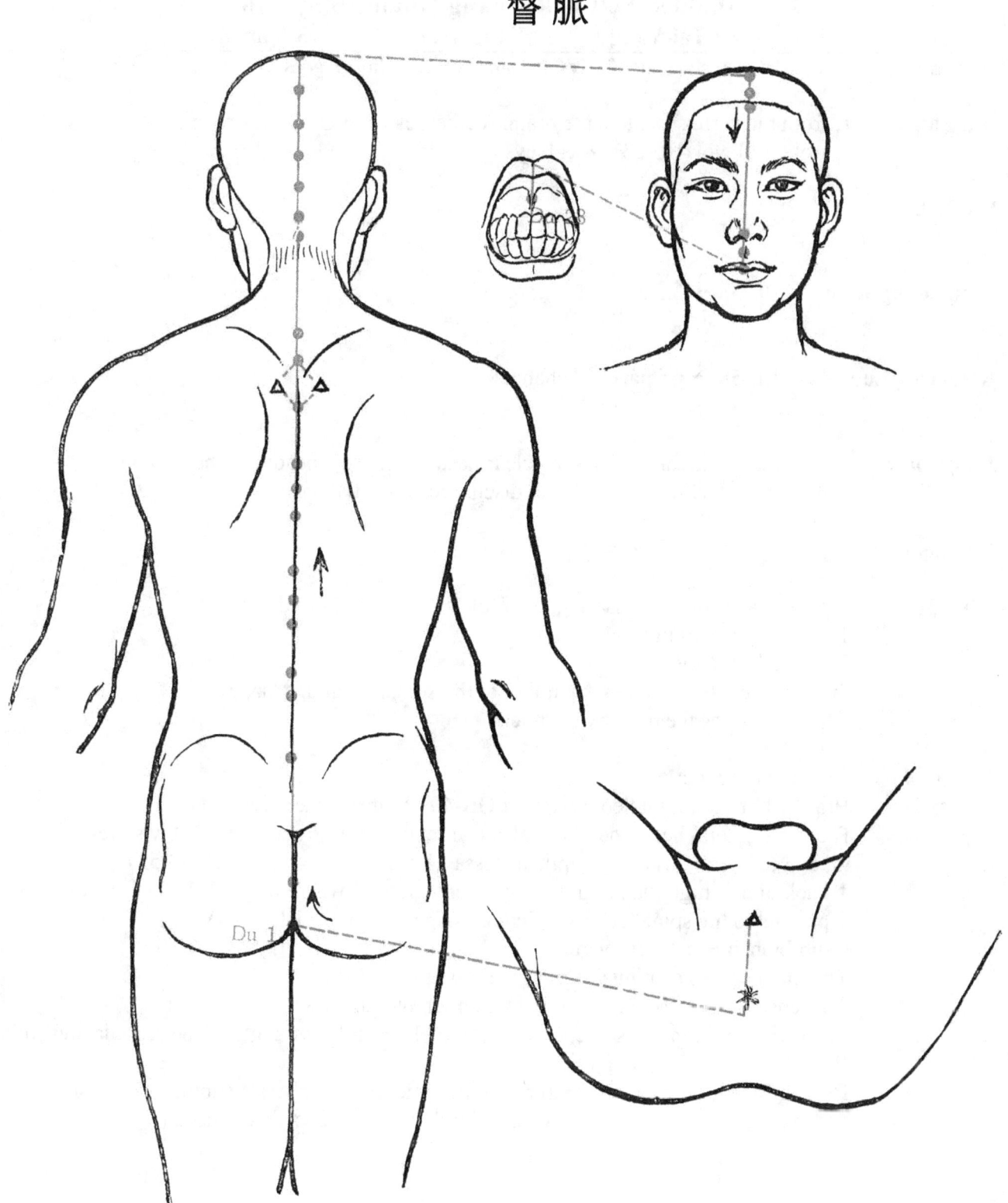

Dū Mài
Solid line is the external channel.   Dashed lines show the internal pathway.

© 1990–2016   Jim Cleaver LAc.

Bladder Network – Páng Guāng Jīng-Luò
Zú Tài-Yáng   Yang-Water   3-5pm

• arrows can be translated in a variety of ways, but simply put: → 'to' or 'goes to', ↑ 'goes up', ↓ 'goes down'

Int. Path: 1. from the vertex ↓ enters the brain, reemerges from GV-17?, or the nape.
         2. from L2 level (BL-23) → kidneys → bladder

Ext. Path:

Connecting Luo: BL-58 → Kd-3

Reservoir Luo: BL-58 → primary Kd channel

Symptoms: *Shi:*   nasal obstruction, clear nasal discharge; headache; back ache
            Xu: chronic clear nasal discharge, sinusitis, epistaxis

Venous Luo:

Divergent: separates at popliteal fossa ↑ gluteal fold/ischium and divides?:
         1. → anus & sacrum
         2. → bladder ↑ kidney ↑ heart
         the main course continues ↑ parallel to the spinal column ↑ nape
         where it rejoins the primary channel.

Sinew: from the little toe:
         Branch 1. ↑ lateral malleolus (ties at GB-40) ↑ lateral knee (ties at GB-34).
         Branch 2. lateral heel ↑ achilles/calcaneal tendon ↑ gastrocnemius follows the
         medial & lateral gastroc ↑ popliteal fossa (Kd-10 – BL-40/54 – BL-39/53)
         ↑ back of the thigh (hamstrings) ↑ buttocks/gluteals where they all rejoin (BL-50 / GB-30)
         ↑ parallel to the spine (erector spinae) ↑ nape ↑ occiput (BL-10/GV-16)
         a sub-branch → root of tongue.
         The main course continues ↑ over the top of the head
         ↓ forehead ↓ nose → inner canthus → upper eyelid.
         Meanwhile, a branch also departs ~ level of T7 → inferior angle of the scapula and splits:
         Branch A. ↑ shoulder (LI-15).
         Branch B. → under the arm → thru armpit → across the chest ↑ supraclavicular fossa
         and splits again: B1. ↑ mastoid (GB-12)   B2. ↑ face ↑ nose (LI-20).

Root: Zhi Yin (BL-67)   **Node:** (eyes) Ming Men = Jing Ming (BL-1)

Jct Pts: **GV-24, GB-15, GV-20, GB-6-7-8, GB-10-11-12, GV-17-16, GV-14 & 13, GB-30**
(14-17 pts)   probably also SI-10, LI-14, GB-23

足太陽膀胱經

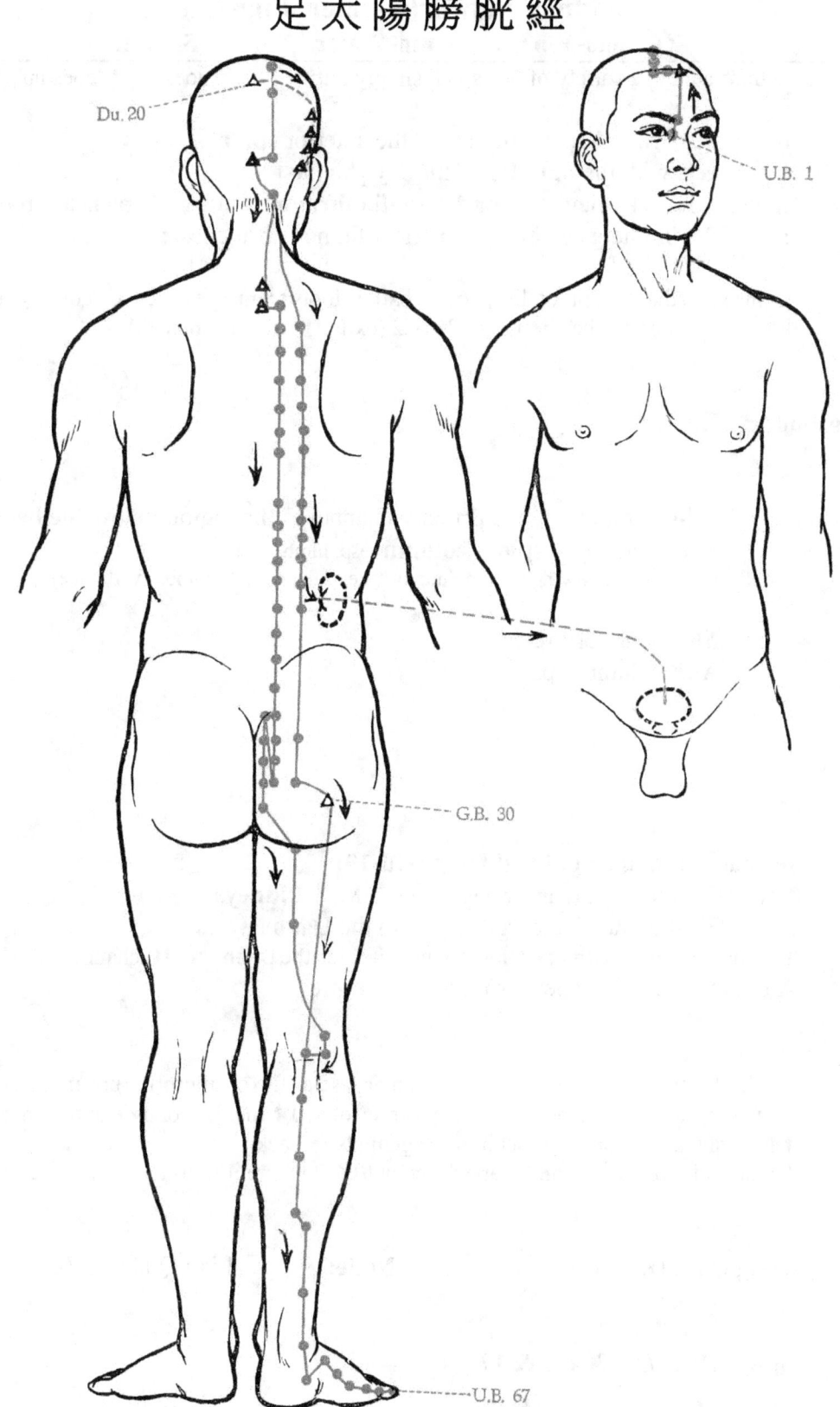

Zú Tài Yáng Páng-Guāng Jīng

Solid line is the external channel.　Dashed lines show the internal pathway.

Kidney Network – Shèn Jīng-Luò
Zú Shǎo-Yīn   Yin-Water   5-7 pm

• arrows can be translated in a variety of ways, but simply put: ➜ 'to' or 'goes to', ↑ 'goes up', ↓ 'goes down'

Int. Path: from coccyx runs ↑ internally along the anterior **spine**
➜ connects with the **bladder & kidney** [**uterus**]
Branch 1 from kidney ➜ **liver** ↑ thru **diaphragm** ➜ **lungs** ↑ trachea ↑ root of **tongue**
Branch 2 from lungs ➜ **heart** & pericardium ➜ thru chest ➜ Pc channel (**Pc-1**).

Ext. Path: begins at medial nail pt. on little toe ➜ ball of foot ➜ emerge at Kd-1 (Yong Quan).
there is a branch on the chest from Kd-22 (exit pt) ➜ Pc-1 (entry pt)

Connecting Luo: Kd-4 ➜ BL-64

Reservoir Luo: Kd-4 ↑ following the primary channel to the region **below the heart** (Pc & Ht)
➜ posteriorly ↓ **spinal column** (esp. lumbar v.)
(perhaps it following the diaphragm & central tendon to lumbar vertebrae)

Symptoms: *Shi:*   urinary retention
           Xu: lumbar pain

Venous Luo:

Divergent: separates from the **popliteal fossa (Kd-10)**
↑ the **BL divergent** (hamstrings: semi-T&M) ↑ **kidneys**.
At L2/GV-4 a branch emerges to begin the Dai mai.
The main course continues ↑ **nape** where it joins the **primary BL** channel (at BL-10)
A branch from the nape ➜ root of the **tongue**.

Sinew: medial & inferior little toe ➜ ball ➜ plantar fascia (flexor digitorum) ➜ medial calcaneus
↑ medial malleolus (joins BL sinew/gastroc/soleus) ↑ medial condyle at the knee
↑ medial thigh (gracilis ➜ ischium) ➜ genitals ➜ back
↑ alongside spinal column ↑ nape ↑ occiput/EOP where it joins again with BL sinew.

Root: Yong Quan (Kd-1)   **Node:**   Lian Quan (CV-23)

Jct Pts: **Sp-6, GV-1, CV-3, 4, 7 & 17**
(6 pts)

       © 1990–2016   *Jim Cleaver LAc.*

足少陰腎經

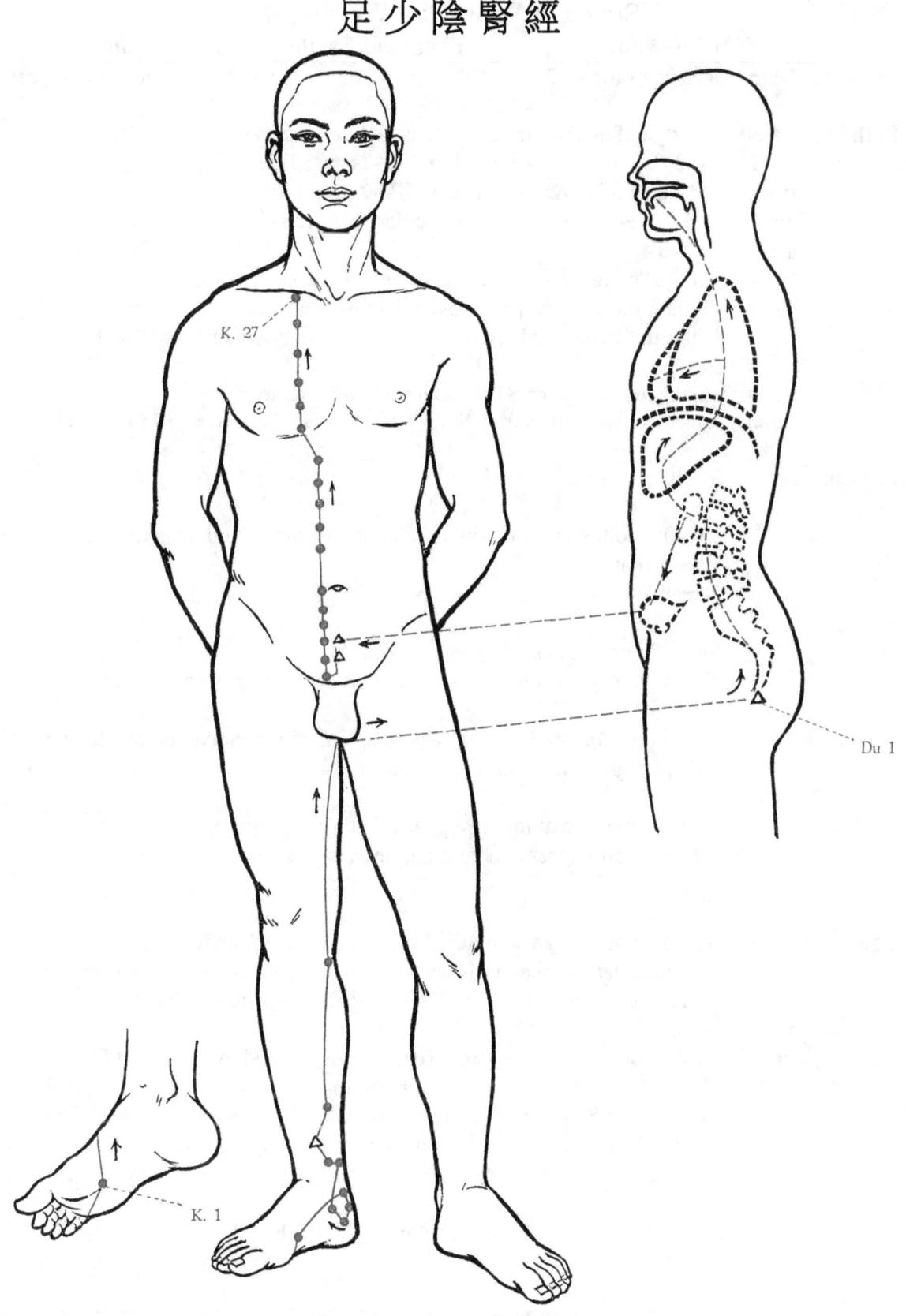

K. 27

Du 1

K. 1

Zú Shǎo/Shào Yīn Shèn Jīng

Solid line is the external channel.   Dashed lines show the internal pathway.

Stomach Network – Wèi Jīng-Luò
Zú Yáng-Míng   Yang-Soil/Earth   7-9 am

• arrows can be translated in a variety of ways, but simply put: → 'to' or 'goes to', ↑ 'goes up', ↓ 'goes down'

Int. Path: LI-20 → bridge of nose → inner canthus (**BL-1**) → ST-1.
(incl. Ext.)   ST-1 ↓ ST-2 & 3 → **GV-26** ↓ ST-4 → **CV-24** → ST-5.
                   from ST-5 ↑ thru ST-6 & 7 to ST-8 → **GV-24**.
                   main path ↓ ST-9-10-11 → supraclavicular fossa (ST-12):
                   a. → C7/**GV-14**
                   b1. ↓ chest ↓ diaphragm ↓ **CV-13 & 12** → stomach → spleen.
                   b2. ↓ pylorus ↓ duodenum [pancreas] ↓ LJiao/intestines,
                        ↓ inguinal groove where it rejoins the primary channel at ST-30.

Ext. Path: a branch on the foot runs from ST-42 (exit pt) → Sp-1 (entry pt)
                   another branch on the leg runs from St-36 ↓ ST-40 ↓ ST-41 area → **3rd toe** lateral nail pt

Connecting Luo: ST-40 → spleen channel (Sp-3)

Reservoir Luo: ST-40 ↑ following the primary channel to supraclavicular fossa and splits:
                   1. → throat
                   2. → C7/GV-14 ↑ nape ↑ occiput → brain

Symptoms: *Shi:*   mental disorders (dian or kuang), epilepsy
                   Xu: wei syndrome (weakness, atrophy, flaccidity) of leg or foot

Great Luo: ST-18 (esp. on the left side) where apical heartbeat can be felt & seen.
                   ↓ diaphragm ↓ stomach   ↑ chest & lungs

Symptoms: *Shi:*   rapid breathing, irregular breathing, dyspnea
                   Xu: chest oppression, angina, heart attack, wheezing, cough

Divergent: separates mid-thigh ↑ inguinal groove (ST-30) ↑ abdominal cavity ↑ spleen
                   → stomach ↑ esophagus ↑ heart ↑ throat ↑ mouth ↑ sides of nose
                   → inner canthus (BL-1) → ST-1 to rejoin the primary channel.

Sinew: 2nd-3rd & 4th toes ↑ dorsum of foot (ext digitorum tendons) ↑ ties at ST-41 then splits:
                   1. ↑ peroneals/fibularis muscles to knee ↑ IT tendon to hip ↑ flank → back → spinal column.
                   2. ↑ tibialis & quads ties at ST-31 → external genitalia ↑ abdomen (rectus abd.) ↑ chest
                        ↑ supraclavicular fossa ↑ neck ↑ jaw ↑ corners of mouth (ST-4) ↑ ties at the nose (LI-19/20)
                   divides: a. → ear   b. ↑ lower eyelid (lower net= ST) ↻ upper eyelid (upper net= BL)

Root: Li Dui (ST-45)   **Node:** Zang Da = Tou Wei (ST-8)

Jct Pts: **LI-20, BL-1, CV-24, GB-3&4, GB-5&6, GV-24, 26/28, GV-14, CV-12 & 13, Sp-1**
(14-16 pts)   also (GB-14, GB-21)

足陽明胃經

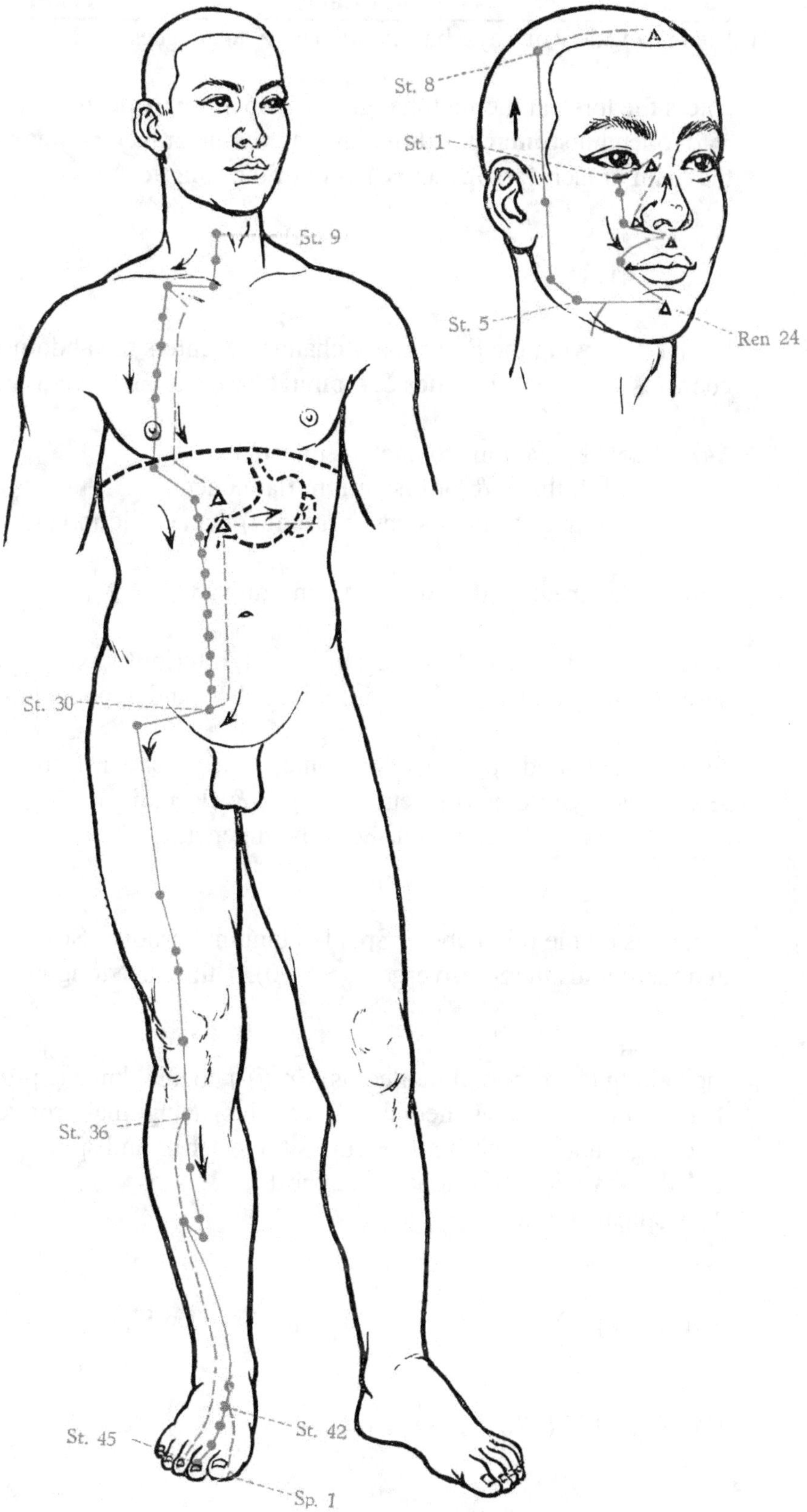

St. 8

St. 1

St. 9

St. 5

Ren 24

St. 30

St. 36

St. 45

St. 42

Sp. 1

Zú Yáng Míng Wèi Jīng

Solid line is the external channel.　Dashed lines show the internal pathway.

© 1990–2016　Jim Cleaver LAc.

Spleen Network – Pí Jīng-Luò

Zú Tài-Yīn	Yin-Soil/Earth	9-11am

• arrows can be translated in a variety of ways, but simply put: ➜ 'to' or 'goes to', ↑ 'goes up', ↓ 'goes down'

Int. Path: enters the torso at the inguinal groove (Sp-12) ➜ **spleen** ➜ [pancreas]
➜ duodenum/**stomach** ↑ thru diaphragm: one branch ➜ **heart**;
the main branch ↑ **esophagus** ↑ root of the **tongue**.

Connecting Luo: Sp-4 ➜ ST-42

Reservoir Luo: Sp-4 ↑ following the Sp primary channel, ↑ enters the abdomen and
connects with the **intestines** & **stomach** [and presumably the pancreas & spleen itself].

Symptoms:
Shi: colicky pain in stomach or intestines
Xu: abd. fullness &/or distention, flatulence
gu zhang (drum distention/ascites), gan (childhood nutritional impairment)

Venous Luo: follows the **great saphenous** v. ↑ femoral v. ↑ iliac ↑ vena cava ➜ splenic

Great Luo: separates at Sp-21 (mid axillary line 6 cun inferior to axilla ~ 7th ICS)
spreads though the lateral costal region, chest and hypochondrium.

Symptoms:
Shi: whole body pain, Bi syndrome, multiple site arthritis
Xu: wei syndrome (muscular atrophy & flaccidity),
weakness of the joints & body in general.

Divergent: separates on the thigh above Sp-11 ↑ inguinal groove (Sp-12)
and there joins the ST divergent (ST-30), ↑ throat, ↑ tongue.

Sinew: medial big toe ↑ medial malleolus (Sp-5) ↑ medial knee (Sp-9)
↑ medial thigh [vastus medialis & sartorius] ↑ inguinal groove (Sp-12/ST-30)
➜ ext. genitals ↑ umbilicus ➜ enters torso ↑ ribs and splits:
1. ↑ disperses into/throughout the chest
2. ➜ spinal column

Root:	Yin Bai (Sp-1)	**Node:**	Tai Shang = Zhong Wan (CV-12)

Jct Pts: CV-3-4, 10 & (17), GB-24, Lr-14, Lu-1
(6-7 pts)

足太陰脾經

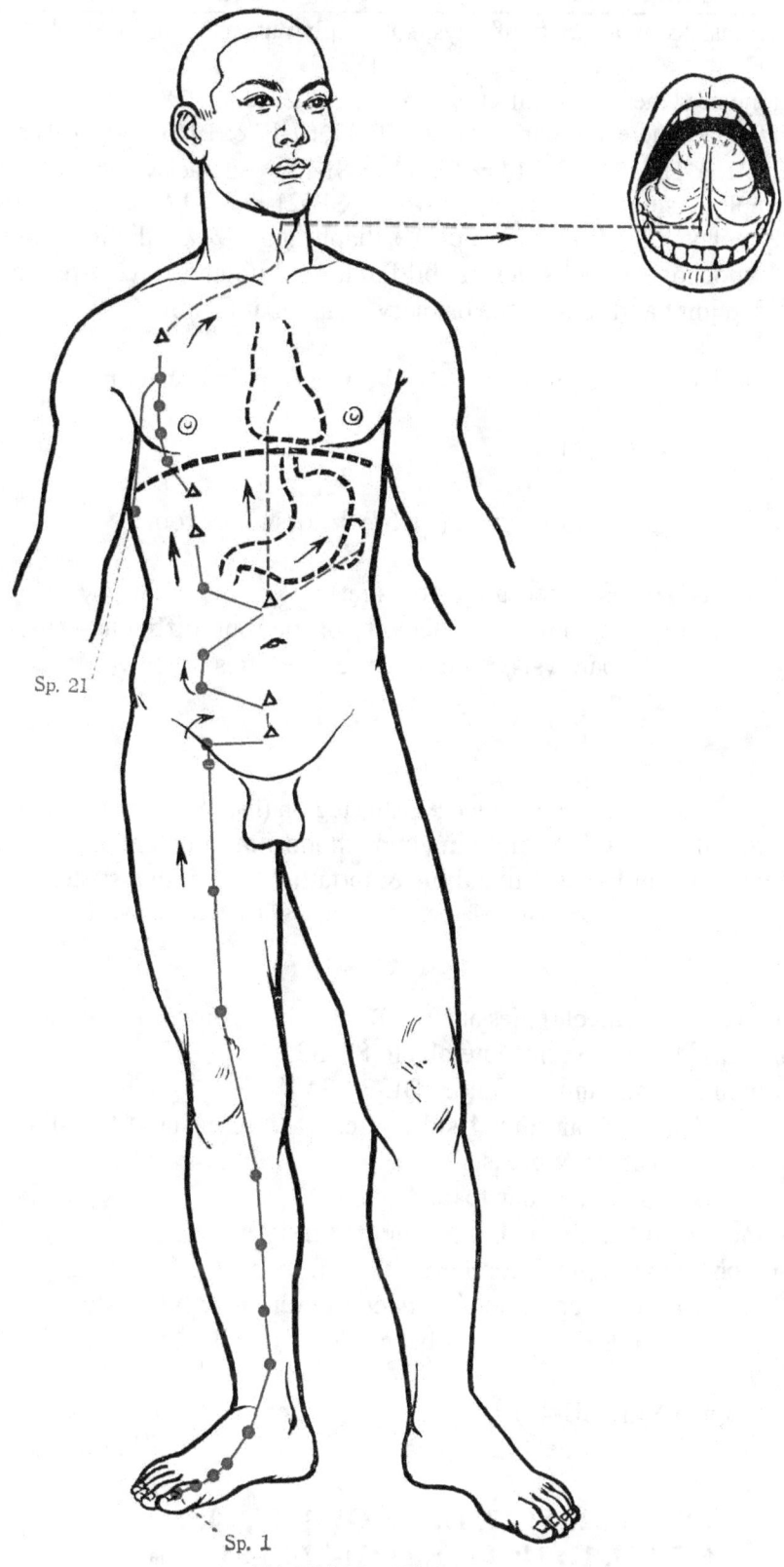

Sp. 21

Sp. 1

Zú Tài Yīn Pí Jīng

Solid line is the external channel.   Dashed lines show the internal pathway.

Gall Bladder Network – Dăn Jīng-Luò

Zú Shăo-Yáng	Yang-Wood	11pm-1am

• arrows can be translated in a variety of ways, but simply put: → 'to' or 'goes to', ↑ 'goes up', ↓ 'goes down'

Ext. Path: on the head there are connections to TB20 & 22 and ST-8.
on the face there are connections to TB-17, SI-17 & 19, ST-5-6 & 9 and BL-1.
GB-21 → TB-15 → GV-14 → BL-11 → SI-12 → supraclavicular fossa (ST-12)
[simple version is: GB-21 → GV-14 & GB-21 → ST-12]

Int. Path: supraclavicular f. ↓ chest (Pc-1) ↓ diaphragm *wraps* the liver and *enters* the GB
↓ hypochondrium ↓ sides of abd/flank ↓ inguinal groove ↓ pubic region/genitals & sacrum
→ hip joint and rejoins the primary channel at GB-30.

Ext. Path: a branch on the foot runs from GB-41 (exit pt) → Lr-1 (entry pt)

Connecting Luo: GB-37 → Lr-3

Reservoir Luo: GB-37 → Lr channel (Lr-5?) ↓ dorsum of foot

Symptoms:
Shi: cold sensations (of feet)
Xu: weakness & flaccidity of the foot, difficulty standing,
paralysis of the lower extremities

Venous Luo:

Divergent: separates at GB-30 → hip joint → pubic region (hair & external genitalia) (connects with Lr channel)
↑ lateral abd/flank ↑ following hypochondrium it enters torso → liver & gall bladder
↑ heart ↑ esophagus ↑ mandible & mouth ↑ face ↑ 'eye-system' → outer canthus (GB-1).
[eye-system includes: lids & lashes, eye muscles, lens, retina, rods & cones, optic nerve → brain]

Sinew: 4th toe ↑ lat. malleolus (ties at GB-40) ↑ fibularis/peroneals to knee (ties at GB-34) ↑ IT band to hip
branch1. follows vastus lateralis to ST-32
branch 2. to sacrum/SI joint & BL-31-34
↑ hypochondrium ↑ sides of chest (intercostals) ↑ axilla
branch 3. to chest & breasts
↑ supraclavicular fossa ↑
branch A. to BL channel & occiput/behind ear,
branch B. to temple & forehead where it meets the 3 arm yang & Yg Qiao mai ~ ST-8),
↑ vertex ∩ over top of head ↓ mandible/ramus & bifurcates:
a. → nose   b. → outer canthus of the eye (GB-1)

Root:	(Zu) Qiao Yin (GB-44)	**Node:**	Chuang Long = Ting Gong (SI-19)
			Window Basket = ear

Jct Pts:
(26 pts)
TB-15, 17, 20, 22; SI-12, 17, 19; GV-1, 14, 20;
ST-5, 6, 7, 8, 9, 12, 34; BL-1, 11, 31-32-33-34 (ba liao)
Lr-1 & 13; Pc-1

足少陽膽經

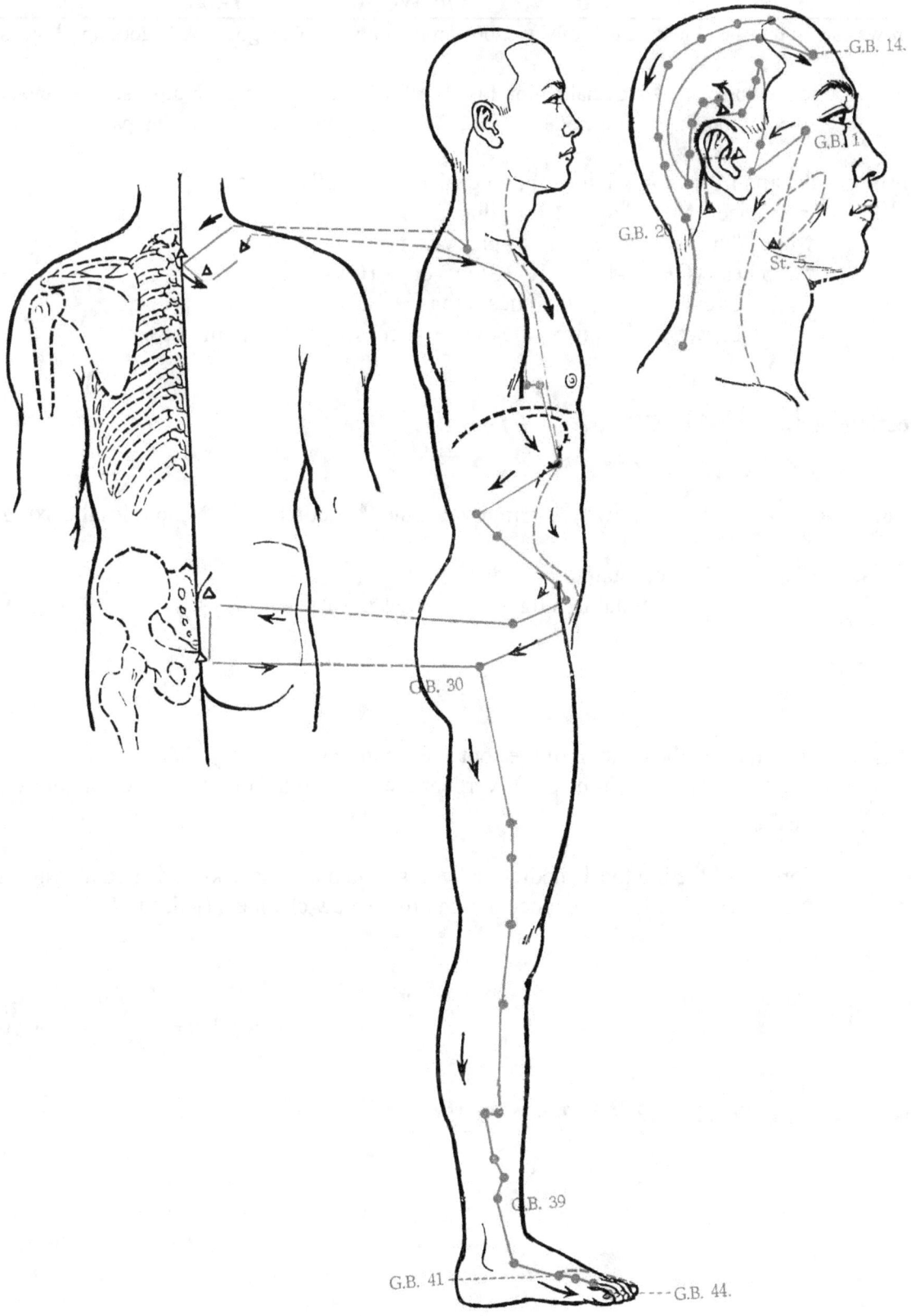

Zú Shǎo/Shào Yáng Dǎn Jīng

Solid line is the external channel.　　Dashed lines show the internal pathway.

　　　© 1990–2016　Jim Cleaver LAc.

Liver Network – Gān Jīng-Luò
Zú Jué-Yīn   Yin-Wood   1-3am

• arrows can be translated in a variety of ways, but simply put: → 'to' or 'goes to', ↑ 'goes up', ↓ 'goes down'

Ext. Path: jct. at Sp-6   ↑ inguinal region Lr-12 → Sp-12 & 13 → Lr-13 & traverses hypochondrium.
branch: ↓ ext. genitals ↑ CV-2-3-4 ↑ Lr-13 → into abd. (see Int. path.)

Int. Path: departs from Sp-13 ↑ into abdomen ↑ liver & gall bladder
→ stomach ↑ esophagus ↑ thru diaphragm
↑ chest/lungs ↑ trachea ↑ naso-pharynx ↑ 'eye-system'
↑ forehead (GB-14-15-16-17-18) → vertex (GV-20).
branch 1.   from chest/lungs → Lu-1.
branch 2.   from the eyes ↓ cheeks ↓ & around the lips.

Connecting Luo: Lr-5 → GB-40

Reservoir Luo: Lr-5 → follows the primary channel ↑ medial thigh ↑ encircles the ext. genitalia.

Symptoms: *Shi:*   constant erection
Xu: genital itching (eczema, candida, vulvitis, herpes etc.)

Venous Luo:

Divergent: separates on the dorsum of the foot ↑ following the primary channel
↑ ext. genitalia and joins GB divergent there which it follows ↑ outer canthus (GB-1).

Sinew: dorsum of the big toe ↑ medial malleolus ↑ medial tibia ↑ knee ↑ medial thigh (adductors)
↑ ext. genitals where it connects with other sinew channels (Kd, Sp, GB).

Root: Da Dun (Lr-1)   **Node:**   Yu Ying = Yu Tang (CV-18)
jueyin luo = Dan/Tan Zhong (CV-17)

Jct Pts: **Sp-6, Sp-12 & 13; CV-2-3-4; Pc-1; GV-20**
(8 pts)

足厥陰肝經

Liv. 14

Liv. 4

Liv. 1

Zú Jué Yīn Gān Jīng

Solid line is the external channel.   Dashed lines show the internal pathway.

Jing Luo – The Complete Channel System – Synopsis of Pathways

經 水 **Jīng Shuǐ**   Channels & Waters / Classic of/on Water(s) Shui is a also generic term for river

(Title of Ling Shu 12, in which the 12 channels are each correlated with a river or body of water,
in the following order: (1st legs then arms, first yang then yin; TY-SY-YM; Ty-Sy-Jy)
NVN p.285   Wu p.579   JNWu p.69   Ki p.176

#	River	River PinYin (Channel)	Translation	Notes and Comments
1.	經	Jīng (BL)	stream(s), **river**(s) underground waterways flowing water	M:1117 river in Gansu that flows into the Wei river (see GB) M:1121 the Jing & the Wei both join the He near Xi'an • distinguish jing & wei = discriminate pros & cons (LS p.579 uses 清 Qing but spells it Jing in the translation)
2.	渭	Wèi (GB)	river in Shanxi (ST w/ water radical)	M:7077 a large tributary of the Huang, in the heart of Zhou territory (see Lu) wei yang = the relationship between uncle & nephew in the Odes
3.	海	Hǎi (ST)	sea, oceans (vast, extensive; an accumulation of things)	M:2014 Qing Hai in NW China is the legendary source of the Yellow R.
4.	湖	Hú (SP)	lake(s) (also Hu-nan & Hu-bei provinces)	M:2168 famous lake in northern Hunan called Dong Ting Hu NVN p.286 Zhang Shi says this is a region of five lakes, (Dong, Ding, Bengze, Zanze with the Sp in the center) Shan Hai Jing refers to a "River Lake"
5.	汝	Rǔ (KD)	two tributaries of the Huai river (see #7)	M:3142
6.	澠	Miǎn (LR)	river in Henan	M:4507 (only key river to flow westward) all others flow eastward apa mǐn
7.	淮	**Huái** (SI)	large river in Henan & northern Anhui	M:2229 (Huai Nan Zi)
8.	洛	Luò (TB)	two tributaries of the Yellow R. (see #10) one in Shanxi, one in Hunan	M:4121 assoc. w/ Yu & the mystic markings revealed to him on the back of a turtle from this river (square of 9) [see Waley Ode 186] same luo as Luoyang = ancient capitol of Eastern Zhou & Eastern Han dynasties (TB-12 = Xiao Luo)
9.	江	**Jiāng** (LI)	the Yang-zi (Chang Jiang)	M:638 rivers in general, esp. the Yangzi / Chang Jiang
10.	河	**Hé** (LU)	the Huang He (Yellow river)	M:2111 streams/brooks, rivers and canals in general (see also He-bei & He-nan provinces)
11.	濟	**Jì** (HT)	a ford, to cross a river	M:459a to ferry across (as in Hex. 63 & 64)
12.	漳	Zhāng (PC)	large tributary of the river Wei in NE Henan	M:188 this also seems to be a two tributary river (one is considered qing the other zhuo)
13.	瀆 / 凟	**Dú**	a ditch, sluice; river	M:6518 a river (one that flows directly into a sea) (Mathews says the first is the correct form; see 6515 below) (however, the latter seems to be the one more commonly used)
14.	四瀆	**Sì Dú**	The 4 Ditches/Rivers	10. He=Lu alt. version } 3. Hai=ST 9. Jiang=LI 4. Hu=Sp 7. Huai=SI 8. Luo=TB 11. Ji=Ht 12. Zhang=Pc

* Si Du = TB-9   瀆 M:6515 = to trouble, annoy, harass   = The 4 Annoyances: head, tooth, ear, aches/tinnitus, dizziness

Illustrations from Antiquity

Circuit One: 地 Dì/Terrestrial
(8 hrs: from 3am to 11am)

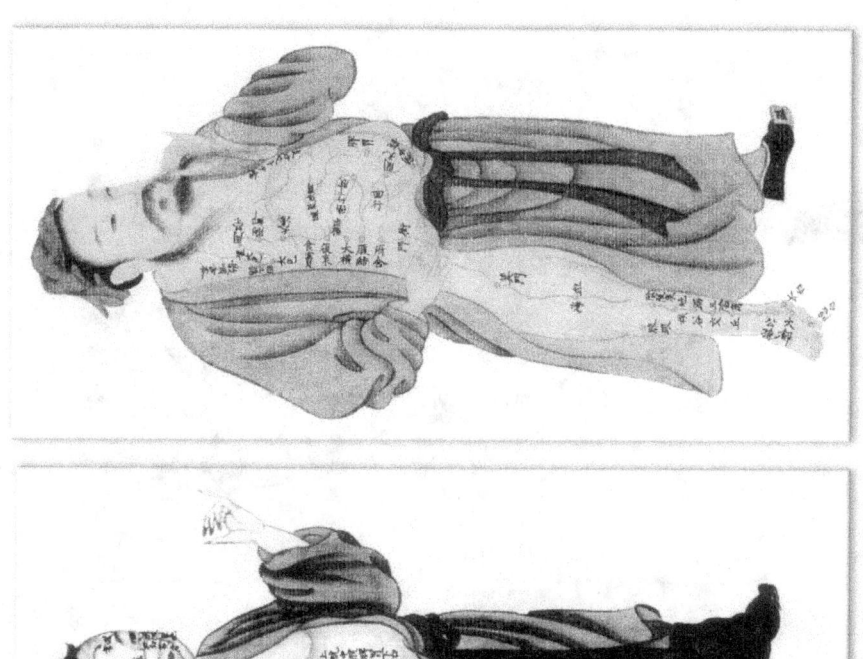

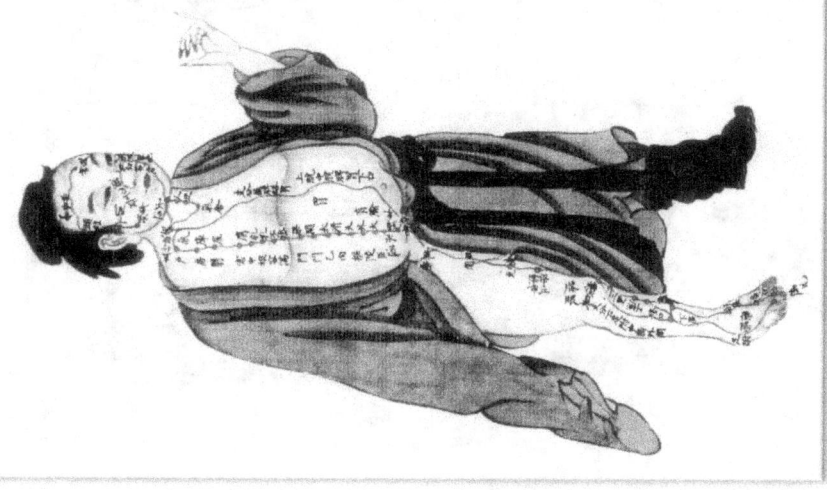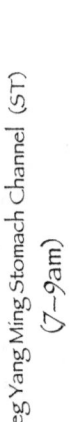

Foot/Leg Tai-Yin Spleen Channel (Sp)
(9–11am)

Foot/Leg Yang-Ming Stomach Channel (ST)
(7–9am)

Hand/Arm Yang-Ming Large Intestine Channel (LI)
(5–7am)

Hand/Arm Tai-Yin Lung Channel (Lu)
(3–5am)

Illustrations from Antiquity

Circuit Two: 天 **Tiān/Celestial**
(8 hrs: from 11am to 7pm)

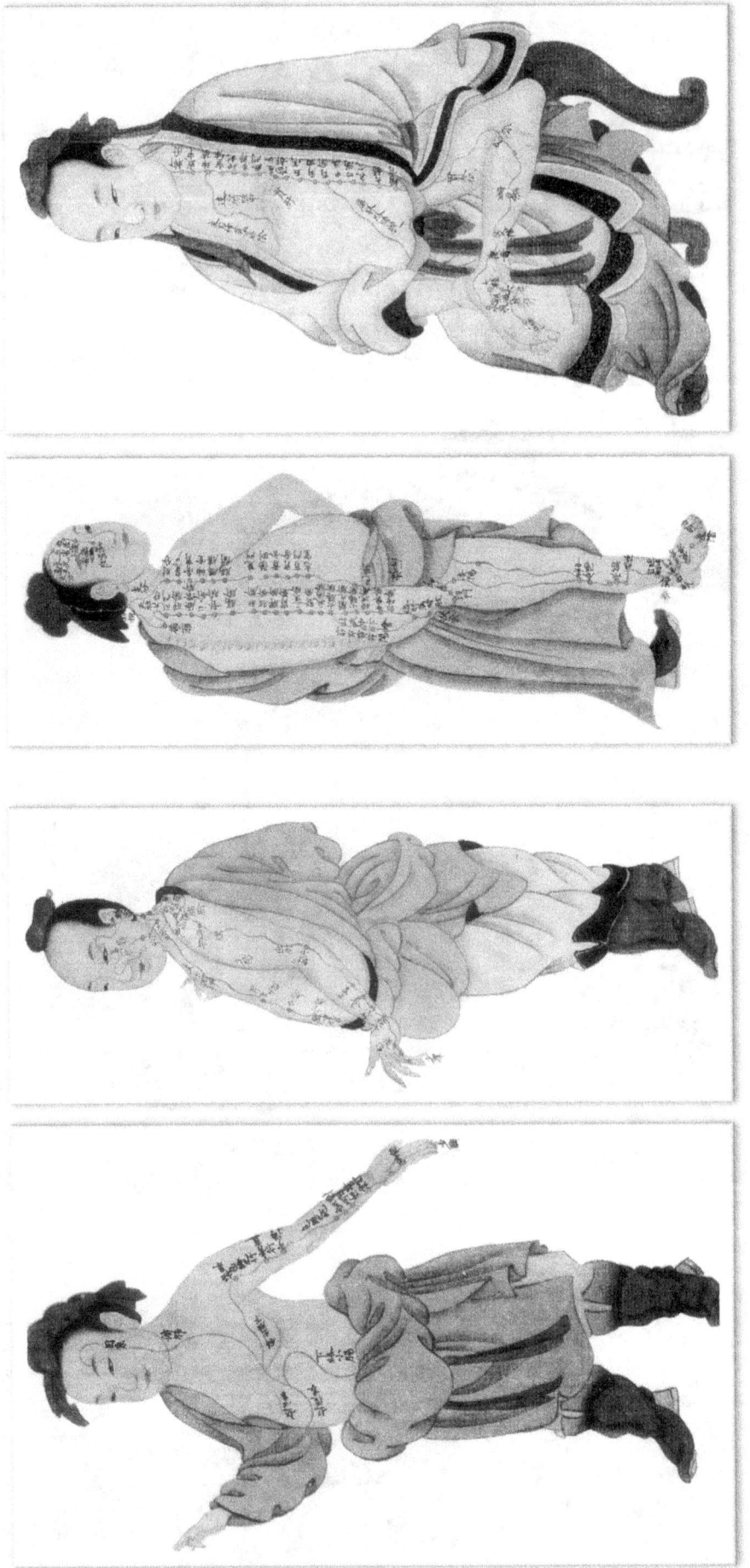

Hand/Arm Shao-Yin Heart Channel (Ht)
(11am–1pm)

Hand/Arm Tai-Yang Small Intestine Channel (SI)
(1–3pm)

Foot/Leg Tai Yang Urinary Bladder Channel (BL)
(3–5pm)

Foot/Leg Shao Yin Kidney Channel (Kd)
(5–7pm)

Illustrations from Antiquity

Circuit Three: 人 **Rén/Human**
(8 hrs: from 7pm to 3am)

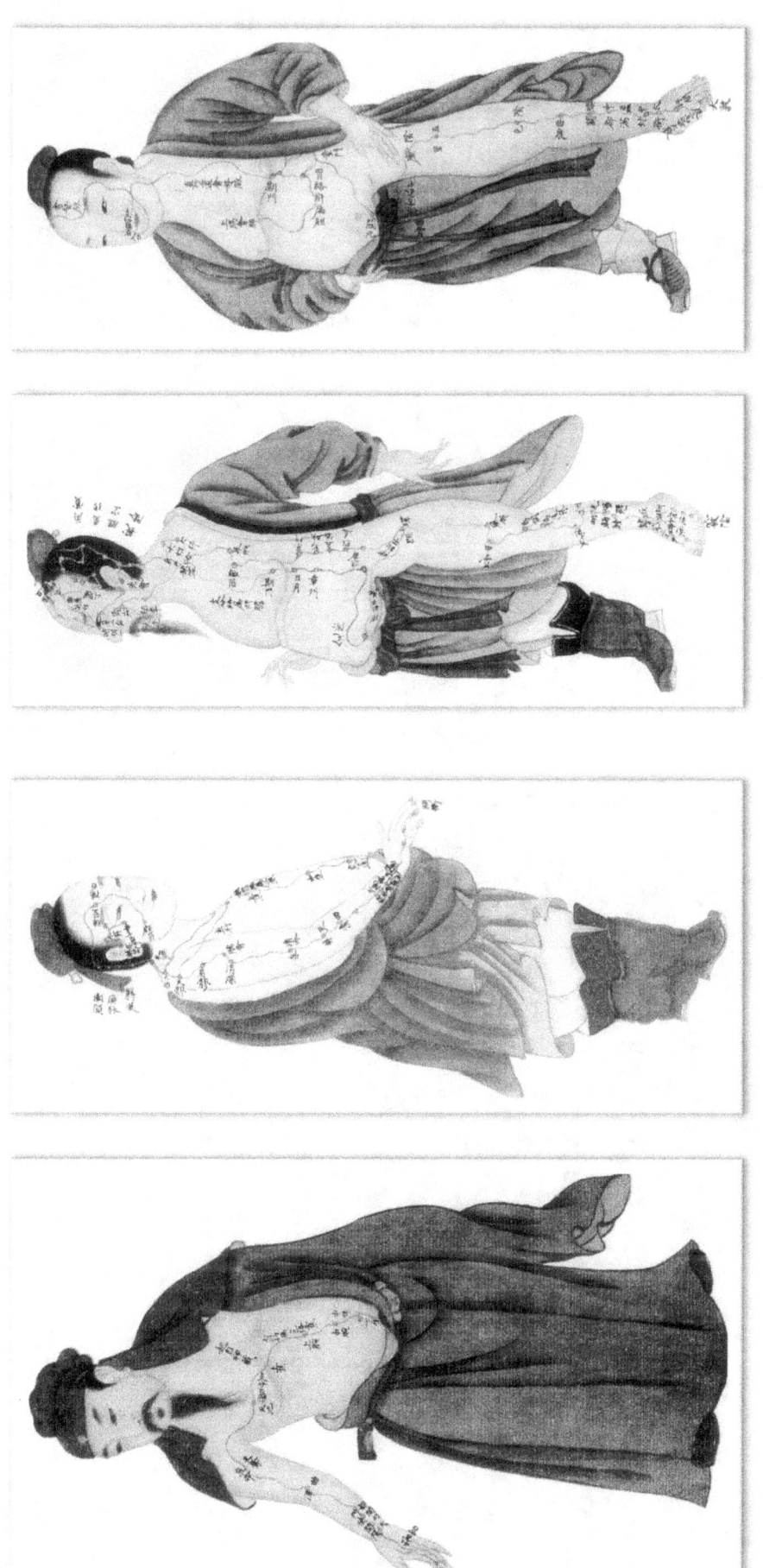

Hand/Arm Jue-Yin Pericardium Channel (Pc)   Hand/Arm Shao-Yang Triple Burner Channel (TB)   Foot/Leg Shao-Yang Gall Bladder Channel (GB)   Foot/Leg Jue-Yin Liver Channel (Lr)
(7–9pm)   (9–11pm)   (11pm–1am)   (1–3am)

Appendix

C

Category Review
Eight & Ten Digit Codes

Think of these like phone numbers to memorize for each channel
(xerox and practice filling these out from memory)

The **8 digits** pertain to the 8 special categories of points on each channel
yuan, luo, xi, and the 5 transport pts (well, <u>brook</u>, stream, river, & sea)

10 digits adds the Mu & Shu points to the above eight,
and are usually not on their organ's channel.
• Only 3 of the 12 Mu pts are on their channel (Lu, Lr, & GB)
• All of the Shu points are on the BL channel (medial/inner column)
• Mu & Shu points are all on the torso/trunk
• All the Mu pts are on the front of the torso (except Kd),
all are in close proximity to their organ.
• All the Shu pts are on the back of the torso (parallel to the spine)
at the level of the sympathetic nerves that innervate their corresponding organs.

	募	腧	原	絡	郄	井	榮	輸	經	合
	Mu	Shu	Yuan	Luo	Xi	J/W	Y/B	S/S	J/R	H/S
HT	CV-14	BL-15	7	5	6	9	8	7	4	3
Arm Shao-yin						wood	fire	soil	metal	water
I. Fire					phase	mù	huǒ	tǔ	jīn	shuǐ
11–1 pm						木	火	土	金	水

	募	腧	原	絡	郄	井	榮	輸	經	合
	Mu	Shu	Yuan	Luo	Xi	J/W	Y/B	S/S	J/R	H/S
PC	CV-17	BL-14	7	6	4	9	8	7	5	3
Arm Jue-yin						wood	fire	soil	metal	water
M. Fire					phase	mù	huǒ	tǔ	jīn	shuǐ
7–9 pm						木	火	土	金	水

	募	腧	原	絡	郄	井	榮	輸	經	合
	Mu	Shu	Yuan	Luo	Xi	J/W	Y/B	S/S	J/R	H/S
LU	Lu-1	BL-13	9	7	6	11	10	9	8	5
Arm Tai-yin						wood	fire	soil	metal	water
Metal					phase	mù	huǒ	tǔ	jīn	shuǐ
3–5 am						木	火	土	金	水

	募	腧	原	絡	郄	井	榮	輸	經	合
	Mu	Shu	Yuan	Luo	Xi	J/W	Y/B	S/S	J/R	H/S
LI	ST-25	BL-25	4	6	7	1	2	3	5	11
Arm Yg-Ming						metal	water	wood	fire	soil
Metal					phase	jīn	shuǐ	mù	huǒ	tǔ
5-7 am						金	水	木	火	土

	募	腧	原	絡	郄	井	榮	輸	經	合
	Mu	Shu	Yuan	Luo	Xi	J/W	Y/B	S/S	J/R	H/S
SI	CV-4	BL-27	4	7	6	1	2	3	5	8
Arm Tai-Yg						metal	water	wood	fire	soil
I. Fire					phase	jīn	shuǐ	mù	huǒ	tǔ
1-3 pm						金	水	木	火	土

	募	腧	原	絡	郄	井	榮	輸	經	合
	Mu	Shu	Yuan	Luo	Xi	J/W	Y/B	S/S	J/R	H/S
TB	CV-5	BL-22	4	5	7	1	2	3	6	10
Arm Shao-Yg						metal	water	wood	fire	soil
M. Fire					phase	jīn	shuǐ	mù	huǒ	tǔ
9-11 pm						金	水	木	火	土

Table IA - Arm Channels – 8 & 10 Digit Memorization (Blanks)

	募	腧	原	絡	郄	井	榮	輸	經	合	
	Mu	Shu	Yuan	Luo	Xi	J/W	Y/B	S/S	J/R	H/S	
											phase
											pinyin
						木	火	土	金	水	

	募	腧	原	絡	郄	井	榮	輸	經	合	
	Mu	Shu	Yuan	Luo	Xi	J/W	Y/B	S/S	J/R	H/S	
											phase
											pinyin
						木	火	土	金	水	

	募	腧	原	絡	郄	井	榮	輸	經	合	
	Mu	Shu	Yuan	Luo	Xi	J/W	Y/B	S/S	J/R	H/S	
											phase
											pinyin
						木	火	土	金	水	

	募	腧	原	絡	郄	井	榮	輸	經	合	
	Mu	Shu	Yuan	Luo	Xi	J/W	Y/B	S/S	J/R	H/S	
											phase
											pinyin
						金	水	木	火	土	

	募	腧	原	絡	郄	井	榮	輸	經	合	
	Mu	Shu	Yuan	Luo	Xi	J/W	Y/B	S/S	J/R	H/S	
											phase
											pinyin
						金	水	木	火	土	

	募	腧	原	絡	郄	井	榮	輸	經	合	
	Mu	Shu	Yuan	Luo	Xi	J/W	Y/B	S/S	J/R	H/S	
											phase
											pinyin
						金	水	木	火	土	

Table IB - Leg Channels – 8 & 10 Digit Memorization (Answers)

	募	腧	原	絡	郄	井	滎	輸	經	合
	Mu	Shu	Yuan	Luo	Xi	J/W	Y/B	S/S	J/R	H/S
BL	CV-3	BL-28	64	58	63	67	66	65	60	54/40
Leg Tai-Yang						metal	water	wood	fire	soil
Water					phase	jīn	shuǐ	mù	huǒ	tǔ
3-5 pm						金	水	木	火	土

	募	腧	原	絡	郄	井	滎	輸	經	合
	Mu	Shu	Yuan	Luo	Xi	J/W	Y/B	S/S	J/R	H/S
Kd	GB-25	BL-23	3	4	5	1	2	3	7	10
Leg Shao-yin						wood	fire	soil	metal	water
Water					phase	mù	huǒ	tǔ	jīn	shuǐ
5–7 pm						木	火	土	金	水

	募	腧	原	絡	郄	井	滎	輸	經	合
	Mu	Shu	Yuan	Luo	Xi	J/W	Y/B	S/S	J/R	H/S
ST	CV-12	BL-21	42	40	34	45	44	43	41	36
Leg Yg-Ming						metal	water	wood	fire	soil
Soil					phase	jīn	shuǐ	mù	huǒ	tǔ
7-9 am						金	水	木	火	土

	募	腧	原	絡	郄	井	滎	輸	經	合
	Mu	Shu	Yuan	Luo	Xi	J/W	Y/B	S/S	J/R	H/S
SP	Lr-13	BL-20	3	4	8	1	2	3	5	9
Leg Tai-yin						wood	fire	soil	metal	water
Soil					phase	mù	huǒ	tǔ	jīn	shuǐ
9–11 am						木	火	土	金	水

	募	腧	原	絡	郄	井	滎	輸	經	合
	Mu	Shu	Yuan	Luo	Xi	J/W	Y/B	S/S	J/R	H/S
GB	GB-24	BL-19	40	37	36	44	43	41*	38	34
Leg Shao-Yg						metal	water	wood	fire	soil
Wood					phase	jīn	shuǐ	mù	huǒ	tǔ
11-1 am						金	水	木	火	土

	募	腧	原	絡	郄	井	滎	輸	經	合
	Mu	Shu	Yuan	Luo	Xi	J/W	Y/B	S/S	J/R	H/S
LR	Lr-14	BL-18	3	5	6	1	2	3	4	8
Leg Jue-yin						wood	fire	soil	metal	water
Wood					phase	mù	huǒ	tǔ	jīn	shuǐ
1–3 am						木	火	土	金	水

© 1990–2016   Jim Cleaver LAc.

Table IB - Leg Channels – 8 & 10 Digit Memorization (Blanks)

	募	腧	原	絡	郄	井	滎	輸	經	合	
	Mu	Shu	Yuan	Luo	Xi	J/W	Y/B	S/S	J/R	H/S	
											phase
											pinyin
						金	水	木	火	土	

	募	腧	原	絡	郄	井	滎	輸	經	合	
	Mu	Shu	Yuan	Luo	Xi	J/W	Y/B	S/S	J/R	H/S	
											phase
											pinyin
						木	火	土	金	水	

	募	腧	原	絡	郄	井	滎	輸	經	合	
	Mu	Shu	Yuan	Luo	Xi	J/W	Y/B	S/S	J/R	H/S	
											phase
											pinyin
						金	水	木	火	土	

	募	腧	原	絡	郄	井	滎	輸	經	合	
	Mu	Shu	Yuan	Luo	Xi	J/W	Y/B	S/S	J/R	H/S	
											phase
											pinyin
						木	火	土	金	水	

	募	腧	原	絡	郄	井	滎	輸	經	合	
	Mu	Shu	Yuan	Luo	Xi	J/W	Y/B	S/S	J/R	H/S	
											phase
											pinyin
						金	水	木	火	土	

	募	腧	原	絡	郄	井	滎	輸	經	合	
	Mu	Shu	Yuan	Luo	Xi	J/W	Y/B	S/S	J/R	H/S	
											phase
											pinyin
						木	火	土	金	水	

Table II – Main Categories & Five Transport-Element Points

Yang Channels		Yin Channels	
Arm/Hand/Shou Tai-Yang	SI	Arm/Hand/Shou Shao-Yin	Ht
Category	Point	Category	Point
front-Mu	CV-4	Mu	CV-14
back-Shu	BL-27	Shu	BL-15
Entry → Exit	1 → 18	Entry → Exit	1 → 9
Yuan-source	4	Yuan	7
Luo-connecting	7	Luo	5
Xi-cleft	6	Xi	6
Jing/Well-Metal	1	J/W-Wood	9 T
Ying/Brook-Water	2 C	Y/B-Fire	8 P
Shu/Stream-Wood	3 T	S/S-Earth	7 D
Jing/River-Fire	5 P	J/R-Metal	4
He/Sea-Earth	8 D	H/S-Water	3 C

Yin Channels		Yang Channels	
Arm/Hand/Shou Jue-Yin	Pc	Arm/Hand/Shou Shao-Yang	TB
Category	Point	Category	Point
Mu	CV-17	Mu	CV-5
Shu	BL-14	Shu	BL-22
Entry → Exit	1 → 8	Entry → Exit	1 → 23
Yuan	7	Yuan	4
Luo	6	Luo	5
Xi	4	Xi	7
J/W-Wood	9 T	J/W-Metal	1
Y/B-Fire	8 P	Y/B-Water	2 C
S/S-Earth	7 D	S/S-Wood	3 T
J/R-Metal	5	J/R-Fire	6 P
H/S-Water	3 C	H/S-Earth	10 D

C = Control pt. T = Tonification/mother pt. P = Phase pt. D = Dispersion/child pt

Leg/Foot/Zu Shao-Yang	GB	Leg/Foot/Zu Jue-Yin	Lr
Category	Point	Category	Point
Mu	GB-24	Mu	Lr-14
Shu	BL-19	Shu	BL-18
Entry → Exit	1 → 41	Entry → Exit	1 → 14
Yuan	40	Yuan	3
Luo	37	Luo	5
Xi	36	Xi	6
J/W-Metal	44 C	J/W-Wood	1 P
Y/B-Water	43 T	Y/B-Fire	2 D
S/S-Wood	41 P	S/S-Earth	3
J/R-Fire	38 D	J/R-Metal	4 C
H/S-Earth	34	H/S-Water	8 T

Leg/Foot/Zu Tai-Yin	Sp	Leg/Foot/Zu Yang-Ming	ST
Category	Point	Category	Point
Mu	Lr-13	Mu	CV-12
Shu	BL-20	Shu	BL-21
Entry → Exit	1 → 21	Entry → Exit	1 → 42
Yuan	3	Yuan	42
Luo	4	Luo	40
Xi	8	Xi	34
J/W-Wood	1 C	J/W-Metal	45 D
Y/B-Fire	2 T	Y/B-Water	44
S/S-Earth	3 P	S/S-Wood	43 C
J/R-Metal	5 D	J/R-Fire	41 T
H/S-Water	9	H/S-Earth	36 P

Leg/Foot/Zu Tai-Yang	BL	Leg/Foot/Zu Shao-Yin:	Kd
Category	Point	Category	Point
Mu	CV-3	Mu	GB-25
Shu	BL-28	Shu	BL-23
Entry → Exit	1 → 67	Entry → Exit	1 → 22
Yuan	64	Yuan	3
Luo	58	Luo	4
Xi	63	Xi	5
J/W-Metal	67 T	J/W-Wood	1 D
Y/B-Water	66 P	Y/B-Fire	2
S/S-Wood	65 D	S/S-Earth	3 C
J/R-Fire	60	J/R-Metal	7 T
H/S-Earth	54 C	H/S-Water	10 P

Arm/Hand/Shou Tai-Yin	Lu	Arm/Hand/Shou Yang-Ming	LI
Category	Point	Category	Point
Mu	Lu-1	Mu	ST-25
Shu	BL-13	Shu	BL-25
Entry → Exit	1 → 7	Entry → Exit	4 → 20
Yuan	9	Yuan	4
Luo	7	Luo	6
Xi	6	Xi	7
J/W-Wood	11	J/W-Metal	1 P
Y/B-Fire	10 C	Y/B-Water	2 D
S/S-Earth	9 T	S/S-Wood	3
J/R-Metal	8 P	J/R-Fire	5 C
H/S-Water	5 D	H/S-Earth	11 T

Table III – Miscellaneous Point Categories

Yang Channels — Arm/Hand/Shou Tai-Yang (SI) / Yin Channels — Arm/Hand/Shou Shao-Yin (Ht)

Category	SI Point	Category	Ht Point
Master Pt: Du mai	SI-3		
alt. Ruler: back of head & neck	SI-3		
Celestial Window	SI-16		
Celestial Window	SI-17		

Yin Channels — Arm/Hand/Shou Jue-Yin (Pc) / Yang Channels — Arm/Hand/Shou Shao-Yang (TB)

Category	Pc Point	Category	TB Point
Celestial Window / alt. CW	Pc-1 / Pc-2	Master Pt: Yang-Wei mai	TB-5
Group Luo: 3 Arm Yin	Pc-5		
Master Pt: Yin-Wei mai	Pc-6	Group Luo: 3 Arm Yang	TB-8
Ruler: chest & diaphragm	Pc-6		
(4th) Ghost pt	Pc-7	Celestial Window	TB-16
(9th) Ghost pt	Pc-8		
9N to Rescue Yang	Pc-8		

Leg/Foot/Zu Shao-Yang (GB) / Leg/Foot/Zu Jue-Yin (Lr)

Category	GB Point	Category	Lr Point
alt. CW	GB-9		
GB Mu pt	GB-24	Infl pt: Zang	Lr-13
Kd Mu pt	GB-25	Sp Mu pt	Lr-13
9N to Rescue Yang	GB-30		
		last pt in Cycle of Qi	Lr-14
Infl pt: Sinews	GB-34		
Xia-He: GB	GB-34		
Xi-cleft for: Yang-Wei mai	GB-35		
Infl pt: Marrow	GB-39		
Group Luo: 3 Leg Yang	GB-39		
Master Pt: Dai mai	GB-41		

Leg/Foot/Zu Tai-Yin (Sp) / Leg/Foot/Zu Yang-Ming (ST)

Category	Sp Point	Category	ST Point
(3rd) Ghost pt	Sp-1	(7th) Ghost pt	ST-6
		Sea of Qi	ST-9
Master Pt: Chong mai	Sp-4	Celestial Window	ST-9
		Great Luo of ST	ST-18
		Sea of Nourishment	ST-30
Ruler: pelvis & lower abd.	Sp-6	Sea of Nourishment	ST-36
Group Luo: 3 Arm Yin	Sp-6	Ruler: abdomen	ST-36
9N to Rescue Yang	Sp-6	9N to Rescue Yang	ST-36
		Xia-He: ST	ST-36
		Xia-He: LI	ST-37
		Xia-He: SI	ST-39
Great Luo of Sp	Sp-21	Sea of Blood	ST-37
		Sea of Blood	ST-39

Leg/Foot/Zu Tai-Yang (BL) / Leg/Foot/Zu Shao-Yin (Kd)

Category	BL Point	Category	Kd Point
Celestial Window	BL-10	9N to Rescue Yang	Kd-1
Sea of Qi	BL-10	9N to Rescue Yang	Kd-3
Infl pt: Bones	BL-11		
Infl pt: Blood	BL-17	Master Pt: Yin-Qiao mai	Kd-6
Xia-He pt: TB	BL-53		
Xia-He pt: BL	BL-54	Xi-cleft for: Yin-Qiao mai	Kd-8
Ruler: back	BL-54	Xi-cleft for: Yin-Wei mai	Kd-9
Xi-cleft for: Yang-Qiao mai	BL-59		
Master Pt: Yang-Qiao mai	BL-62	2nd Ht Mu pt	Kd-25
(5th) Ghost pt	BL-62		

Arm/Hand/Shou Tai-Yin (Lu) / Arm/Hand/Shou Yang-Ming (LI)

Category	Lu Point	Category	LI Point
first pt in Cycle of Qi	Lu-1	Ruler: face & mouth	LI-4
		9N to Rescue Yang	LI-4
Celestial Window	Lu-3		
		Xia-He analog: SI	LI-8
Master Pt: Ren mai	Lu-7	Xia-He analog: LI	LI-9
Ruler: back of head & neck	Lu-7	Xia-He analog: ST	LI-10
Influential pt: pulse & bl. vessels	Lu-9	(12th) Ghost pt	LI-11
(2nd) Ghost pt	Lu-11	Celestial Window	LI-18

Miscellaneous Categories on Ren & Du

Du Mai	*GV*
Category	*Point*
Luo	*GV-1*
Sea of Qi *(alt. to BL-10)*	*GV-15*
9N to Rescue Yang	*GV-15*
Celestial Window	*GV-16*
Sea of Marrow	*GV-16* *GV-20*
(6th) **Ghost** *pt*	*GV-16*
(10th) **Ghost** *pt*	*GV-23*
(1st) **Ghost** *pt*	*GV-26*
GV pt for Kd (L2)	*GV-4*
GV pt for Sp (T11)	*GV-6*
GV pt for Lr (T9)	*GV-8*
GV pt for Ht (T5)	*GV-11*
GV pt for Lu (T3)	*GV-12*
GV pt for Yang (C7)	*GV-14*

Ren Mai	**CV**
Category	**Point**
Luo alt. Luo	**CV-15** **CV-1**
Sea of Qi	**CV-17**
9N to Rescue Yang	**CV-12**
Celestial Window	**CV-22**
Infl pt: Fu **Infl pt**: Qi	**CV-12** **CV-17**
(11th) **Ghost** pt	**CV-1**
(8th) **Ghost** pt	**CV-24**
(13th) **Ghost** pt	Hai Quan
Mu pt for BL	**CV-3**
Mu pt for SI	**CV-4**
Mu pt for TB	**CV-5**
Mu pt for ST	**CV-12**
Mu pt for HT	**CV-14**
Mu pt for PC	**CV-17**

Organ Mu & Shu Pts
(organized by Burner: 3 upper, 4 middle, 5 lower)

Back Shu	Organ	Front Mu
BL-13	Lu	LU-1
BL-14	Pc	CV-17
BL-15	Ht	CV-14
BL-18	Lr	LR-14
BL-19	GB	GB-24
BL-20	Sp	LR-13
BL-21	ST	CV-12
BL-22	TB	CV-5
BL-23	Kd	GB-25
BL-25	LI	ST-25
BL-27	SI	CV-4
BL-28	BL	CV-3

Table VI – Vertebral Levels – Du Mai & Jia-Ji Points

+ Bladder (Inner & Outer Columns) Back Shu and their Correspondences (+ Mu Pts)

post. midline Vertebral level & GV	0.5 – 0.75 cun Jia Ji & Ba Liao (sacral foramen)	1.5 cun Inner BL Back Shu	3 cun Outer BL • Jim's # • Shanghai / Beijing #	Organs + other Correspondences	Front Mu Pt
– C7 – GV-14	*Ding Chuan*		*SI-15 (2 cun)* *Jian Zhong Shu*		
– T1 – GV-13	*Jia Ji 1*	**BL-11** Da Zhu	*SI-14* *Jian Wai Shu*	Bones	
T2 Ø	*Jia Ji 2*	**BL-12** Feng Men	BL-12a / 36/41 Fu Fen	Wind	
– T3 – GV-12	*Jia Ji 3*	**BL-13** Fei Shu	BL-13a / 37/42 Po Hu	**Lu**	**Lu-1** Zhong Fu
T4 Ø	*Jia Ji 4*	**BL-14** Jue-Yin Shu	BL-14a / 38/43 Gao Huang Shu	**Pc**	**CV-17** Dan Zhong
– T5 – GV-11	*Jia Ji 5*	**BL-15** Xin Shu	BL-15a / 39/44 Shen Tang	**Ht**	**CV-14** Ju Que
– T6 – GV-10	*Jia Ji 6*	**BL-16** Du Shu	BL-16a / 40/45 Yi Xi	GV	
– T7 – GV-9	*Jia Ji 7*	**BL-17** Ge Shu	**BL-17a / 41/46** Ge Guan	Diaphragm Blood	
T8 Ø	*Jia Ji 8*	*Yi Shu* *Wei Wan Xia Shu*		Pancreas	
– T9 – GV-8	*Jia Ji 9*	**BL-18** Gan Shu	BL-18a / 42/47 Hun Men	**Lr**	**Lr-14** Qi Men
– T10 – GV-7	*Jia Ji 10*	**BL-19** Dan Shu	BL-19a / 43/48 Yang Gang	**GB**	**GB-24** Ri Yue
– T11 – GV-6	*Jia Ji 11*	**BL-20** Pi Shu	BL-20a / 44/49 Yi She	**Sp**	**Lr-13** Zhang Men
T12 Ø	*Jia Ji 12*	**BL-21** Wei Shu	BL-21a / 45/50 Wei Cang	**ST**	**CV-12** Zhong Wan
– L1 – GV-5	*Jia Ji 13*	**BL-22** San Jiao Shu	BL-22a / 46/51 Huang Men	**TB**	**CV-5** Shi men
– L2 – GV-4	*Jia Ji 14*	**BL-23** Shen Shu	BL-23a / 47/52 Zhi Shi	**Kd**	**GB-25** Jing Men
L3 Ø	*Jia Ji 15*	**BL-24** Qi Hai Shu		CV-6	
– L4 – GV-3	*Jia Ji 16*	**BL-25** Da Chang Shu		**LI**	**ST-25** Tian Shu
L5 Ø	*Jia Ji 17*	**BL-26** Guan Yuan Shu		CV-4	
S1 Ø	**BL-31** Shang Liao	**BL-27** Xiao Chang Shu		**SI**	**CV-4** Guan Yuan
S2 Ø	**BL-32** Ci Liao	**BL-28** Pang Guang Shu	BL-28a / 48/53 Bao Huang	**BL**	**CV-3** Zhong Ji
S3 Ø	**BL-33** Zhong Liao	**BL-29** Zhong Lu Shu		backbone & sacrum	
– S4 – GV-2	**BL-34** Xia Liao	**BL-30** Bai Huan Shu	BL-30a / 49/54 Zhi Bian	anus & rectum	
coccyx GV-1	**BL-35** Hui Yang				

Table VII – Command Points

The Eight 'Points of Command' for Each Channel
(These are also known as Command Pts and Antique Pts)

* Because the shu/stream & yuan/source pts (columns III & IV) are the same on yin channels, therefore only 7 different pts, making a total of 90 distinct pts, for the 96 "points of command". 5 Transport Pts + 3 Yuan-Luo-Xi for each channel.

** Note the regularity/predictability of 4 of the 5 Transport Points (Columns I - II - III & VIII).
But the irregularity of the category related to columns V-VI-VII, wherein the J/R , Luo & Xi points mix it up. See details below.

*** Note the two exceptions in (**Bold**) on the GB and ST channels.

My System of Channel Abbreviations: 2 letters for each: 1 cap +1 lower case for one word Yin chan.; 2 caps for two word Yang.

Distal	⇨	⇨	⇨	⇨	⇨	⇨	⇨	➡	Proximal
~location:	nail base	MP joint	hand/foot	wrist/ankle	fore-arm/leg	fore-arm/leg	fore-arm/leg	elbow/knee	
Col:	**I**	**II**	**III**	**IV**	**V**	**VI**	**VII**	**VIII**	
Cat:	**J/W**	**Y/B**	**S/S**	**Yuan**	*varies*	*varies*	*varies*	**H/S**	**ARM**
Ht	9	8	7	7 Y	6 (X)	5 (L)	4 (J/R)	3	*elbow*
Pc	9	8	7	7 Y	6 (L)	5 (J/R)	4 (X)	3	"
Lu	11	10	9	9 Y	8 (J/R)	7 (L)	6 (X)	5	"
LI	1	2	3	4 Y	5 (J/R)	6 (L)	7 (X)	11	"
TB	1	2	3	4 Y	5 (L)	6 (J/R)	7 (X)	10	"
SI	1	2	3	4 Y	5 (J/R)	6 (X)	7 (L)	8	"
									LEG
UB/BL	67	66	65	64 Y	63 (X)	60 (J/R)	58 (L)	54	*knee*
GB	44	43	**(41)**	40 Y	38 (J/R)	37 (L)	36 (X)	34	"
ST	45	44	43	42 Y	41 (J/R)	40 (L)	–	36	**34 (X)**
Kd	1	2	3	3 Y	4 (L)	5 (X)	7 (J/R)	10	"
Lr	1	2	3	3 Y	4 (J/R)	5 (L)	6 (X)	8	"
Sp	1	2	3	3 Y	4 (L)	5 (J/R)	8 (X)	9	"
				J/R	= 6	= 4	= 2		
			Analysis:	**Luo**	= 4	= 6	= 2		
				Xi	= 2	= 2	= 7+1		

Key: Col: = Column   Cat: = Category

J/W = Jing/well (lit. 'a well' is here more like the western sense of a spring, where water emerges, **welling** up from underground)
         (the next category is more like a babbling brook, and smaller than a stream, hence my choice there)

Y/B = Ying/brook - ying should probably be spelled & pronounced xíng = brook, (see p.23)
    yíng is actually a slightly different character with 'fire' on the bottom instead of 'water' and means to shimmer & sparkle
    while yǒng = to gush/turbulent (see Kd-1) is also used and adds the dimension of movement, (babbling adds sound as well).

S/S = Shu/stream

J/R = Jing/river

H/S = He/sea/uniting (here the water metaphor is a river's confluence with the sea, but 'He' means 'to unite, while sea=hai)

Y   = Yuan/source

L   = Luo/connecting/network

X   = Xi/cleft

Highlights of This Text

- Topically specific, this book focuses on point locations, categories & names

- Designed specifically for students and teachers of point location

- Lightweight and easy to carry to class or clinic

- The Introductory section surveys all pertinent aspects of Eastern energetic anatomy in logical table format

- Convenient one subject per page format
  Each channel includes 4 topic pages:

  a) the external course of the channel in a clear linear narrative

  b) concise, accurate point location descriptions, crafted for memorization

  c) an illustration of the entire channel on the facing page
     one illustration allows viewing the whole channel as well as each point in context
     all points on the illustration are named in pinyin as well as numbered

  d) synoptic table of all point categories and their point names with
     original translations designed to highlight their medical meaning

- Important Chinese characters are included throughout the text
   including characters of point names for all points in categories

- Extraordinary Vessels chapter

- NCCAOM 54 Extra Points chapter

- Both numbering systems for the Bladder channel, plus
   Jim's alternative system which facilitates understanding as well as memorization

- Appendices include:
  A. Regional tables showing the relative position of points across channels
  B. Synopsis of all internal pathways, where they go, and what they connect
  C. Blank tables to copy for self-quizzing purposes

- Comprehensive tables for all point category information

Other Books by Jim Cleaver

* THE ACUPUNCTURE SERIES

Vol.	Title/Subject	# of Pages	
I.	Acu-Point **Location** Handbook	235 pages	(this book)
II.	Acu-Point **Actions** Handbook	364 pages	
III.	Acu-Point **Combining Strategies**	165 pages	
IV.	Acupuncture **Treatment Protocols**	194 pages	
V.	Acu-Point **Name** Character Workbook	189 pages	
VI.	Acu-Point **Name** Reference Guide	95 pages	

* Acuuncture Related Topics

• **Zang-Fu**: Functions and **Patterns**	98 pages	(Diagnostics)

* Chinese Medical Classics - Translation Workbooks

Translation workbooks provide the Chinese characters of the text in full form/traditional characters
 (vs. simplified characters), with pin-yin transliteration, including tone marks.
The texts are arranged sentence by sentence, with space underneath to experiment with your own translation.

• Huang Di Nei Jing **Su Wen**	5 Volumes	(~215 pages each)
• Huang Di Nei Jing **Ling Shu**	4 Volumes	(~195 pages each)
• Su Wen **Vocabulary** (Top 1000 characters)	162 pages	
(all the characters that occur 5x or more)		
• **Nan Jing** Translation Workbook	246 pages	

* Chinese Philosophical Classics - Translation Workbooks

• **Zhou Yi** / **Yi Jing** Translation Workbook	333 pages
• **Dao De Jing** / **Lao Zi** Translation Workbook	222 pages
• **Zhuang Zi** Inner Chapters (1-7)	274 pages
• **Sun Zi** (Master Sun's Classic on Military Strategy)	150 pages

About the Author

Jim Cleaver has devoted much of the last forty years to teaching many aspects of Chinese medicine, and has held positions at Five Branches Institute in Santa Cruz, CA., The Oregon College of Oriental Medicine, and the last 22 years at National College/University of Natural Medicine in Portland, OR.

Using his books students, teachers, and practitioners will all benefit from his depth of experience in both clinic and classroom. As a classroom tool and an office reference, this book is an invaluable resource.

Now retired from academics, Jim is making available some of the many books he created for his classes and students during his teaching career. These cover a wide range of topics related to Chinese Medicine, especially acupuncture, as well as the Yi-Jing and Chinese philosophical classics.

Jim also maintains a private practice, and has taught Tai-Ji & Qi-Gong classes since 1992.

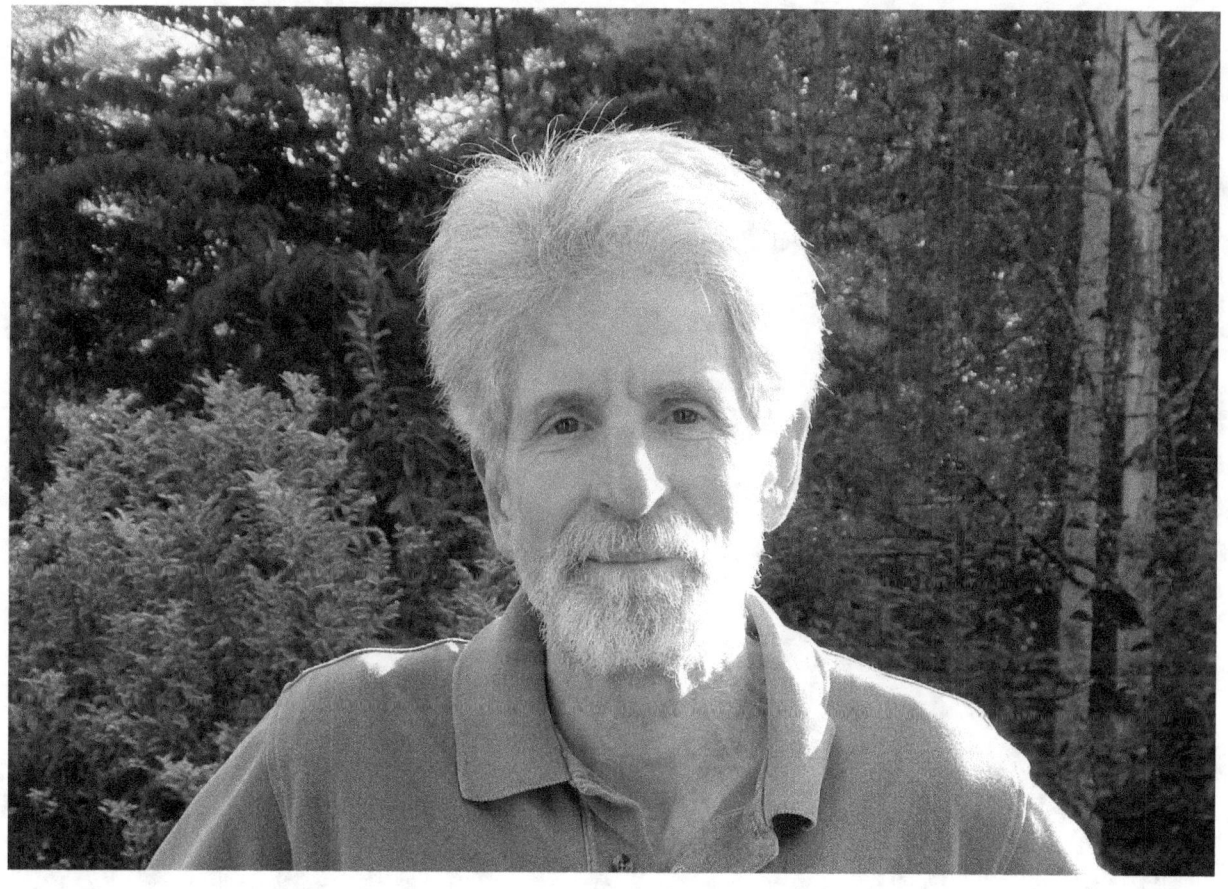

* cover photographs and design by Jim

www.ingramcontent.com/pod-product-compliance
Lightning Source LLC
Chambersburg PA
CBHW081555220526

45468CB00010B/2668